Revision Notes in Psychiatry

BASANT K. PURI MA MB BChir MRCPsych
Consultant Psychiatrist
MR Unit, Imperial College School of Medicine
Hammersmith Hospital
London, UK

ANNE D. HALL BA MB BCh MRCPsych
Consultant Psychiatrist
South Kensington and Chelsea Mental Health Centre
Chelsea & Westminster Hospital
London, UK

A member of the Hodder Headline Group
LONDON • SYDNEY • AUCKLAND
Co-published in the USA by Oxford University Press, Inc., New York

First published in Great Britain in 1998 by
Arnold, a member of the Hodder Headline Group,
338 Euston Road, London NW1 3BH
http://www.arnoldpublishers.com

Co-published in the United States of America by
Oxford University Press, Inc.,
198 Madison Avenue, New York, NY 10016
Oxford is a registered trademark of Oxford University Press

Whilst the advice and information in this book is believed to be true and
accurate at the date of going to press, neither the authors nor the publisher
can accept any legal responsibility or liability for any errors or omissions
that may be made. In particular (but without limiting the generality of the
preceding disclaimer) every effort has been made to check drug dosages;
however it is still possible that errors have been missed. Furthermore,
dosage schedules are constantly being revised and new side-effects
recognized. For these reasons the reader is strongly urged to consult the
drug companies' printed instructions before administering any of the drugs
recommended in this book.

British Library Cataloguing in Publication Data
A catalogue record for this book is available from the Library of Congress

Library of Congress Cataloging-in-Publication Data
Puri, Basant K.
Revision notes in psychiatry/by Basant K. Puri, Anne D. Hall.
p.   cm.
Includes bibliographical references and index.
1. Psychiatry–Handbooks, manuals, etc.   I. Hall, Anne D., 1962–
II. Title.
[DNLM: 1. Psychiatry.   2. Mental Disorders.   WM 100 P9898r 1997]
RC456.P87   1997
616.89–dc21
DNLM/DLC   97-30185
for Library of Congress   CIP

ISBN 0 340 66227 1

2 3 4 5 6 7 8 9 10

Publisher: Georgina Bentliff
Production Editor: James Rabson
Production Controller: Rose James
Cover designer: Terry Griffiths

Typeset in Garamond and Optima by J&L Composition Ltd, Filey, North Yorkshire
Printed and bound in Great Britain by J W Arrowsmith, Bristol

Contents

Preface

This book aims to provide detailed revision notes covering all the important basic sciences and clinical topics required for postgraduate psychiatry examinations. To this end, the current syllabus for both parts of the examinations for the Membership of the Royal College of Psychiatrists has been followed closely. It should be emphasized, however, that this book is not meant to be a replacement for either wider reading, or, more importantly, clerking and following-up patients.

BKP
ADH

1
Basic psychology

LEARNING THEORY

Definition of learning

Learning is a change in behaviour as a result of prior experience. It does not include behaviour change caused by maturation or temporary conditions (e.g. drug effects or fatigue).

Learning may occur through associations being made between two or more phenomena. Two forms of such **associative learning** are recognized: classical conditioning and operant conditioning. **Cognitive learning** is a more complex process in which current perceptions are interpreted in the context of previous information in order to solve unfamiliar problems. Evidence that learning can also take place through the observation and imitation of others has led to the development of the **observational learning theory.**

Classical conditioning

Classical conditioning (respondent learning) was first described by Pavlov in 1927. Following several repetitions of pairing of light (or a bell sounding) followed by the presentation of food to a dog it was found that just switching on the light led to salivation. The dog had been conditioned to associate the light with food. Food was acting as the **unconditioned stimulus**, eliciting the reflex response of salivation without new learning being involved. The response to the unconditioned stimulus is known as the **unconditioned response**. The light would normally not have elicited the response of salivation, but was now a **conditioned stimulus** that had elicited the response through its association with an unconditioned stimulus. The **conditioned response** is the learned or acquired response to a conditioned stimulus. Thus, in Pavlov's experiments, salivation was both an unconditioned response before conditioning, and a conditioned response after conditioning.

The **acquisition** stage of conditioning is the period during which the association is being acquired between the conditioned stimulus and the unconditioned stimulus with which it is being paired. In **delayed conditioning** the onset of the conditioned stimulus precedes that of the unconditioned stimulus and the conditioned stimulus continues until the response occurs. Delayed conditioning is optimal when the delay between the onset of the two stimuli is around half a second.

SIMULTANEOUS CONDITIONING In **simultaneous conditioning** the onset of both stimuli is simultaneous and the conditioned stimulus continues until the response occurs. It is less successful than delayed conditioning.

```
US ◄--► CS
 |       |
UR      CR
```

Fig. 1.1

TRACE CONDITIONING   In **trace conditioning** the conditioned stimulus ends before the onset of the unconditioned stimulus and the conditioning becomes less effective as the delay between the two increases.

EXTINCTION   This is the gradual disappearance of a conditioned response and occurs when the conditioned stimulus is repeatedly presented without the unconditioned stimulus. It does not entail the complete loss of the conditioned stimulus. Following extinction, if an experimental animal is allowed to rest, a weaker conditioned response re-emerges. This is known as **partial recovery**.

GENERALIZATION   This is the process whereby once a conditioned response has been established to a given stimulus, that response can also be evoked by other stimuli that are similar to the original conditioned stimulus.

DISCRIMINATION   This is the differential recognition of and response to two or more similar stimuli.

INCUBATION   This is the increase in strength of conditioned responses resulting from repeated brief exposure to the conditioned stimulus.

STIMULUS PREPAREDNESS   This refers to the fact that some stimuli are more likely to become conditioned stimuli than are others.

LITTLE ALBERT   In 1920 Watson and Rayner described the experimental induction of a phobia, using classical conditioning, in an 11–month-old boy known as Little Albert. Following several episodes of pairing in which the presentation of a white rat was accompanied by a loud noise, the boy developed a fear of the rat in the absence of the frightening noise. This was then repeated with a rabbit, and then generalized to any furry mammal.

Operant conditioning (instrumental learning)

This is particularly associated with Skinner (1938) although much of the groundwork for the underlying theory was carried out by Thorndike (1911). A voluntary behaviour is engaged in because its occurrence is **reinforced** by being rewarded. Such behaviour is independent of stimuli and was termed **operant behaviour** by Skinner. An alternative type of behaviour termed **respondent behaviour** by Skinner refers to behaviour that is dependent on known stimuli.

Thorndike described experiments in which hungry cats were placed in puzzle boxes. By chance, in time a cat would effect an escape, for example by pressing on a lever, and reach some visible food outside the box. Less time would be needed to carry out the same behaviour in later trials. This is **trial-and-error learning** or behaviour. Thorndike's **law of effect** holds that voluntary behaviour that is paired with subsequent reward is strengthened.

Operant conditioning can be demonstrated using a Skinner box in which, for example, every time the animal presses a lever a pellet of food is released. If hungry rats are placed in it, random trial-and-error learning leads to the lever being pressed, the **conditioned response**, to obtain the reinforcing stimulus of the reward of food pellets. If, after many repetitions of this pairing, the conditioned response is no longer reinforced, then the conditioned response abates; that is, **extinction** occurs. Following extinction, if the animal is allowed to rest, a weaker conditioned response can re-emerge; this is **partial recovery**. **Discrimination** can also occur.

A **positive reinforcer** is a reinforcing reward stimulus (e.g. food and water, money in humans) which increases the probability of occurrence of the operant behaviour, while a **negative reinforcer** is an aversive stimulus (e.g. an electric shock, fear) whose removal increases the probability of occurrence of the operant behaviour. For example, a Skinner box may be arranged so that in order to avoid an aversive stimulus, the animal must press a lever. Learning this response is called **avoidance conditioning**. **Escape conditioning** is a variety of negative reinforcement in which the response learnt provides complete escape from the aversive stimulus (very resistant to extinction).

Punishment is the situation that occurs if an aversive stimulus is presented whenever a given behaviour occurs, thereby reducing the probability of occurrence of this response. The removal of the aversive stimulus then allows it to act as a negative reinforcer rather than a punisher.

Primary reinforcement is that occurring through reduction of needs deriving from basic drives (e.g. food and drink).

Secondary reinforcement is that deriving from association with primary reinforcers (e.g. money, tokens).

Different **schedules of reinforcement** can be used:

- In **continuous reinforcement** reinforcement takes place following every conditioned response. This leads to the maximum response rate.
- In **partial reinforcement** only some of the conditioned responses are reinforced.
    - In a **fixed interval** schedule, reinforcement occurs after a fixed interval of time. It is poor at maintaining the conditioned response; the maximum response rate typically occurs only when the reinforcement is expected.
    - In a **variable interval** schedule, reinforcement occurs after variable intervals. It is very good at maintaining the conditioned response.
    - In a **fixed ratio** schedule, reinforcement occurs after a fixed number of responses. It is good at maintaining a high response rate.
    - In a **variable ratio** schedule, reinforcement occurs after a variable number of responses. It is very good at maintaining a high response rate.

Clinical applications of associative learning

RECIPROCAL INHIBITION   This holds that relaxation inhibits anxiety so that the two are mutually exclusive (Wolpe 1950) and in fact does not hold true. It can be used in treating conditions associated with anticipatory anxiety (e.g. phobias). Patients identify increasingly greater anxiety evoking stimuli, to form an **anxiety hierarchy**. During **systematic desensitization** the patient is successfully exposed (in reality or in imagination) to these stimuli in the hierarchy, beginning with the least anxiety evoking one, each exposure being paired with relaxation.

HABITUATION   Habituation is an important component of the behavioural treatment of obsessive-compulsive disorder using exposure and response prevention. The ultimate aim of exposure techniques is to reduce the discomfort associated with the eliciting stimuli through habituation.

CHAINING   In chaining the components of a more complex desired behaviour are first taught and then connected in order to teach the latter. It can be used, for example, in people with learning difficulties.

SHAPING   In shaping, successively closer approximations to the desired behaviour are reinforced in order to achieve the latter. It finds application clinically in the management of behavioural disturbances in people with learning difficulties.

Cognitive learning

The notion of a mental model of reality is central to the cognitive approach to psychology. Cognition involves the reception, organization, and utilization of information. Cognitive learning is an active form of learning in which mental cognitive structures (**cognitive maps**) are formed. These allow mental images to be formed which allow meaning and structure to be given to the internal and external environment.

Cognitive learning can occur in the following ways:

- **Insight learning** – the learning occurs apparently out of the blue, because of an understanding of the relationship between various elements relevant to a problem.
- **Latent learning** – cognitive learning takes place but is not manifested except in certain circumstances such as the need to satisfy a basic drive.

Observational learning (vicarious learning/modelling (Bandura))

This is the learning of behaviours and skills that can occur by observation without direct reinforcement.

OPTIMAL CONDITIONS FOR OBSERVATIONAL LEARNING

1   The subject sees that the behaviour observed is being reinforced.
2   Perceived similarity – the subject must believe that they can emit the response necessary to obtain reinforcement (self-efficacy).

VISUAL AND AUDITORY PERCEPTION

Perception is an active process involving the awareness and interpretation of sensations received through sensory organs.

ABSOLUTE THRESHOLD   This is the minimum energy required to activate the sensory organ.

DIFFERENCE THRESHOLD   The difference threshold of two sources of a sensory modality is the minimum difference that has to exist between the intensities of the two sources to allow them to be perceived separately.

WEBER'S LAW   The increase in stimulus intensity needed to allow two sources of intensity to be perceived as being different is directly proportional to the value of the baseline intensity.

FECHNER'S LAW   Weber's law is only an approximation which fails to hold over a large range of stimulus intensity. A better, though again not perfect, approximation is provided by Fechner's law which holds that sensory perception is a logarithmic function of stimulus intensity.

SIGNAL DETECTION THEORY   This holds that perception does not depend solely on stimulus intensity but is also a function of biophysical factors and psychological factors such as motivation, previous experiences, and expectations.

Perceptual organization

Perception is an active process in which there is a search for meaning.

A number of perceptual phenomena are described in Gestalt psychology:

- The whole perception is different from the sum of its parts.
- Law of simplicity: the percept corresponds to the simplest stimulation interpretation.
- Law of closure: partial outlines are perceived as whole.
- Law of continuity: e.g. interrupted lines are seen as continuous.
- Law of similarity: like items are grouped together.
- Law of proximity: adjacent items are grouped together.
- Figure ground differentiation: patterns are perceived as figures differentiated from their background with contours and boundaries, thus simulating objects. (This is not confined to visual stimuli – e.g. hearing a particular conversation over a background noise.)

OBJECT CONSTANCY

This is the tendency to perceive objects as unchanged under different conditions:

- Shape constancy: the perception of an object's shape is constant regardless of the viewing angle.
- Size constancy: the perception of an object's size is constant regardless of the viewing distance.
- Lightness/colour constancy: the perception of an object's shade/colour is constant regardless of the lighting conditions.
- Location constancy: the perception of an object's spatial position is constant regardless of the viewer's movement.

DEPTH PERCEPTION

A three-dimensional visual perception is formed from two-dimensional retinal images as a result of multiple cues such as binocular vision and convergence, relative size and brightness, motion parallax, object interposition, and linear perspective.

PERCEPTUAL SET

This is a motivational state of mind in which certain aspects of stimuli are perceived according to expectation. This can be associated with a change in the perception threshold. The way in which stimuli are perceived is influenced by personality and individual values, and past experiences.

RELEVANCE OF PERCEPTUAL THEORY TO PSYCHOPATHOLOGY

Illusions are misperceptions of real stimuli that are influenced by the perceptual set and suggest an active search for meaning.

In schizophrenia, depersonalization, derealization, temporal lobe epilepsy and acute brain syndromes, there is disturbance of perception, particularly depth perception and perceptual constancy.

DEVELOPMENT OF VISUAL PERCEPTION

The development of human visual perception is an illustration of a constitutional-environmental interaction. In general complex visual stimuli (e.g. human faces) are preferred.

Birth: there is the ability to discriminate brightness and to carry out eye tracking; visual acuity is impaired and focusing is fixed at 0.2 m.

- 2 months: depth perception (as evidenced by visual cliff experiments)
- 4 months: accommodation and colour vision
- 6 months: 6:6 acuity

Visual scanning, tracking and fixating and figure ground discrimination are believed to be innate. Size and shape constancy, depth perception, and shape discrimination are believed to be learnt.

INFORMATION PROCESSING AND ATTENTION

Information processing
Information processing is concerned with the way in which external signals arriving at the sense organs are converted into meaningful perceptual experiences.

DATA-DRIVEN PROCESSING   The processing is initiated by the arrival of data. The simplest scheme for classifying and recognizing patterns is template matching, in which recognition is achieved by matching the external signal against the internal template.

CONCEPTUALLY DRIVEN PROCESSING   This applies when data input is incomplete. The processing starts with the conceptualization of what might be present and then looks for confirmatory evidence, thereby biasing the processing mechanisms to give the expected results. Conceptually driven data (schema) are essential to perception. However, they can lead to misperceptions.

Attention
Attention is an intensive process in which information selection takes place. Types include:

- Selective/focused attention: one type of information is attended to while additional distracting information is ignored e.g. the cocktail party effect. In dichotic listening studies in which subjects attend to one channel, evidence indicates that the unattended channel is still being processed and the listener can switch rapidly if it is appropriate.
- Divided attention: at least two sources of information are attended to simultaneously. Performance is inefficient. Loss of performance is called dual-task interference.
- Sustained attention: the environment is monitored over a long period of time. Performance deteriorates with time.
- Controlled attention: effort is required. It has been suggested that a defect of controlled attention might underlie symptoms of schizophrenia.
- Automatic attention: the subject becomes skilled at a task and therefore little conscious effort is required.
- Stroop effect: automatic process is so ingrained that it interferes with controlled processing.

MEMORY

Memory comprises encoding/registration, storage and retrieval of information.

Encoding/registration
This is the transformation of physical information into a code that memory can accept.

Storage
This is the retention of encoded information. Memory storage can be considered to be made up of: sensory memory, short-term memory and long-term memory.

SENSORY MEMORY   Sensory information is retained in an unprocessed form in peripheral receptors. It has a large capacity.

Sensory memory is a very short-lived (fade time 0.5 s) trace of the sensory input. Visual input is briefly retained as a mental image called an **icon**; this is known as an iconic memory. The sensory memory for auditory information is called an **echoic** memory, while that for information from touch is called a **haptic** memory.

It gives an accurate account of the environment as experienced by the sensory system. It holds a representation of the stimulus so that parts of it can be attended to, processed, and transferred into more permanent memory stores.

SHORT-TERM (PRIMARY/WORKING) MEMORY   Those aspects of sensory information that are the object of active attention are transferred into a temporary working memory called the short-term memory.

Encoding is mainly acoustic; visual encoding rapidly fades.

This is the memory used temporarily to hold a telephone number, for example, until dialled. It is lost in 20 s unless rehearsed. It consists of a small finite number (7 ± 2) of registers which can be filled only by data entering one at a time.

The displacement principle: when the registers are full the addition of a new datum leads to the displacement and loss of an existing one.

Chunking: this increases the amount of information stored in short-term memory by allowing one entry to cover several items. While the number of chunks is restricted, their content is not. With the help of long-term memory new material can be recoded, thereby increasing the content of chunks.

- Primacy effect: the probability of correctly recalling an item of information is greater if it is one of the first items to be encountered, even if more than seven items have been presented.
- Recency effect: the probability of correctly recalling an item of information is increased if it is one of the most recent items to be encountered.

Those items which have an intermediate serial position are least likely to be recalled accurately, and this overall phenomenon is referred to as the serial position effect. Whereas the recency effect can be accounted for in terms of the comparatively short interval of time elapsing before recall, the primary effect is more difficult to explain, and may be caused by greater rehearsal of these first items.

Rehearsal is not as necessary in approximately 5 per cent of children possessing a photographic memory, known in psychology as eidetic imagery, in whom a detailed visual image can be retained for over half a minute.

Verbal short-term memory is stored in the left hemisphere and visual in the right.

Retrieval is effortless and error free.

LONG-TERM (SECONDARY) MEMORY   This stores information more or less permanently. Theoretically it may have unlimited capacity, although there may be limitations on retrieval.

- Semantic memory: verbal information is stored in terms of meaning rather than exact words. It is easier to remember words paired with meanings and the recall of synonymous words to those in a given list. Therefore semantic encoding is a more efficient way than simple rehearsal of transferring information from the short-term memory to the long-term one.
- Episodic memory: this is long-term memory for events. It provides a continually changing and updated record of autobiographical material.

Input and retrieval take longer and are more effortful than for short-term memory. Some motivation is required to encode information into long-term memory. Schizophrenia and depression affect memory at this level.

Visuomotor knowledge and motor skills are also aspects of the organization of long-term memory.

RETRIEVAL

This is the recovery of information from memory when needed.

Retrieval of information from the long-term memory is error prone but is improved by using an hierarchical network to organize the information storage.

Emotional factors can influence retrieval from long-term memory in the following ways:

- Emotionally charged situations are rehearsed and organized more than non-emotionally charged ones. Retrieval is facilitated.
- Negative emotions and anxiety hinder retrieval.
- Retrieval of events and emotions is more likely to be successful if it occurs in the same context as that in which the original events and emotions occurred; this is known as **state-dependent learning.**
- Repression of emotionally charged material hinders retrieval.

FORGETTING

Forgetting from long-term memory is believed usually to be the result of retrieval failure rather than storage failure. This explains both why hypnosis can recover forgotten memories and the 'tip of the tongue' experience.

INTERFERENCE THEORY   Proactive interference/inhibition: previous learning is likely to impair subsequent learning.

Retroactive interference/inhibition: new learning is likely to impair previous learning.

Forgetting by interference is item dependent.

DECAY THEORY   Memories fade with time.

The longer the item remains in the memory system, the weaker its strength. New material has a high-trace strength while older has a low-trace strength.

Forgetting by decay is time dependent.

MOTIVATION

EXTRINSIC MOTIVATION THEORIES

Theories based on instincts were replaced by a **drive reduction theory** in which the motivation of behaviour is to reduce the level of arousal associated with a **basic drive** (biological drive e.g. hunger and thirst) in order to maintain homeostatic control of the internal somatic environment.

Hull developed a theory in which **primary biological drives** are activated by needs which arise from homeostatic imbalance acting via brain receptors. An example is provided by hypothalamic systems and satiety. In rat experiments, the hypothalamic ventromedial nucleus acts as a satiety centre, with hyperphagia occurring if it is ablated, while the lateral hypothalamus contains a hunger centre, with aphagia occurring if it is ablated.

Mowrer developed the notion of **secondary drives** (e.g. anxiety) which result from generalization and conditioning.

INTRINSIC MOTIVATION THEORIES

Whereas extrinsic theories require reduction of drive externally, intrinsic theories propose that the activity engaged in has its own intrinsic reward.

OPTIMAL AROUSAL   An example is offered by optimal arousal, in which the subject attains an optimal level of arousal to achieve optimal performance. In general a moderate level of arousal leads to an optimum degree of alertness and interest, and therefore to a comparatively high efficiency of performance. High and low arousal lead to reduced performance and are described in the inverted U-shape of the Yerkes–Dodson curve.

COGNITIVE DISSONANCE   According to this theory, first formulated by Festinger, discomfort occurs when two or more cognitions are held but are inconsistent with each other. The individual is motivated to achieve cognitive consistency and may change one or more of the cognitions.

ATTITUDE-DISCREPANT BEHAVIOUR   When attitude and behaviour are inconsistent (attitude-discrepant behaviour), the alteration of attitude helps to bring about cognitive consistency.

NEED FOR ACHIEVEMENT (nAch)   McClelland formulated a need for achievement (nAch) to explain pleasure resulting from mastery.

MASLOW'S HIERARCHY OF NEEDS

This unified theory, relating to self-actualization, integrates both extrinsic and intrinsic theories of motivation. A hierarchy of needs is described in which those with survival importance take precedence over others: self-actualization (highest), autonomy, self-esteem, love and belonging, safety, and physical needs (lowest).

EMOTION

Types of emotion
An emotion is a mental feeling or affection having cognitive, physiological and social concomitants. Plutchik has classified them into eight **primary emotions**: disgust, anger, anticipation, joy, acceptance, fear, surprise and sadness. Any two adjacent emotions can give rise to a **secondary emotion**. For example, the secondary emotion of love is derived from the primary emotions of joy and acceptance. Similarly, submission results from acceptance and fear, disappointment from surprise and sadness, contempt from disgust and anger, and so on.

Components of emotional response
The main components of emotional response are:

- subjective awareness
- physiological changes
- behaviour

James–Lange theory
According to this theory the experience of emotion is secondary to the somatic responses (e.g. sweating, increased cardiac rate, increased arousal) to the perception of given emotionally important events. For example, if an arachnophobe becomes aroused, experiences the increased activity of the sympathetic nervous system and runs away after seeing a spider, the feelings of anxiety and fear are the result of the increased sympathetic activity and running away, and not primarily because of the emotion-evoking stimulus.

Cannon criticized this theory. It was argued that similar physiological changes can accompany different emotions. Also, pharmacologically-induced simulation of such physiological changes is usually not accompanied by these emotions. The experience of emotions can be shown to be independent of somatic responses, sometimes occurring before the somatic responses.

Cannon–Bard theory

This holds that following the perception of an emotionally important event both the somatic responses and the experience of emotion occur together. In neuro-physiological terms, the perceived stimulus undergoes thalamic processing, and signals are then relayed to both the cerebral cortex, leading to the experience of emotion, and other parts of the body, such as the autonomic nervous system, leading to somatic responses.

This theory can be criticized on the basis of the observation that there are stimuli, e.g. sudden danger, which can lead to increased sympathetic activity before the emotion is experienced. Conversely, the experience of emotions sometimes occurs before the somatic response.

Schachter's cognitive labelling theory

According to this theory the conscious experience of an emotion is a function of the stimulus, of somatic or physiological responses, and of cognitive factors such as the cognitive appraisal of the situation and input from long-term memory. The influence of cognitive factors on the conscious experience of emotion was demonstrated in an experiment by Schachter and Singer (1962) in which subjects were injected with adrenaline. Their cognitive appraisal of the current situation, based on the observation of others, influenced the conscious experience of emotion. Thus cognitive cues were important in their interpretation of arousal.

STRESS

Stress results when demand exceeds resources. An individual's response to a stressful event situation is affected by biological susceptibility and personality characteristics.

Physiological and psychological aspects

Physiological effects of stress include: physical disorders (ulcers, cardiac disease and hypertension); and immune response changes. Other physical disorders have also been attributed to emotional stress, e.g. migraine, eczema, asthma and allergies.

Situational factors

These include life events, daily hassles/uplifts, conflict and trauma (see Chapter 29 on neurotic, stress-related and somatoform disorders).

LIFE EVENTS   These are changes in a person's life that require readjustment. They are ranked in order from most to least stressful. The most stressful include: the death of a spouse; divorce; marital separation; jail term; the death of a close family member; personal illness; and marriage. The scale has been found to be universally applicable to people in both underdeveloped and Western countries. Many conditions, both physical and mental, show an excess of life events in the months preceding the onset.

Vulnerability and invulnerability

Type A behaviour is related to increased proneness to heart disease. Such behaviour includes: competitiveness; striving for achievement; time urgency; difficulty relaxing; impatience; and anger.

It is possible to modify such behaviour.

Type B individuals do not exhibit the above characteristics; e.g. they can relax more easily and are slow to anger.

Stress-resistant people are those who view change as a challenge, and feel they have more control over events.

Coping mechanisms

Although the following mechanisms, used to cope with stress, are conscious, they relate to unconscious defence mechanisms too (given in parentheses): concentration only on the current task (denial); empathy (projection); logical analysis (rationalization); objectivity (isolation); playfulness (regression); substitution of other thoughts for disturbing ones (reaction formation); suppression of inappropriate feelings (repression).

Learned helplessness

Seligman found that dogs given unavoidable electric shocks suffered a number of phenomena which he considered were similar to depression, such as reduced appetite, disturbed sleep and reduced sex drive. He called this **learned helplessness.**

The cognitive theory of depression is based largely on this concept. Further work has found that individuals who believe that they have no personal control over events are much more likely to develop learned helplessness, whereas those who believe that nobody could have controlled the outcome are unlikely to do so. Thus a person's attribution of what is occurring influences the likelihood of developing major depression in cognitive terms.

Locus of control

Rotter differentiated those who see their lives as being under their own control (internal locus of control) from those who see their lives as being controlled externally (external locus of control).

BIBLIOGRAPHY

Atkinson, R.L., Atkinson, R.C. and Smith, E.E. 1990: *Introduction to psychology.* 10th edn. San Diego: Harcourt Brace Jovanovich.

Bandura, A. and Walters, R.H. 1963: *Social learning and personality development.* New York: Holt, Rinehart & Winston.

Hill, P. 1992: *Basic sciences: psychology.* Lecture handout, Guildford: MRCPsych Revision Course.

Spear, P.D., Penrod, S.D. and Baker, T.B 1988: *Psychology: perspectives on behaviour.* New York: John Wiley.

Wolpe, J. 1958: *Psychotherapy by Reciprocal Inhibition.* Stanford: Stanford University Press.

2
Social psychology

ATTITUDES

Definition
The definition of an attitude has been given variously as: 'a mental and neural state of readiness, organized through experience, exerting a directive or dynamic influence upon the individual's response to all objects and situations with which it is related' (Allport); and 'an enduring organization of motivational, emotional, perceptual, and cognitive processes with respect to some aspect of the individual's world' (Krech and Crutchfield). They are mutually consistent and internally consistent.

Components
Attitudes are based on **beliefs**, a tendency to **behave in an observable way**, and also have **affective** components which are the most resistant to change. A change in one of these three components leads to changes in the other two.

When predicting behaviour, situational variables must be taken into account. Otherwise measured attitudes are poor predictors of behaviour.

MEASUREMENT

Thurstone scale
This is a dichotomous scale indicating agreement/disagreement with presented and previously ranked statements.

Disadvantages: different response patterns may result in the same mean score; the setup is unwieldy; and the ranking may be biased.

Likert scale
This is a five-point scale indicating the level of agreement with presented statements.

Advantages: increased sensitivity compared with dichotomous Thurstone scale; more easily administered.

Disadvantages: different response patterns may result in the same mean score.

Semantic differential scale
This is a bipolar visual analogue scale.

Advantages: ease of use; good test-retest reliability.

Disadvantages: positional response bias may occur; no consistent meaning is attributed to a midpoint mark.

ATTITUDE CHANGE

A change in one of the three components of attitude leads to changes in the other two.

The origin of attitudes can be by means of the processes of learning: classical conditioning, operant conditioning, and observational learning. Superimposed on these are cognitive processes such as appraisal and modification in the light of new information.

Attitudes can be modified by either central pathways, entailing the consideration of new information, or by peripheral pathways involving the presentation of cues. Advertising uses both pathways.

The **balance theory** of Heider holds that each individual attempts to organize their attitudes, perceptions, and beliefs so that they are in harmony or balance with each other.

PERSUASIVE COMMUNICATION

The factors to consider are those concerned with the communicator, the recipient and the message being communicated.

Communicator
The characteristics of persuasive communicators include: attractiveness and audience identification with the communicator; credibility; expertise; genuine motivation; being an opinion leader; non-verbal communication; and views of reference groups.

Recipient
High self-esteem and intelligence of the recipient increase the likelihood that complex communications will be persuasive.

Message
Message repetition can be a persuasive influence leading to attitude change. Explicit messages are more persuasive for the less intelligent recipient and implicit messages for the more intelligent recipient.

Interactive personal discussions are more persuasive than mass media communication. One-sided communications are more persuasive for those who are less intelligent and/or already favourably disposed to the message. Two-sided presentations are more effective with intelligent and neutral recipients.

A low anxiety recipient is more influenced by a high fear message, and vice versa.

COGNITIVE CONSISTENCY AND DISSONANCE

When cognitive dissonance occurs, the individual feels uncomfortable, may experience increased arousal, and is motivated to achieve cognitive consistency. This may occur by changing one or more of the cognitions involved in the dissonant relationship, changing the behaviour which is inconsistent with the cognition(s), or adding new cognitions which are consonant with pre-existing ones. Cognitive consistency can also be achieved, when attitude and behaviour are inconsistent (attitude discrepant behaviour), by altering attitude.

SELF-PSYCHOLOGY

SELF-CONCEPT

This is a set of attitudes that the individual holds about himself/herself. It does not necessarily correspond to reality. Self-theory was developed by Rogers.

Self-esteem
This is one's own evaluation of self-worth and feeling accepted by others. Those lacking in self-esteem have feelings of worthlessness, alienation and lack of

acceptance by others, whereas those with high self-esteem are more socially active, less prejudiced, more risk-taking and warmer in social relationships. It is learned and so may change with experience.

Self-image
Self-image is a set of beliefs held about oneself, based on achievements and social interactions, which influences personal meaning and behaviour.

SELF-PERCEPTION THEORY

An individual infers what their attitude must be by observation of their own behaviour, in a similar way to how other people infer their behaviour.

Self-perception theory provides a better explanation than cognitive dissonance theory for behaviour that lies within the general range of behaviours acceptable to the individual.

INTERPERSONAL ISSUES

INTERPERSONAL ATTRACTION

In general, humans seek the company of others, to whom they are attracted. In difficult situations this may allow assessment by social comparisons, taking note of the opinions of others (**social comparison theory** (Festinger)). An alternative theory is that seeking the company of others leads to **arousal reduction** (Epley).

Theories of interpersonal attraction include:

- Reinforcement theory: reciprocal reinforcement of the attractions occurs with rewards in both directions (Newcomb). Conversely, punishments diminish the probability of interpersonal attraction.
- Social exchange theory: people prefer relationships that appear to offer an optimum cost-benefit ratio (Homans).
- Equity theory: the preferred relationships are those in which each feels that the cost-benefit ratio of the relationship for each person is approximately equal (Hatfield and Traupmann).
- Proxemics: relates to interpersonal space/body buffer zone.

Factors predisposing to interpersonal attraction include proximity, familiarity, similarity of interests and values, exposure, perceived competence, reciprocal liking and self-disclosure and physical attractiveness. Similarity is more important than complimentarity although the latter increases in importance with time.

According to the **matching hypothesis**, pairing occurs such that individuals seek others who have a similar level of physical attractiveness.

Attribution theory (Heider)
This deals with the rules people use to infer the causes of observed behaviour.

- Internal or dispositional attribution: the inference that the person is primarily responsible for their behaviour.
- External or situational attribution: the inference that the cause of a behaviour is external to the person.
- Primary (fundamental) attribution error: a bias towards dispositional rather than situational attribution when inferring the cause of other people's behaviour.

SOCIAL INFLUENCE

LEADERSHIP

Lewin *et al.* distinguished between the following leadership styles:

- Autocratic: abandon task in leader's absence; good for situations of urgency.
- Democratic: yields greater productivity unless a highly original product is required.
- *Laissez-faire*: appropriate for creative, open-ended, person-oriented tasks.

SOCIAL FACILITATION

This refers to the way in which tasks and responses are facilitated when carried out in the presence of others (Allport; Harlow). To occur, the others do not necessarily have to be engaging in the same task. Facilitation also occurs if the others are simply observing; this has been called the **audience effect** (Dashiell).

SOCIAL POWER

French and Raven described the following five types of social power:

- Authority: power derived from role
- Reward: power derived from ability to allocate resources
- Coercive: power to punish
- Referent: charismatic and liked by others
- Expert: power derived from skill, knowledge and experience

Conformity

Two types of conformity to the actions and opinions of others have been identified (Duetsch and Gerard):

- **Informational** social influence: an individual conforms to the consensual opinion and behaviour of the group both publicly and in their own thoughts (evident with ambiguous stimuli).
- **Normative** social influence: situations in which an individual publicly conforms to the consensual opinion and behaviour of the group but has a different view in their own mind. The individual conforms to the group under social pressure to avoid **social rejection.**

Self-reliant, intelligent, expressive, socially effective individuals are least vulnerable to group pressure.

Obedience to authority

Milgram found that most subjects would obey an experimenter's orders to administer what they believed to be increasingly powerful electrical shocks to others, right up to the maximum voltage available. Factors that increased the rate of obedience included the presence of the experimenter, the belief that the prior agreement was binding on the subject, and increasing distance from the apparently suffering person.

INTERGROUP BEHAVIOUR

Stereotypes
A stereotype is an overgeneralized inference about a person or a group of people in which they are all assumed to possess particular traits or characteristics.

The use of schemata (working stereotypes) is inevitable until further experience either refines or discredits them. Many stereotypes are benign but may be resistant to change. However, stereotypes can become self-perpetuating and self-fulfilling.

Prejudice
This refers to the prejudgement of others that is not amenable to discussion and is resistant to change.

Prejudiced individuals may behave in ways that create stereotyped behaviour which sustains their prejudice.

REDUCING PREJUDICE   Cook showed that the following conditions need to be satisfied in order to reduce prejudice:

- equal status
- the potential for personal acquaintance
- exposure to non-stereotypic individuals
- a social environment favouring equality
- cooperative effort

AGGRESSION

Aggression is behaviour intended to harm others.

- Hostile aggression: the sole intent is to inflict injury
- Instrumental aggression: the intention is to obtain reward or inflict suffering

Explanations
PSYCHOANALYTIC   Aggression is viewed as a basic instinct.

SOCIAL LEARNING THEORY   Aggression is viewed as a learned response. It is learned through observation, imitation and operant conditioning.

OPERANT CONDITIONING   Positive reinforcers can include victim suffering and material gains. The consequences of aggression play an important role in shaping future behaviour.

ETHOLOGY   Some ethologists believe that humans and animals are innately aggressive. Animal studies show that certain behaviours inhibit aggression:

- maintaining a distance
- evoking a social response incompatible with aggression
- familiarity

FRUSTRATION–AGGRESSION HYPOTHESIS   This proposes that preventing a person reaching their goal induces an aggressive drive resulting in behaviour intended to harm the one causing the frustration. Expressing this aggression reduces the aggressive drive.

AROUSAL   Emotional arousal can increase aggression.

Influence of television
It is known that children imitate observed aggression. Some studies suggest a relationship between exposure to violence on television and aggressive behaviour

in boys, but not in girls. It may be that this is because aggressive behaviour in boys, but not in girls, is socially reinforced.

The ways in which filmed violence may increase aggressive behaviour include:

- teaching aggressive styles of conduct
- increasing arousal
- desensitizing people to violence
- reducing restraint on aggressive behaviour
- distorting views about conflict resolution

INTERPERSONAL COOPERATION

Altruism

This is a higher defence mechanism in which the individual deals with emotional conflict or internal or external stressors by dedication to meeting the needs of others. Unlike the self-sacrifice sometimes characteristic of reaction formation, the individual receives gratification either vicariously or from the response of others (DSM-IV).

BIBLIOGRAPHY

Atkinson, R.L., Atkinson, R.C. and Smith, E.E. 1990: *Introduction to psychology.* 10th edn. San Diego: Harcourt Brace Jovanovich.

Bandura, A. and Walters, R.H 1963: *Social learning and personality development.* New York: Holt, Rinehart & Winston.

Hill, P. 1992: *Basic sciences: psychology.* Lecture handout, Guildford: MRCPsych Revision Course.

Spear, P.D., Penrod, S.D. and Baker, T.B. 1988: *Psychology: perspectives on behaviour.* New York: John Wiley.

3
Neuropsychology

MEMORY

Sensory memory
The anatomical correlate of iconic memory is probably the visual association cortex, while that of echoic memory is probably the auditory association cortex.

Short-term memory
The anatomical correlate of auditory verbal short-term memory is the left (dominant) parietal lobe, while that of visual verbal short-term memory is possibly the left temporo-occipital area. That of non-verbal short-term memory is possibly the right (non-dominant) temporal lobe.

Long-term memory
Long-term memory can be considered to be made up of explicit and implicit memory.

EXPLICIT MEMORY   This requires a deliberate act of recollection and can be reported verbally. It includes declarative memory and episodic memory, which are probably stored separately, since it is possible to lose one type of memory while retaining the other. **Declarative** memory involves knowledge of facts whereas **episodic** memory involves memory of autobiographical events. Explicit memory involves the medial temporal lobes, particularly the hippocampus, the entorhinal cortex, the subiculum and the parahippocampal cortex. Damage to these structures results in an inability to store new memory. Memory probably passes from medial temporal lobe structures after a few weeks/months to longer term storage in the cortex.

IMPLICIT MEMORY   This is recalled automatically without effort and is learnt slowly through repetition. It is not readily amenable to verbal reporting. It comprises **procedural** knowledge: that is, knowing **how**. Its storage requires functioning of the cerebellum, amygdala and specific sensory and motor systems used in the learned task. For example, the basal ganglia are involved in learning motor skills. Classical and operant learning involve implicit memory.

LANGUAGE

Cerebral dominance
Cerebral dominance for language is as follows:

- In 99 per cent of right-handers the left cerebral hemisphere is dominant.
- In 60 per cent of left-handers the left cerebral hemisphere is dominant.

In early life there is plasticity for cerebral dominance for language before the functions are established.

Speech and language areas

BROCA'S AREA   This is the motor speech area, occupying the opercular and triangular zones of the inferior frontal gyrus (BA 44 and 45). It is involved in coordinating the organs of speech to produce coherent sounds. In lesions confined to this area in the dominant hemisphere, speech comprehesion is intact and the muscles involved in speech production work normally, but the production of speech is affected.

WERNICKE'S AREA   This is the sensory speech and language area, occupying the posterior part of the auditory association cortex (BA 42 and 22) of the superior temporal gyrus. It is usually larger in the left hemisphere. It is involved in making sense of speech and language.

ANGULAR GYRUS   This part of the brain (BA 39) has abundant connections with the somatosensory, visual, and auditory association cortices. Lesions here produce an inability to read or write.

Pathways

Understanding spoken language (hearing):   Spoken word → Auditory cortex → Auditory association cortex → Wernicke's area → Hear and comprehend speech.

Understanding written language (reading):   Written word → Visual cortex → Visual association cortex → Angular gyrus → Wernicke's area → Read and comprehend.

Speaking: Thought/cognition → Wernicke's area → Broca's area → Motor speech areas → Speech.

Writing: Thought/cognition → Wernicke's area → Angular gyrus → Motor areas → Write.

Dysphasias

Damage to those brain areas involved with speech and language results in dysphasia; the type of dysphasia is determined by the areas of the brain involved.

Receptive dysphasia: damage to Wernicke's area disrupts the ability to comprehend language, either written or spoken. In addition to loss of comprehension, the person is also unaware that their dysphasic speech is difficult for others to follow. Speech is normal in rhythm and intonation (because Broca's area is intact), but the content is abnormal. The words used have lost their meaning; empty words (e.g. 'thing', 'it') and paraphrasias are used liberally. Thus damage to Wernicke's area results in a **fluent receptive dysphasia**.

Expressive dysphasia: damage to Broca's area results in loss of rhythm, intonation and grammatical aspects of speech. Comprehension is normal (because Wernicke's area is intact) and the person is aware that their speech is difficult for others to follow, resulting in distress and frustration. Speech is slow and hesitant, often lacking the connecting words. Speech sounds agrammatical and articulation may be crude, probably because of the close proximity of Broca's area to motor areas. Thus damage to Broca's area results in **dysfluent expressive dysphasia**.

Conduction dysphasia: damage to the arcuate fasciculus results in a conduction dysphasia in which the person cannot repeat what is said to them. Their comprehension and verbal fluency remain intact.

Global dysphasia: results from global left hemispheric dysfunction, and shows a combination of all the above.

PERCEPTION

Perception relates to the means by which the brain makes representations of the external environment.

Agnosia is the inability to interpret and recognize the significance of sensory information, which does not result from impairment of the sensory pathways, mental deterioration, disorders of consciousness and attention or, in the case of an object, a lack of familiarity with the object.

Visual perception

- Shape, colour and spatial orientation: occipital lobes
  Lesions at this level result in pseudoagnosia
- Visuospatial elements drawn together into complete percepts (objects seen as a whole): right parietal lobe. Meaning not yet attributed to the objects
  Lesions at this level result in apperceptive agnosia
- Meaning of object then accessed from the left parietal lobe (which itself accesses meaning from semantic memory): parieto-occipital areas
  Lesions at this level result in associative agnosia

Other agnosias

Prosopagnosia is an inability to recognize faces. In advanced Alzheimer's disease a patient may misidentify their own mirrored reflection, the **mirror sign**.

In **agnosia for colours** the patient is unable correctly to name colours, although colour sense is still present.

In **simultanagnosia** the patient is unable to recognize the overall meaning of a picture whereas its individual details are understood.

Agraphognosia or agraphaesthesia is tested by asking the patient to identify, with closed eyes, numbers or letters traced on their palm; this disorder is present if the patient is unable to identify such writing.

In **anosognosia** there is a lack of awareness of disease, particularly of hemiplegia (most often following a right parietal lesion).

Autotopagnosia is the inability to name, recognize or point on command to parts of the body.

In **astereognosia** objects cannot be recognized by palpation.

In **finger agnosia** the patient is unable to recognize individual fingers.

Topographical disorientation can be tested using a locomotor map-reading task in which the patient is asked to trace out a given route by foot.

In **hemisomatognosis or hemidepersonalization** the patient feels that a limb (which in fact is present) is missing.

Apraxias

Apraxia is an inability to perform purposive volitional acts, which does not result from paresis, incoordination, sensory loss or involuntary movements.

Constructional apraxia is closely associated with **visuospatial agnosia**. There is an inability to construct a figure.

In **dressing apraxia** there is an inability to dress.

In **ideomotor apraxia** there is an inability to carry out progressively difficult tasks.

In **ideational apraxia** there is an inability to carry out a coordinated sequence of actions.

Frontal lobe functions

PREFRONTAL CORTEX

- Problem-solving
- Perceptual judgement
- Memory
- Programming and planning of sequences of behaviour
- Verbal regulation
- Level of response emission
- Adaptability of response pattern
- Tertiary level of motor control

FRONTAL EYE FIELDS

- Voluntary eye movements

MOTOR AND PREMOTOR CORTEX

- Primary and secondary levels of motor control
- Design fluency

BROCA'S AREA

- Expressive speech

ORBITAL CORTEX

- Personality
- Social behaviour

FRONTAL LOBE LESIONS   These cause:

- personality change: disinhibition, reduced social and ethical control, sexual indiscretions, poor judgement, elevated mood, lack of concern for the feelings of other people and irritability
- perseveration
- utilization behaviour
- pallilalia
- impairment of attention, concentration and initiative
- aspontaneity, slowed psychomotor activity
- motor Jacksonian fits
- urinary incontinence
- contralateral spastic paresis
- aphasia
- primary motor aphasia
- motor agraphia
- anosmia
- ipsilateral optic atrophy

Gerstmann's syndrome

This is caused by dominant parietal lobe lesions and consists of:

- dyscalculia
- agraphia
- finger agnosia
- right-left disorientation

BIBLIOGRAPHY

Atkinson, R.L., Atkinson, R.C. and Smith, E.E. 1990: *Introduction to psychology.* 10th edn. San Diego: Harcourt Brace Jovanovich.

4
Psychological assessment

PRINCIPLES OF MEASUREMENT

Interviews
Sources of error include:

- Response set: the tendency always to agree or to disagree with the questions asked.
- Bias towards the centre: the tendency always to avoid extreme responses. As a result, there is an excess choice of middle responses.
- Extreme responding: the opposite tendency of selecting extreme responses.
- Social desirability: the subject makes a choice of responses that he or she believes the interviewer desires. May be reduced through the inclusion of lie scales or the forced-choice technique.
- Defensiveness: the subject avoids giving too much self-related information.
- Halo effect: the observer allows their preconception to influence the responses.
- Hawthorne effect: interviewer alters the situation by their presence.

Self-predictions
This is a direct method of measuring behaviour in which the subject is asked to give their own prediction concerning the behaviour under question. It can be combined with self-recording.

Psychophysiological techniques
These involve the direct use of physiological measurements in assessing behaviour.

Naturalistic observations
These involve the assessment of behaviour as it occurs with minimum interference by the observer. In time-sampling techniques the subject is observed during given time intervals at given times of the day or night.

Naturalistic observations are used in the functional analysis of problem behaviours. This method is sometimes referred to as ABC (for Antecedents, Behaviours, Consequences).

Scaling
This refers to the conversion of raw data into types of scores more readily understood, e.g. ranks, (per)centiles and standardized scores.

Norm-referencing
A norm is an average, common or standard performance under specified conditions. A test may be standardized to this norm.

Criterion-referencing
A criterion is a set of scores against which a predictive test's success can be compared.

INTELLIGENCE

Aptitude
This is the raw or potential ability of an individual.

Attainment
This is the result of learning.

Mental age scale
The concept of the mental age (MA) was devised by Binet as the average intellectual ability, as measured by the level of problem-solving and reasoning. The scale was devised such that the average range of scores corresponds to the chronological age (CA).

For children with a higher than average level of intelligence, MA > CA.

For children with a lower than average level of intelligence, MA < CA.

The Stanford–Binet test can be applied to each year, up to the age of 15.

Intelligence quotient (IQ)
This is the ratio of the mental age to the chronological age, expressed as a percentage:

$$IQ = (MA/CA) \times 100$$

By convention, intelligence has a normal distribution with a mean of 100 and a standard deviation of 15.

There is a natural decline in intellectual ability with age. Performance IQ falls off with age more quickly than verbal IQ: the verbal-performance discrepancy. This decline is taken into account when raw scores are converted into IQ equivalents. Thus, although raw abilities decline with age, measured IQ remains constant.

Wechsler Adult Intelligence Scale: Revised (WAIS-R)
This well-standardized test gives both a verbal IQ and a performance IQ, and consists of 11 subtests:

Verbal		*Performance*	
	■ information		■ picture completion
	■ comprehension		■ block design
	■ arithmetic		■ picture arrangement
	■ similarities		■ object assembly
	■ digit span		■ digit symbol
	■ vocabulary		

The verbal and performance scores are added together to produce a full scale IQ. The WAIS has a relatively high reliability and validity.

Weschler Intelligence Scale for Children: Revised (WISC-R)
This is a modified version of the WAIS for children between the ages of five and 15 years.

Weschler Preschool and Primary Scale of Intelligence (WPPSI)
This is a modified version of the WAIS for children between the ages of four and six years and six months.

Group ability tests
Unlike the above, these can be used by one examiner to assess the intellectual ability and aptitude of a group of people, e.g. the Armed Services Vocational Aptitude Battery (ASVAB).

Nature–nurture
Potential intelligence (aptitude) is inherited, but environmental factors influence the fulfilment of potential (attainment).

Cultural influences
Tests of attainment can give rise to discrepant results when applied to people from different cultures. It is thought that tests measuring aptitude, e.g. Raven's matrices, are less prone to such influences.

PSYCHOMETRIC METHODS OF ASSESSING PERSONALITY

Objective tests
The items presented have limited responses.

MINNESOTA MULTIPHASIC PERSONALITY INVENTORY (MMPI)   This is a standardized self-report personality inventory, consisting of around 550 statements concerning attitudes, emotional reactions, physical symptoms, psychological symptoms and previous experiences presented in a true/false/cannot say format.

CALIFORNIA PSYCHOLOGICAL INVENTORY (CPI)   This allows the measurement of 18 traits that are part of normal personality, such as achievement, dominance, self-acceptance and sociability.

EYSENCK PERSONALITY QUESTIONNAIRE (EPQ)   This contains 90 items in true/false format. Subjects are rated on the following dimensions: extraversion; introversion; and neuroticism.

HOSTILITY AND DIRECTION OF HOSTILITY QUESTIONNAIRE (HDHQ)   This is used to measure relationships that could be affected by personality status.

In general, because of evidence that mental state markedly affects the scoring of questionnaires, they have been replaced by interview schedules and other observer ratings.

Projective tests
The presented items have no one correct answer, instead taking the form of ambiguous stimuli, upon which the subject projects their personality. Their reliability and validity have not been established: for example, the Rorschach Inkblot Test, Thematic Apperception Test (TAT) and Sentence Completion Test (SCT).

BIBLIOGRAPHY

Atkinson, R.L., Atkinson, R.C. and Smith, E.E. 1990: *Introduction to psychology*, 10th edn. San Diego: Harcourt Brace Jovanovich.

5
Human development

CONCEPTUALIZING DEVELOPMENT

Basic concepts
Human development involves an interaction between nature and nurture.

Stage theories propose that development occurs in a progressive sequence reflecting maturation. Examples include Piaget's cognitive stages; Freud's psychosexual stages; and Kohlberg's stage theory. Maturation refers to the orderly changes in behaviour that result from biological development and whose timing and form are relatively independent of external experience. Maturational tasks are influenced by biological growth; the drive for independence; and other people's general expectations.

Gene–environment interactions
These interactions determine all psychological characteristics, such as intelligence. Genetic factors determine the inherited potential, while environmental factors determine the degree to which this potential is fulfilled.

With respect to intelligence, while it is generally agreed that there is a genetic component to intelligence, there is disagreement about the degree of environmental influence on it. The correlation coefficient for IQ between MZ twins is 0.86 compared with 0.60 for DZ twins. Using factor analysis, Spearman identified a general factor, g, and a specific factor, s, of intelligence; it was proposed that the level of g was associated with how intelligent the individual was.

Historical models
The historical developmental models of Freud and Erikson are described in Chapter 33 on Personality Disorders. Social-learning models lay emphasis on the way in which environmental influences affect subsequent behaviour. The most influential theory of cognitive development is that of Piaget (see below).

ATTACHMENT AND BONDING

ATTACHMENT THEORY
This comes from the work of Bowlby. **Attachment** refers to the tendency of infants to remain close to certain people (attachment figures) with whom they share strong positive emotional ties. Monotropic attachment is when the attachment is one individual, usually the mother. Polytropic attachment is less common. Attachment usually takes place from infant to mother. In contrast,

neonatal-maternal **bonding** takes place in the opposite direction. Both processes can start immediately after birth.

Some behaviourists consider attachment to result from the mother acting as a conditioned reinforcer.

This theory was challenged by Harlow who, using cuddly and wire artificial surrogate mothers and infant rhesus monkeys, found that attachment is a function of the requirement to be in contact with a soft object (contact comfort), which provides security. Other studies have found that warm or rocking artificial surrogate mothers are preferred to colder or still surrogates, respectively.

Lorenz considered attachment to result from imprinting whereby geese, during a critical period soon after hatching, persistently follow the first nearby moving object encountered. There is no evidence that imprinting occurs in primates.

Bowlby considered infant attachment to take place in the context of a warm, intimate and continuous relationship with the caregiver in which there is reciprocal satisfaction. The attachment process takes an average of six months to become fully established. Bonding is stronger if there is tactile contact as soon as possible after birth. The mother's attachment behaviour is reinforced by infant smiling, movement, and crying. **Attachment behaviours** are the signs of distress shown by the child when separated from their attachment figure, and include:

- crying when the caregiver (usually the mother) leaves the room
- attempting to follow her
- clinging hard when distressed
- hugging her
- being more playful and talkative in her company
- using her as a secure base from which exploration can take place

These start to occur at about the age of six months and decrease visibly by three years. Prior to this age separation is tolerated without distress.

Attachment abnormalities

INSECURE ATTACHMENT   There is chronic clinginess and ambivalence towards the mother. Clinically this may be relevant as it may be a precursor to:

- childhood emotional disorders (including school refusal)
- disorders (such as agoraphobia) starting in adolescence and adulthood

AVOIDANT ATTACHMENT   A distance is kept from the mother, who may sometimes be ignored. Clinically, avoidant attachment caused by rejection by the mother may be relevant as it may be a precursor to:

- poor social functioning in later life (including aggression)

Separation anxiety

This is the fear an infant shows of being separated from their caregiver. Holding a comfort object or transitional object (Winnicott) may help with separation.

The rate of disappearance of separation anxiety varies with the child's:

- experiences of previous separations (real or threatened)
- handling by mother
- perception of whether mother will die or depart
- temperament

Acute separation reaction

After starting to form attachments, around six months to two years of age, separation from the mother leads to the following reactions:

- first, **protest**: including crying and searching behaviour
- second, **despair**: apathy and misery with an apparent belief that the mother may not return
- finally, **detachment**: emotionally distant from (and indifferent to) the mother.

Stranger anxiety
This refers to a fear of strangers shown by infants usually between the ages of eight months and one year. It is not necessarily part of attachment behaviour and may occur independently of separation anxiety.

Maternal deprivation
Following a failure to form adequate attachments, for example because of prolonged maternal separation or rejecting parents, the effects of maternal deprivation may include:

- developmental language delay
- indiscriminate affection-seeking
- shallow relationships
- enuresis
- aggression
- lack of empathy
- social disinhibition
- attention-seeking and overactivity in school
- poor growth: deprivation dwarfism

FAMILY RELATIONSHIPS AND PARENTING PRACTICE

Child-rearing practice
Table 5.1 (after Baumrind, 1967) shows how the parents of three groups of children have been found to score on the four dimensions of:

- control: by the parents of the child's activities and behaviour
- maturity demands: of the child to act at their ability level
- communication: clarity of parent–child communication
- nurturance: parental nurturance towards the child

The three groups of children were:

Group I: the most mature and competent
Group II: moderately self-controlled and self-reliant but somewhat withdrawn
   and distrustful
Group III: the most immature and dependent

Table 5.1   The way in which parents of three groups of children score on the dimensions of control, maturity demands, communication and nurturance

	Control	Maturity demands	Communication	Nurturance
Group I	↑ ↑	↑ ↑	↑ ↑	↑ ↑
Group II	↑	→	↓	↓ ↓
Group III	↓ ↓	↓ ↓	↓ ↓	↑

Family structure

In the UK and US, around 25 per cent of children are not living with both biological parents by the age of 16 years. If orthodox families are defined as those nuclear families in which there are two parents with a small number of children, then non-orthodox family structures may or may not be relevant so far as the healthy psychosocial development of the child is concerned:

SINGLE PARENTS ↑ behavioural and emotional problems (particularly if no other support)

EXTENDED FAMILY Not harmful

TWO LESBIAN PARENTS Not harmful

LARGE FAMILY SIZE ↑ behavioural and educational problems
↓ intelligence

Ordinal position in family

The oldest child has a slight advantage in intellectual development. This also applies to only children.

Twins show delayed language development.

Distorted family function

Dysfunctional families may manifest:

- discord
- overprotection: of the child(ren) by the parents
- rejection: of the child(ren)
- enmeshment: parents may be overinvolved in their children's feelings and lives
- disengagement: parents may be underinvolved in their children's feelings and lives
- triangulation: exclusive alliances are formed within the family; e.g. father/daughter (although this may, for example, be helpful in preventing the father from leaving home)
- communication difficulties: e.g. ambiguous or incongruous communications
- myths: created within the families

Marital conflicts may cause the parents to need to have a child with a problem who can act as a scapegoat (until they leave home).

Impact of bereavement

The death of a parent leads to initial bereavement reactions, which may include prolonged sadness, crying and irritability during childhood, and:

- young children: ↑ functional enuresis
  ↑ temper tantrums
- older children (especially girls): ↑ sleep disturbance
  ↑ clear-cut depressive reactions
- school performance: impaired (may be only temporary)

Impact of parental divorce

Parental divorce is associated with an increased rate of disturbance in children (greater than following parental bereavement). Protective factors include:

- amicable arrangements for access following the divorce
- good parental relationship with the child
- good relationships of the child with other siblings
- the child's temperament

Impact of intrafamilial abuse

SEXUAL ABUSE   Child sexual abuse is 'the involvement of dependent, developmentally immature children and adolescents in sexual activities that they do not fully comprehend, are unable to give informed consent to, and that violate the social taboos of family roles'(Schechter and Roberge 1976).

The findings of a study by Cosentino *et al.* (1995) suggest that sexual abuse in preadolescent girls is associated with sexual behaviour problems. This study compared a group of sexually abused girls, aged six to 12 years, with two demographically comparable control groups, girls from a child psychiatry outpatient department, and girls from a general paediatric clinic. Compared to both control groups, sexually abused girls manifested more sexual behaviour problems: masturbating openly and excessively, exposing their genitals, indiscriminately hugging and kissing strange adults and children, and attempting to insert objects into their genitals. Abuse by fathers or stepfathers involving intercourse was associated with particularly marked sexual behaviour disturbances. There was a subgroup of sexually abused girls who tended to force sexual activities on siblings and peers. All these girls had experienced prolonged sexual abuse (more than two years) involving physical force which was perpetrated by a parent.

Recognized sequelae of sexual abuse include:

- anxiety states and anxiety-related symptoms (e.g. sleep disturbance, nightmares, psychosomatic complaints, and hypervigilance), re-enactments of the victimization, and post-traumatic stress disorder (Goodwin 1985; Green 1985)
- depression (Gaensbauer and Sands 1979; Sgroi 1982)
- dissociation (Kluft 1985)
- paranoid reactions and mistrust (Green 1978; Herman 1981)
- excessive reliance on primitive defence mechanisms (e.g. denial, projection, dissociation, and splitting) (Green 1978)
- borderline personality disorder (especially in females) (Herman *et al.* 1989)
- inability to control sexual impulses (precocious sexual play with high sexual arousal) (Cosentino *et al.* 1995; Friedrich and Reams 1987; Yates 1982)
- weakened gender identity (a tendency to reject their maleness or femaleness) (Aiosa-Karpas *et al.* 1991)
- ↑ incidence of homosexuality (Finkelhor 1984)
- ↑ incidence of molesting children (the cycle of abuse may continue: there is a high incidence of sexual abuse in the backgrounds of male and female child molesters) (McCarty 1986; Seghorn *et al.* 1987)
- drug and alcohol abuse (Herman 1981)
- eating disorders (Oppenheimer *et al.* 1985)

PHYSICAL ABUSE/NON-ACCIDENTAL INJURY   Non-accidental injury can be defined as occurring 'when an adult inflicts a physical injury on a child more severe than that which is culturally acceptable' (Graham 1991).

The recognized sequelae of physical abuse (which overlap with those of sexual abuse) include:

- anxiety states and anxiety-related symptoms (e.g. sleep disturbance, nightmares, psychosomatic complaints, and hypervigilance), re-enactments of the victimization, and post-traumatic stress disorder (Goodwin 1985; Green 1985)
- depression (Gaensbauer and Sands 1979; Sgroi 1982)
- dissociation (Kluft 1985; Putnam 1985)

- paranoid reactions and mistrust (Green 1978; Herman 1981)
- excessive reliance on primitive defence mechanisms (e.g. denial, projection, dissociation, and splitting) (Green 1978)
- borderline personality disorder (especially in females) (Herman *et al*. 1989)
- aggressive and destructive behaviour at home and school (George and Main 1979; Green 1978)
- cognitive and developmental impairment (Elmer and Gregg 1967; Oates 1986)
- delayed language development (Martin 1972)
- neurological impairment (Green *et al*. 1981)
- abusive behaviour with their own children (the cycle of abuse may continue) (Steele 1983)

TEMPERAMENT

Temperament can be defined as early appearing, biologically rooted, basic personality dimensions (Zuckerman 1991).

Individual temperamental differences
In the New York Longitudinal Study, Thomas and Chess (Chess and Thomas 1984; Thomas and Chess 1977) identified the following nine categories of temperament describing how children behave in daily life situations:

1 Activity level
2 Rhythmicity (regularity of biological functions)
3 Approach or withdrawal to new situations
4 Adaptability in new or altered situations
5 Sensory threshhold of responsiveness to stimuli
6 Intensity of reaction
7 Quality of mood
8 Distractibility
9 Attention span/persistence

In terms of the impact of individual temperamental differences on parent-child relationships, the above nine categories have been found to cluster as follows:

- **easy child** pattern: characterized by regularity, positive approach responses to new stimuli, high adaptability to change, and expressions of mood that are mild/moderate in intensity and predominantly positive
- **difficult child** pattern: characterized by irregularity in biological functions, negative withdrawal responses to new situations, non-adaptability or slow adaptability to change, and intense, frequently negative expressions of mood
- **slow-to-warm-up child**: characterized by a combination of negative responses of mild intensity to new situations with slow adaptability after repeated contact

ORIGINS, TYPOLOGIES AND STABILITY OF TEMPERAMENT

Medieval personality theorists relied on a temperament typology based on the balance of the humours, but twentieth-century theorists have put the strongest emphasis on environmental causation models. Acceptance of the concept of biologically rooted personality dimensions is a fairly recent stage in the history of scientific psychology and psychiatry (Bates *et al.* 1995); important points to note are:

- Temperament is a theoretical construct: it is more useful to think of specific dimensions of temperament, e.g. activity level, sociability, negative emotionality, or distractibility. Temperament concepts can be defined at the following three levels (Bates 1989):

  1 as patterns of surface behaviour
  2 as a pattern of nervous system responses
  3 as having inborn genetic roots

- There is an increased understanding of the biological processes involved in temperament. Since concepts of temperament typically focus on individual differences in emotion, attention, and activity (Bates 1989), the neural basis of temperament can be thought of as emerging from the brain systems supporting emotion, attention, and activity:

  1 limbic structures
  2 association cortex
  3 motor cortical areas

- Environmental influences affect how the biological bases of temperament are expressed. For example, Gunnar (1994) showed how sensitive, responsive caregivers could enhance otherwise highly inhibited preschoolers' likelihood of approaching novel stimuli.
- Concepts of temperament can be useful in helping people solve problems. When the processes of linkage between temperament and the evolution of character and personality are better understood, this should assist prevention and treatment.

The stability of temperament and its relationship to the evolution of character and personality have been demonstrated in a number of studies. Characteristics of temperament in infants and preschool-age children predict adjustment in middle childhood and adolescence. For example, Caspi and Silva (1995) showed how temperamental qualities at the age of three years predict personality traits in young adulthood. In an unselected sample of over 800 subjects, five temperament groups (Undercontrolled, Inhibited, Confident, Reserved, and Well-adjusted) were identified when the children were aged three years. These groups were reassessed at 18. As young adults, Undercontrolled children scored high on measures of impulsivity, danger-seeking, aggression, and interpersonal alienation; Inhibited children scored low on measures of impulsivity, danger-seeking, aggression, and social potency; Confident children scored high on impulsivity; Reserved children scored low on social potency; and Well-adjusted children continued to exhibit normative behaviours.

PIAGET'S MODEL OF COGNITIVE DEVELOPMENT

Piaget believed that infantile and childhood intellectual development involve interactions with the outside world (e.g. through play). These lead to:

- new cognitive structures (**schemes**) are constructed incorporating new information
- in the presence of suitable existing schemes

- **assimilation**: new information is incorporated into appropriate existing schemes
- **accommodation**: modification of existing scheme(s)

Piaget identified four stages of cognitive development.

Sensorimotor stage

This is the first stage and occurs from birth to two years of age.

Circular reactions are repeated voluntary motor activities, e.g. shaking a toy, occurring from around two months.

- Primary circular reactions: from two to five months (approximately), when they have no apparent purpose
- Secondary circular reactions: from five to nine months (approximately), experimentation and purposeful behaviour is gradually manifested.
- Tertiary circular reactions: from one year to 18 months (approximately), include the creation of original behaviour patterns and the purposeful quest for novel experiences.

During this stage the infant comes to distinguish themselves from the environment. Thought processes exhibit **egocentrism**, in which the infant believes that everything happens in relation to them.

Until around six months the infant believes that an object hidden from view no longer exists. **Object permanence** is fully developed after around the age of 18 months.

Preoperational stage

This is the second stage and occurs from age two to seven years. During this stage the child learns to use the symbols of language.

Thought processes exhibited during this stage include:

- **animism**: life, thoughts and feelings are attributed to all objects, including inanimate ones
- **artificialism**: natural events are attributed to the action of people
- **authoritarian morality**: it is believed that wrongdoing, including breaking the rules of a game, should be punished according to the degree of the damage caused, whether accidental or not, rather than according to motive; negative events are perceived as punishments
- **creationism**: a teleological approach is taken in which, for example, stars and the moon exists in order to provide light at night
- **egocentrism**: as in the sensorimotor stage
- **finalism**: all things have a purpose
- **precausal reasoning**: based on internal schemes rather than the results of observation so that, for example, the same volume of liquid poured from one container to another with a different height and diameter may be considered to have changed volume
- **syncretism**: everything is believed to be connected with everything else

Concrete operational stage

This is the third stage and occurs from age seven to around 12–14 years. During this stage the child demonstrates logical thought processes and more subjective moral judgements.

An understanding of the **laws of conservation** of, initially, number and volume, and then weight, is normally achieved. Reversibility and some aspects of classification are mastered.

Formal operational stage

This is the final stage and occurs from the age of around 12–14 years onwards. It is characterized by the achievement of being able to think in the **abstract**, including the ability systematically to test hypotheses.

LANGUAGE DEVELOPMENT

Language can be defined as the sum of the skills required to communicate verbally (Graham 1991).

Normal childhood development

In the first hours postnatally, the baby learns to distinguish their mother's voice.

By three to four months babbling occurs.

By eight months repetitive babbling occurs.

By one year the baby has usually acquired the equivalent designations 'Mama', 'Dada', (no matter what language the parent speaks) and one additional word.

By 18 months a 20– to 50–word vocabulary is expressed in single word.

By two years, two- or three-word utterances can be strung together with some understanding of grammar. These are telegraphic utterances omitting grammatical morphemes (small units of meaning signifying the plural, for example).

At an average age of three years, the child can usually understand a request containing three parts.

Environmental influences and communicative competence

BILINGUAL HOME   Not a disadvantage unless there is another cause of slowed language development.

FAMILY SIZE   Larger family size is associated with slower speech development.

PREGNANCY   Intrauterine growth retardation is associated with slower language development. Prolonged second stage labour is associated with slower language development.

SEX   Early language development in girls is slightly greater than in boys.

SOCIAL CLASS   Being middle-class is associated with relatively faster language development.

STIMULATION   Although the capacity for language and grammar may be built-in, speech and language are not achieved in the usual manner if children are deaf or are not spoken to.

TWINS   Being a twin is associated with slower speech development.

MORAL DEVELOPMENT

KOHLBERG'S STAGE THEORY

Kohlberg presented a set of stories, each containing a moral dilemma, to various individuals of various ages and backgrounds. Questions were posed concerning the moral dilemmas. On the basis of the reasons given for the answers Kohlberg formulated a theory of moral development consisting of six developmental stages of moral judgement categorized into three Levels (I to III).

Preconventional morality (Level I)

This is the level at which the moral judgements of children up to the age of seven years mainly lie.

STAGE 1: PUNISHMENT ORIENTATION   Rules are obeyed in order to avoid punishment.

STAGE 2: REWARD ORIENTATION   Rules are conformed to in order to be rewarded.

Conventional morality (Level II)

This is the level at which most moral judgements of children lie by the age of 13 years.

STAGE 3: GOOD-BOY/GOOD-GIRL ORIENTATION   Rules are conformed to in order to avoid the disapproval of others.

STAGE 4: AUTHORITY ORIENTATION   Laws and social rules are upheld in order to avoid the censure of authorities and because of guilt about not doing one's duty.

Postconventional morality (Level III)

This level, which may never be reached even in adulthood, requires individuals to have achieved the later stages of Piaget's formal operational stage.

STAGE 5: SOCIAL CONTRACT ORIENTATION   Actions are guided by principles generally agreed to be essential for public welfare. These principles are upheld in order to maintain the respect of peers and self-respect.

STAGE 6: ETHICAL PRINCIPLE ORIENTATION   Actions are guided by principles chosen oneself, usually emphasizing dignity, equality and justice. These principles are upheld in order to avoid self-condemnation.

RELATIONSHIP TO THE DEVELOPMENT OF SOCIAL PERSPECTIVE-TAKING

Social perspective-taking is the ability to take the perspective of others. It is a skill that may be seen at the following levels:

- perceptual role-taking: the ability to take into account how a perceptual array appears to another person when their perspective differs from that of oneself
- cognitive role-taking: the ability to take into account the thoughts of another person when they differ from those of oneself
- affective role-taking: the ability to take into account the feelings of another person when they differ from those of oneself

In addition to being necessary to being able to emphathize with others, social perspective-taking was considered by Kohlberg as being necessary to develop the higher stages of moral reasoning.

DEVELOPMENT OF FEARS IN CHILDHOOD AND ADOLESCENCE

Definition

Fear is an unpleasant emotional state (a feeling of apprehension, tension or uneasiness) caused by a realistic current or impending danger that is recognized at a conscious level. It differs from anxiety in that in the latter the cause is vague or not as understandable. However, fear and anxiety are terms that are often used interchangeably.

Development with age

The types of fear that develop in childhood and adolescence differ with age (Marks 1987):

- six months: fear of novel stimuli begins (such as fear of strangers), reaching a peak at 18 months to two years
- six to eight months: fear of heights begins, and becomes worse when walking starts
- three to five years: common fears are those of animals, the dark, and 'monsters'
- six to 11 years: fear of shameful social situations (such as ridicule) begins
- adolescence: fear of death, failure, social gatherings (such as parties) and thermonuclear war may be particularly evident.

Possible aetiological and maintenance mechanisms

UNCONSCIOUS CONFLICT   Sigmund Freud (1926/1959) suggested that psychological anxiety is a signal phenomenon and that neurotic anxiety starts as the remembrance of realistic anxiety/fear related to a real danger. Each stage of life was considered to have age-appropriate determinants of anxiety/fear, including, with increasing age:

- fear of birth
- fear of separation from the mother
- fear of castration
- fear of the superego: fear of its anger or punishment
- fear of the superego: fear of its loss of love
- fear of the superego: fear of death

LEARNED RESPONSE   Fear/anxiety may become associated with particular situations by means of learning.

LACK OF CONTROL   Fear/anxiety may occur when an individual feels helpless in a situation beyond their control.

SEXUAL DEVELOPMENT

Sex determination

Sex determination is primarily as a result of the sex chromosomes (XX female and XY male). Gonad formation is first indicated in the embryo by the appearance of an area of thickened epithelium on the medial aspect of the mesonephric ridge during week five. Factors affecting subsequent differentiation of the genital organs into male ones (epididymis, ductus (vas) deferens, ejaculatory ducts, penis, and scrotum) or female ones (fallopian tubes, uterus, clitoris, and vagina) during ontogeny include:

- **Y chromosome**: In mammals, testis determination is under the control of the testis-determining factor borne by the Y chromosome. SRY, a gene cloned from the sex-determining region of the human Y chromosome, has been equated with the testis-determining factor in humans.
- **Degree of ripeness of the ovum at fertilization**: Over-ripeness of the ovum at fertilization is associated with a reduced number of primordial germ cells. This in turns leads to a masculinizing effect on genetic females.
- **Endocrine actions**: Androgens and oestrogens can modify the process of sexual differentiation, while in twin pregnancy with fetuses of opposite sex

and anastomosed placental circulations, the genetically male fetus may have a masculinizing effect on the genetically female fetus. A genetically female fetus may also be masculinized (and be born with either ambiguous or male genitalia) by fetal androgen from another source (e.g. in congenital adrenal (suprarenal) hyperplasia). Similarly, a genetically male fetus with a Y chromosome and testes may develop female genitalia in the absence of fetal androgen (e.g. in enzyme deficiency) or if androgen receptors are defective (e.g. in androgen insensitivity syndrome).

Changes at puberty

Puberty consists of a series of physical and physiological changes which convert a child into an adult who is capable of sexual reproduction.

PHYSICAL CHANGES   These include:

- growth spurt
- change in body proportion
- development of sexual organs
- development of secondary sexual characteristics

Tanner described a standardized system for recording breast, pubic hair and genital maturation.

ONSET IN GIRLS   In 95 per cent onset occurs between nine and 13 years. The first sign is:

- breast formation: in 80 per cent
- pubic hair growth: in 20 per cent

In Western countries menarche occurs at a mean age of 13.5 years.

ONSET IN BOYS   In 95 per cent onset occurs between 9.5 and 13.5 years. The first sign is usually testicular and scrotal enlargement, followed by growth of the penis and pubic hair. On average, the first ejaculation occurs at around 13 years.

PHYSIOLOGICAL CHANGES   A raising of the threshold for gonadohypothalamic negative feedback precedes the onset of puberty. An increase in suprarenal androgen release (adrenarche) usually begins between the ages of six and eight years; these hormones lead to the growth of sexual hair and skeletal maturation.

Gender identity

This is an individual's perception and self-awareness with respect to gender. It is usually established by the age of three or four years and usually remains firmly established thereafter.

Gender/sex typing

This is the process by which individuals acquire a sense of gender and gender-related cultural traits appropriate to the society and age into which they are born. It usually begins at an early age with male and female infants being treated differently, for example with respect to the choice of their clothing.

Gender role

This is the type of behaviour that an individual engages in that identifies them as being male or female, for example with respect to the type of clothes worn and the use of cosmetics.

Sexual behaviour

SEXUAL DRIVE   This is the need to achieve sexual pleasure through genital stimulation. It exists from birth to middle childhood and increases again during adolescence as a result of increased androgen secretion.

CHILDHOOD SEXUALITY   This may manifest itself in normal children as:

- sex play in infancy
- erections in boys
- vaginal lubrication in girls
- masturbation: which may involve orgasm
- exploratory encounters with other children

MASTURBATION   This is the predominant mode of sexual expression for most adolescent males and probably fewer adolescent females.

Sexual orientation

This is the erotic attraction that an individual feels. Its shaping is a developmental process associated with certain patterns of childhood experience and activity. Superimposed on this, there are arguments for and against the theory that human sexual orientation is biologically determined.

HOMOSEXUALITY   This term is associated with the following behavioural dimensions:

- sexual fantasy
- sexual activity
- sense of identity
- social role

The first of these is the most important dimension in assessing homosexual orientation. If present, it does not necessarily imply sexual activity with others, as in individuals who are homosexual in orientation and celibate.

It should be noted that there is no nonhuman mammalian species in which predominant or exclusive homosexuality occurs in the way it does in humans.

MODERN ARGUMENTS IN FAVOUR OF BIOLOGICAL DETERMINISM

- *Endocrine.* On the basis of rat and human experiments, Dorner (1986, 1989) has hypothesized that 21-hydroxylase deficiency represents a genetic predisposition to female homosexuality in heterozygous forms (homozygous forms lead to congenital adrenal hyperplasia) while in males 21-hydroxylase deficiency and/or prenatal stress leads to an overall inhibition in the effects of androgen on brain differentiation and to male homosexuality. Among their experiments on humans, Dorner and colleagues studied the effects of oestrogen infusion on LH secretion and reported that in contrast to heterosexual men, homosexual men manifest a positive oestrogen feedback effect on LH secretion, which was said to provide evidence that homosexual men have a predominantly female-differentiated brain. Furthermore, as a result of ACTH provocation tests on the suprarenal (adrenal) glands, Dorner reported that female homosexuals display significantly increased ratios of 17α-hydroxyprogesterone/cortisol and androstenedione/cortisol after ACTH stimulation compared with female heterosexual control subjects.
- **Neuroanatomical.** LeVay (1991) reported histological differences in the interstitial nuclei of the anterior hypothalamus between homosexual and heterosexual men, suggesting that sexual orientation may be mediated by the central nervous system. The anterior hypothalamus of the brain is known to participate in the regulation of male-typical sexual behaviour. The volumes of four cell groups in this region (interstitial nuclei of the anterior hypothalamus (INAH) 1, 2, 3, and 4) were measured in postmortem tissue from three subject groups: women, men who were presumed to be heterosexual, and homosexual men. No differences were found between the groups in the

volumes of INAH 1, 2, or 4. As had been previously reported, INAH 3 was found to be more than twice as large in the heterosexual men as in the women. It was also, however, more than twice as large in the heterosexual men as in the homosexual men. This finding indicates that INAH is dimorphic with sexual orientation, at least in men. A second neuroanatomical difference was reported by Allen and Gorski (1992): on the basis of the examination of 90 postmortem brains, it was found that the midsagittal plane of the anterior commissure in homosexual men was 18 per cent larger than in heterosexual women and 34 per cent larger than in heterosexual men. This finding of a difference in a structure not known to be related to reproductive functions supports the hypothesis that factors operating early in development differentiate sexually dimorphic structures and functions of the brain in a global fashion.

- **Genetic.** Bailey and Pillard (1991) found evidence of heritability of homo-sexuality in a study of monozygotic and dizygotic twins. Homosexual male probands with monozygotic cotwins, dizygotic cotwins, or adoptive brothers were recruited. Of the relatives whose sexual orientation could be rated, 52 per cent (29/56) of monozygotic cotwins, 22 per cent (12/54) of dizygotic cotwins, and 11 per cent (6/57) of adoptive brothers were homosexual. Childhood gender nonconformity did not appear to be an indicator of genetic loading for homosexuality. In a second genetic study Hamer *et al.* (1993) reported a linkage between DNA markers on the X chromosome and male sexual orientation. Pedigree and linkage analyses on 114 families of homo-sexual men were carried out. Increased rates of homosexual orientation were found in the maternal uncles and male cousins of these subjects, but not in their fathers or paternal relatives, suggesting the possibility of sex-linked transmission in a portion of the population. DNA linkage analysis of a selected group of 40 families in which there were two gay brothers and no indication of nonmaternal transmission revealed a correlation between homo-sexual orientation and the inheritance of polymorphic markers on the X chromosome in approximately 64 per cent of the sib-pairs tested. The linkage to markers on Xq28 had a multipoint lod score of 4.0.

ARGUMENTS AGAINST BIOLOGICAL DETERMINISM

- **Endocrine.** Gooren *et al.* (1990) have argued that oestrogen feedback cannot be used to assess the status of brain differentiation in primates in the same way as it can in the rat. For example, sexual differentiation of the control of LH secretion occurs in the mouse, hamster, and guinea pig but not in primates. Among their experiments on humans, Gooren *et al.* studied directly the control of LH secretion in homosexuals and transsexuals compared with heterosexuals. Following oestrogen exposure, the response of LH to LHRH was not positive in male homosexuals, transsexuals, and heterosexuals; it was positive in female homosexuals, transsexuals (prior to treatment), and hetero-sexuals; moreover, a positive LH response to oestrogen infusion in homo-sexual men was not found.

- **Neuroanatomical.** LeVay (1991) pointed out that his sample contained no homosexual women and that AIDS patients may constitute an unrepresenta-tive sample of gay men. Moreover, some presumed heterosexual men had relatively small INAH 3 nuclei (within the homosexual range) and some presumed homosexual men had relatively large INAH 3 nuclei (within the heterosexual range). The effect might have resulted from AIDS (although there was no effect of AIDS on the volume of the three other INAH nuclei

examined and the size difference in INAH 3 was present when the homosexual men were compared with heterosexual AIDS patients).

- **Genetic**. King (1993) has pointed out that the result of Hamer *et al.* (1993) is
preliminary. Their evidence is based on a small, highly selected group of gay
men. The result is purely statistical. The gene is hypothetical and has not been
cloned, and the linkage has been observed in only one series of families.

ADOLESCENCE

Adolescence is a time of transitions, representing a developmental phase between
middle childhood/latency and adulthood, but its boundaries are difficult to
demarcate clearly. In his model of cognitive development, Piaget viewed adolescence as the final, formal operational stage of development; the adolescent has a
greater capacity to focus on themselves. The pubertal changes of adolescence
have been considered above.

Conflict with parents and authority

Theories of why conflict between adolescents and parents and other authority
figures often occur include:

COGNITIVE DEVELOPMENTAL MODELS   The adolescent has newly acquired powers
of hypothetical reasoning which enable them to consider and articulate alterna-
tives to the *status quo*.

ERIKSON'S STAGES OF PSYCHOSOCIAL DEVELOPMENT   In his fifth psychosocial
developmental stage (identity versus role confusion), Erikson considered adolescence to be a time of identity formation during which the individual pursues
personal autonomy. This pursuit is associated with the potential for conflict with
parents and other authority figures.

ETHOLOGICAL AND SOCIOBIOLOGICAL MODELS   Conflict at the time of pubertal
changes is considered to be adaptive, prompting the individual to spend more
time with their peers. It forms part of the status realignments of entry into
adulthood.

SOCIAL LEARNING THEORY   Adolescents may be considered to have experienced
vicarious exposure to problem-solving occurring via conflict. Witnessing their
parents giving in to their children's conflictual demands may be considered to
provide intermittent reinforcement to the children.

EQUITY THEORY   According to equity theory the preferred relationships, particularly those of an intimate nature, between any two given people are those in
which each feels that the cost-benefit ratio of the relationship for each person is
approximately equal. It has been argued that the amount of emotional investment
of both the adolescent and the parent(s) in their relationship means they both
wish to preserve it. As the adolescent pursues autonomy, this can lead to
occasional conflicts, but these are usually not fervent enough to destroy the
relationship.

SEPARATION–INDIVIDUATION   It has been argued that adolescence can be considered to represent a second separation–individuation phase, in which continued
biological, motor, and social development now allow the adolescent to move away
from a dependent relationship with the parent(s) to take their own place in
society. However, social and psychological pulls towards dependency mean that
the separation–individuation may entail ambivalence and conflict.

Affective stability and 'turmoil'

Successive developments in the psychological understanding of affective stability and 'turmoil' in adolescence have been provided by Anna Freud, Erikson and Offer and Offer.

ANNA FREUD   A rapid oscillation between excess and asceticism during adolescence was described by Anna Freud (1936/1946). Affective instability and behaviour swings were considered to be caused by:

- the drives stimulated by sexual maturity
- pubertal endocrine changes
- the instability of the newly stressed defences of the ego against these drives.

ERIKSON   Erikson (1959) characterized adolescence as manifesting 'adolescent turmoil' and a maladaptive, temporary state of 'identity diffusion', which he implied all adolescents passed through.

OFFER AND OFFER   Offer and Offer (1975) showed that, in general, adolescence is a time of less turmoil and upheaval than previously thought. They studied a cohort of American males who had been aged 14 years in 1962. Sixty-one of these adolescents were studied intensively and followed-up into adulthood. They came mainly from intact families, and there were no serious drug problems or major delinquent activity. Seventy-four per cent went to college during the first year after high school graduation. They showed no significant difference in basic values from that of their parents.

Normal and abnormal adolescent development

OFFER AND OFFER   Offer and Offer (1975) identified the following three adolescent developmental routes (the percentages given are those of the sample of adolescents they studied; the remaining 21 per cent could not be classified easily, but were closer to the first two categories than to the third one):

- **Continuous growth** (23 per cent). Eriksonian intimacy was achieved and shame and guilt could be displayed. Major separation, death, and severe illness were less frequent. Their parents encouraged independence.
- **Surgent growth** (35 per cent). The adolescents in this group were 'late-bloomers'. They were more likely than the first group to have frequent depressive and anxious moments. Although often successful, they were less introspective and not as action-oriented as the first group. There were more areas of disagreement with their parents.
- **Tumultuous growth** (21 per cent). Recurrent self-doubt and conflict with their families occurred in this group. Their backgrounds were less stable than in the first two groups. The arts, humanities, and social sciences were preferred to professional and business careers.

BLOCK AND HAAN   Block and Haan (1971) used factor analysis to isolate the following groups among a cohort of 84 male adolescents studied longitudinally to adulthood:

- ego-resilient adolescents
- belated adjustors: similar to the surgent group of Offer and Offer
- vulnerable overcontrollers
- anomic extroverts: less inner life and relatively uncertain values
- unsettled undercontrollers: given to impulsivity

A similar cohort of 86 females was divided into:

- female prototype
- cognitive type: individuals tend to be intellectualized in the way problems are negotiated
- hyperfeminine repressors: similar to hysterical personality disorder
- dominating narcissists
- vulnerable undercontrollers
- lonely independents

ADAPTATIONS IN ADULT LIFE

Pairing

Even in Western countries, it appears that there are a number of constraints which govern the choice of mate in much the same way as elders or parents do in arranged marriages.

HOMOGAMOUS MATE SELECTION   Pairing tends to occur within the same socio-economic, religious and cultural group (Eshelman 1985).

REINFORCEMENT THEORY   People are attracted to those who reinforce the attraction with rewards. This process is a reciprocal one with rewards also passing in the opposite direction and further reinforcing the interpersonal attraction (Newcomb 1956).

SOCIAL EXCHANGE THEORY   People have a preference for relationships that appear to offer an optimum cost-benefit ratio: maximum benefits such as love with minimum costs such as time spent with each other (Homans 1961).

EQUITY THEORY   As mentioned above, this is a modification of the social exchange theory in which the preferred relationships, particularly of an intimate nature, between two people are those in which each feels that the cost-benefit ratio of the relationship for each person is approximately equal (Hatfield and Traupmann 1981).

MATCHING HYPOTHESIS   According to this hypothesis heterosexual pairing tends to occur in such a way that, although ideally a person would prefer to pair with the most attractive people (Huston 1973), in practice individuals seek to pair with others who have a similar level of physical attractiveness rather than the most attractive (Berscheid and Walster 1974). This is felt by the individual to lead to a greater probability of acceptance by the other person, a lower probability of rejection, and a lower probability of losing the partner to another person in the future.

CULTURAL DIFFERENCES   People in Asian and African countries tend to value homekeeping potential and a desire for home and children in mate selection, while people in Western countries tend to value love, character and emotional maturity. Chastity is rated very highly in some countries (e.g. India and China) and very low in others (e.g. Australia, New Zealand, North America, South America, and Scandinavia) (Buss *et al.* 1990).

CROSS-CULTURAL CONSTANCIES   Across cultures, men prefer mates who are physically attractive, while women prefer mates who show ambition, industriousness and other signs of earning power potential (Buss *et al.* 1990).

Parenting

Parenting is a complex, dyadic process that is influenced by a range of factors, including:

- cultural beliefs of the parent about child-rearing (Maccoby and Martin 1983)
- genetic-temperamental characteristics of the parent (that is, genetic factors influencing the provision of parenting) (Perusse *et al.* 1994)
- genetic-temperamental characteristics of the child (that is, genetic factors influencing the elicitation of parenting) (Bell 1968).

Furthermore, reporting bias is likely, with parents stressing the similarity with which they treat their children, and children emphasizing the differences in parental treatment that they perceive (Plomin *et al.* 1994).

Abusive parenting is a strong predictor of later psychopathology. On the other hand, parental warmth and support buffers children against externalizing and antisocial behaviour (Hetherington and Clingempeel 1992) and is positively associated with a child's self-esteem (Bell and Bell 1983).

Grief, mourning and bereavement

DEFINITIONS

- **grief**: those psychological and emotional processes, expressed both internally and externally, that accompany bereavement
- **mourning**: those culture-bound social and cognitive processes through which we must pass in order that grief is resolved, allowing us to return to more normal functioning; it is often used, less strictly, as being synonymous with grief
- **bereavement**: a term that can apply to any loss event, from the loss of a relative by death to unemployment, divorce or the loss of a pet; it refers to being in the state of mourning

NORMAL GRIEF   The symptomatology of normal grief may include:

- initial shock and disbelief: 'a feeling of numbness'
- increasing awareness of the loss is associated with painful emotions of sadness and anger
- anger may be denied
- irritability
- somatic distress: may include sleep disturbance, early morning waking, tearfulness, loss of appetite, weight loss, loss of libido, anhedonia
- identification phenomena: the mannerisms and characteristics of the deceased may be taken on

In 1944 Lindemann read to the centenary meeting of the American Psychiatric Association the results of his study of 101 bereaved individuals, many of whom had lost loved ones in the tragic Cocoanut Grove nightclub fire in Boston, MA. He identified the following five points as being pathognomonic of acute grief:

- somatic distress
- preoccupation with the image of the deceased
- guilt
- hostile reactions
- loss of patterns of conduct

Note that grief is not seen in babies if a parent/caregiver dies before the development of attachment behaviour.

BEREAVEMENT   Parkes described the following five stages of bereavement:

- alarm
- numbness

- pining for the deceased: illusions or hallucinations of the deceased may occur
- depression
- recovery and reorganization

MORBID GRIEF REACTIONS   Lindemann described the following morbid grief reactions:

- delay of reaction
- distorted reactions: subclassified into:

    - overactivity without a sense of loss
    - the acquisition of symptoms belonging to the last illness of the deceased
    - a recognized medical disease
    - alteration in relationship to friends and relatives
    - furious hostility against specific persons
    - loss of affectivity
    - a lasting loss of patterns of social interaction
    - activities attain a colouring detrimental to social and economic existence
    - agitated depression

DIFFERENTIATING BETWEEN BEREAVEMENT AND A DEPRESSIVE EPISODE   The diagnosis of Major Depressive Disorder in DSM-IV is generally not given unless the symptoms are still present two months after the loss. However, the presence of certain symptoms that are not characteristic of a normal grief reaction may be helpful in differentiating bereavement from a Major Depressive Episode:

- guilt about things other than actions taken or not taken by the survivor at the time of the death
- thoughts of death other than the survivor feeling that they would be better off dead or should have died with the deceased person
- morbid preoccupation with worthlessness
- marked psychomotor retardation
- prolonged and marked functional impairment
- hallucinatory experiences other than thinking that they can hear the voice of, or transiently see the image of, the deceased person

Freud (1917/1957) differentiated between normal grief and the depressive response by the presence of shame and guilt in the latter. Yearning for the lost object was considered to be part of the normal response to loss. It was overcome gradually as the mental representation was decathected.

NORMAL AGEING

Physical aspects
HEALTH   In general, most elderly people in Western countries enjoy good health, in spite of the changes that occur in body systems with increasing age.
CEREBRAL CHANGES   Blessed *et al.* (1968) found no histological evidence of dementia in the brains of 28 non demented individuals. Evidence of cerebral atrophy was absent or slight in the majority, and brain mass and ventricular size did not differ significantly from those of younger adults (Tomlinson *et al.* 1968).

Social aspects
STEREOTYPING   Old age is generally a stigmatized period. For instance, people are complimented for looking younger than their chronological age.

EMPTY NEST SYNDROME   Before the onset of old age parents usually witness their children leaving home, particularly in Western countries. The difficulties some parents encounter on being left on their own has been described as the empty nest syndrome.

Ego integrity versus despair

This is Erikson's eighth and final stage of psychosocial development, occurring in old age.

EGO INTEGRITY   Successful resolution of the psychosocial crisis of this age leads to an integrated view of one's life, its meaning, its achievements (both for self and others, including future generations), and the ways in which difficulties were coped with. There is an acceptance of our mortality, a feeling that our life has been lived in a satisfactory way, and a readiness to face death.

DESPAIR   The alternative is despair, both on reflection of how life has been lived and the way in which others have been treated, and also on looking to the future and the sense of transience that is felt on facing the end of life. Rather than having a sense of contentment and completion, there is despair at the prospect of death.

Cognitive aspects

Before the late 1960s it was generally believed that the normal ageing brain degenerates and that this is accompanied by intellectual deterioration. By the 1970s this view had been challenged on the basis of new research. Thus Schaie (1974) wrote:

> The presumed universal decline in adult intelligence is at best a methodological artifact and at worst a popular misunderstanding of the relation between individual development and sociocultural change . . . the major findng . . . in the area of intellectual functioning is the demolishing of [the belief in] serious intellectual decrement in the aged.

Although the elderly do not generally perform as well as younger subjects on cognitive tasks dependent on processing speed, old age is not necessarily associated with a large decline in intellectual ability (Durkin 1995). Reasons for this include:

- different abilities contribute to intellectual behaviour, so that a reduction in one (e.g. processing speed) may be compensated for by an increase in another (e.g. experience-based judgement)
- cross-sectional comparisons of different age groups may confound age differences with cohort effects
- changes in performance with age may be offset by practice
- crystallized intelligence (the ability to store and manipulate learned information) increases through adulthood and often remains high into old age

DEATH AND DYING

Definitions

TIMELY DEATH   This refers to the situation in which the expected life expectancy is approximately equal to the actual length of time lived.

UNTIMELY DEATH   This refers to the situation in which the actual length of time lived is significantly less than the expected life expectancy, as a result of one of the following:

- premature death at a young age
- sudden unexpected death
- violent/accidental death

UNINTENDED DEATH   This refers to the situation in which death is unintended, usually occurring as a result of pathological processes or trauma.

INTENDED DEATH   This refers to the situation in which death is intended by the deceased, who played a part in their suicide.

SUBINTENDED DEATH   This refers to the situation in which the deceased may have manifested an unconscious desire to bring about their death, for example by facilitating the onset of death through psychoactive substance abuse.

Impending death

If it is believed that one's death is near, an individual may pass through the following five stages that are similar to those recognized as occurring in the terminally ill (Kübler-Ross 1969):

- shock and denial: the diagnosis may be disbelieved and another opinion sought; this first stage may never be passed
- anger: the person may be angry and wonder why this has happened to them
- bargaining: the person may, for example, try to negotiate with God
- depression: the symptomatology of a depressive episode is manifested
- acceptance: the person may finally come to terms with their mortality and understand the inevitability of death

BIBLIOGRAPHY

Aiosa-Karpas, C.J., Karpas, R., Pelcovitz, D. *et al.* 1991: Gender identification and sex role attribution in sexually abused adolescent females. *Journal of the American Academy of Child and Adolescent Psychiatry* 30, 266–71.

Allen, L.S. and Gorski, R.A. 1992: Sexual orientation and the size of the anterior commissure in the human brain. *Proceedings of the National Academy of Sciences* 85, 7199–202.

Bailey, J.M. and Pillard, R.C. 1991: A genetic study of male sexual orientation. *Archives of General Psychiatry* 48, 1089–96.

Bates, J.E. 1989: Concepts and measures of temperament. In Kohnstamm, G.A., Bates, J.E. and Rothbart, M.K. (eds) *Temperament in childhood.* New York: Wiley.

Bates, J.E., Wachs, T.D. and VandenBos, G.R. 1995: Trends in research on temperament. *Psychiatric Services* 46, 661–3.

Baumrind, D. 1967: Child care practices anteceding three patterns of pre-school behavior. *Genetic Psychology Monographs* 75, 43–88.

Bell, R.Q. 1968: A reinterpretation of the direction of effects in studies of socialization. *Psychological Review* 75, 81–95.

Bell, D.C. and Bell, L.G. 1983: Parental validation and support in the development of adolescent daughters. In Grotevant, M.D. (ed.) *Adolescent development in the family.* San Francisco: Jossey Bass.

Berscheid, E. and Walster, E. 1974: Physical attractiveness. In Berkowitz, L. (ed.), *Advances in experimental social psychology.* New York: Academic Press.

Blessed, G., Tomlinson, B.E. and Roth, M. 1968: The association between quantitative measures of dementia and of senile change in the cerebral grey matter of elderly subjects. *British Journal of Psychiatry* 114, 797–811.

Block, J. and Haan, N. 1971: *Lives through time.* Berkeley, CA: Bancroft Books.

Buss, D.M. *et al.* 1990: International preferences in selecting mates: a study of 37 cultures. *Journal of Cross-Cultural Psychology* 21, 5–47.

Caspi, A. and Silva, P.A. 1995: Temperamental qualities at age three predict personality traits in young adulthood: longitudinal evidence from a birth cohort. *Child Development* 66, 486–98.

Chess, S. and Thomas, A. 1984: *Origins and evolution of behavior disorders: from infancy to early adult life.* New York: Brunner/Mazel.

Cosentino, C.E., Meyer-Bahlburg, H.F.I., Nat, D.R. *et al.* 1995: Sexual behavior problems and psychopathology symptoms in sexually abused girls. *Journal of the American Academy of Child and Adolescent Psychiatry* 34, 1033–42.

Dorner, G. 1986: Hormone-dependent brain development and preventative medicine. *Monographs in Neural Sciences* 12, 17–27.

Dorner, G. 1989: Hormone-dependent brain development and neuroendocrine prophylaxis. *Experimental and Clinical Endocrinology* 94, 4–22.

Durkin, K. 1995: *Developmental social psychology.* Cambridge, MA: Blackwell.

Elmer, E. and Gregg, C.S. 1967: Developmental characteristics of abused children. *Pediatrics* 40, 596–602.

Erikson, E. 1959: *Growth and crises of the healthy personality.* New York: International Universities Press.

Eshelman, J.R. 1985: One should marry a person of the same religion, race, ethnicity, and social class. In Feldman, H. and Feldman, M. (eds), *Current controversies in marriage and the family.* Newbury Park, CA: Sage.

Finkelhor, D. 1984: *Child sexual abuse: new theory and research.* New York: Free Press.

Freud, A. 1936/1946: *The ego and the mechanisms of defence* (translated by C. Baines). New York: International Universities Press.

Freud, S. 1917/1957: Mourning and melancholia (1917). In *Standard edition of the complete psychological works of Sigmund Freud, Vol. 14* (translated and edited by J. Strachey). London: Hogarth Press.

Freud, S. 1926/1959: Inhibitions, symptoms and anxiety. In *Standard edition of the complete psychological works of Sigmund Freud, Vol. 20* (translated and edited by J. Strachey). London: Hogarth Press.

Friedrich, W. and Reams, R. 1987: Course of psychological symptoms in sexually abused young children. *Psychotherapy* 24, 160–71.

Gaensbauer, T. and Sands, K. 1979: Regulation of emotional expression in infants from two contrasting environments. *Journal of the American Academy of Child Psychiatry* 21, 167–71.

George, C. and Main, M. 1979: Social interactions and young abused children: approach, avoidance, and aggression. *Child Development* 50, 306–19.

Goodwin, J. 1985: Post-traumatic symptoms in incest victims. In Eth, S. and Pynoos, R. S. (eds), *Post-traumatic stress disorder in children.* Washington, DC: American Psychiatric Press.

Gooren, L., Fliers, E. and Courtney, K. 1990: Biological determinants of sexual orientation. *Annual Review of Sex Research* 1, 175–96.

Graham, P. 1991: *Child psychiatry: a developmental approach*, 2nd edn, Oxford: Oxford University Press.

Green, A.H. 1978: Psychiatric treatment of abused children. *Journal of the American Academy of Child Psychiatry* 17, 356–71.

Green, A.H. 1985: Children traumatized by physical abuse. In Eth, S. and Pynoos, R.S. (eds), *Post-traumatic stress disorder in children.* Washington, DC: American Psychiatric Press.

Green, A.H., Voeller, K., Gaines, R. *et al.* 1981: Neurological impairment in battered children. *Child Abuse and Neglect* 5, 129–34.

Gunnar, M.R. 1994: Psychoendocrine studies of temperament and stress in early childhood: expanding current models. In Bates, J.E. and Wachs, T.D. (eds), *Temperament: individual differences at the interface of biology and behavior.* Washington, DC: American Psychological Association.

Hamer, D.H., Hu, S., Magnuson, V.L., Hu, N. and Pattatucci, A.M. 1993: A linkage between DNA markers on the X chromosome and male sexual orientation. *Science* 261, 321–7.

Hatfield, E. and Traupmann, J. 1981: Intimate relationships: a perspective from equity theory. In Duck, S. and Gilmour, R. (eds), *Personal relationships*, Vol. 1. New York: Academic Press.

Herman, J. 1981: *Father–daughter incest.* Cambridge, MA: Harvard University Press.

Herman, J., Perry, J.C. and van der Kolk, B. 1989: Childhood trauma in borderline personality disorder. *American Journal of Psychiatry* 146, 490–5.

Hetherington, E.M. and Clingempeel, W.G. 1992: Coping with marital transitions: a family system's perspective. *Monographs of the Society of Research into Child Development* 57 (serial no. 227).

Homans, G.C. 1961: *Social behavior: its elementary forms.* New York: Harcourt Brace.

Huston, T.L. 1973: Ambiguity of acceptance, social desirability and dating choice. *Journal of Experimental Social Psychology* 9, 32.

King, M.-C. 1993: Human genetics: sexual orientation and the X [news and views]. *Nature* 364, 288–9.

Kluft, R. 1985: *Childhood antecedents of multiple personality.* Washington, DC: American Psychiatric Press.

Kübler-Ross, E. 1969: *On death and dying.* New York: Macmillan.

LeVay, S. 1991: A difference in hypothalamic structure between heterosexual and homosexual men. *Science* 253, 1034–7.

McCarty, L. 1986: Mother–child incest: characteristics of the offender. *Child Welfare* 65, 447–58.

Maccoby, E.E. and Martin, J.A. 1983: Socialization in the context of the family: parent–child interaction. In Mussen, P.H. (ed.) *Handbook of child psychology, Vol IV: socialization, personality, and social development.* New York: John Wiley.

Marks, I. 1987: The development of normal fear: a review. *Journal of Child Psychology and Psychiatry* 28, 667–98.

Martin, H.P. 1972: The child and his development. In Kempe, C.H. and Helfer, R.E. (eds), *Helping the battered child and his family.* Philadelphia, PA: Lippincott.

Newcomb, T. 1956: The prediction of interpersonal attraction. *American Psychologist* 11, 575.

Oates, K. 1986: *Child abuse and neglect: what happens eventually?* New York: Brunner/Mazel.

Offer, B. and Offer, J.B. 1975: *From teenage to young manhood: a psychological study.* New York: Basic Books.

Oppenheimer, R., Howells, K., Palmer, L. *et al.* 1985: Adverse sexual experiences in childhood and clinical eating disorders: A preliminary description. *Journal of Psychosomatic Research* 19, 157–61.

Perusse, D., Neale, M.C,, Heath, A.C. and Eaves, L.J. 1994: Human parental behavior: evidence for genetic influence and potential implication for gene–culture transmission. *Behavioral Genetics* 24, 327–35.

Plomin, R., Reiss, D., Hetherington, E.M. and Howe, G.W. 1994: Nature and nurture: genetic contributions to measures of the family environment. *Developmental Psychology* 30, 32–43.

Schaie, K.W. 1974: Translations in gerontology – from lab to life. Intellectual functioning. *American Psychologist* 29, 802–7.

Schechter, M.D. and Roberge, L. 1976: Sexual exploitation. In Helfer, R.E. and Kempe, C.H. (eds), *Child abuse and neglect: the family and the community.* Cambridge, MA: Ballinger.

Seghorn, T.K., Prentky, R.A. and Boucher, R.J. 1987: Child sexual abuse in the lives of sexually aggressive offenders. *Journal of the American Academy of Child and Adolescent Psychiatry* 26, 262–7.

Sgroi, S. 1982: *Handbook of clinical intervention in child sexual abuse.* Lexington, MA: Lexington Books.

Steele, B.F. 1983: The effect of abuse and neglect on psychological development. In Call, J.D., Galenson, E. and Tyson, K.L. (eds), *Frontiers of infant psychiatry.* New York: Basic Books.

Thomas, A. and Chess, S. 1977: *Temperament and development.* New York: Brunner/Mazel.

Tomlinson, B.E., Blessed, G. and Roth, M. 1968: Observations on the brains of non-demented old people. *Journal of the Neurological Science*s 7, 331–56.

Yates, A. 1982: Children eroticized by incest. *American Journal of Psychiatry* 139, 482–5.

Zuckerman, M. 1991: *Psychobiology of personality.* New York: Cambridge.

6

Principles of evaluation and psychometrics

BASIC CONCEPTS

Types of data

QUALITATIVE   Qualitative variables refer to attributes that can be categorized such that the categories do not have a numerical relationship with each other, e.g. eye colour.

QUANTITATIVE   Quantitative variables refer to numerically represented data. These can be of the following types:

- **discrete** quantitative variables: these can only take on known fixed values, e.g. the number of new patients seen each week in a psychiatric outpatient department
- **continuous** quantitative variables: these can take on any value in a defined range, e.g. the height of psychiatric inpatients

Scales of measurement

Table 6.1 summarizes the properties of different types of measurement scale.

Sampling methods

SIMPLE RANDOM SAMPLING   A **simple random sample** is one chosen from a given population such that every possible sample of the same size has the same probability of being chosen.

SYSTEMATIC SAMPLING   This type of sampling saves time and effort. Common examples include:

- **Periodic sampling**: Every nth member of the population is chosen. This may not always lead to a random choice because of an unforeseen underlying pattern.
- **Using random numbers**: Using random numbers can be a better method than periodic sampling for ensuring random choice. Random numbers, obtained, for example, from a computer program, a scientific calculator with a (pseudo)random number generator, or a table of random numbers, can be used to choose every nth member of the population.
- **Stratified random sampling**: A given population is stratified before random samples are chosen from each stratum. This can be useful when studying a disease that varies with respect to sex and age, for example.

Table 6.1 Types of measurement scale

Property	Nominal	Ordinal	Interval	Ratio
Categories mutually exclusive	✓	✓	✓	✓
Categories logically ordered		✓	✓	✓
Equal distance between adjacent categories			✓	✓
True zero point				✓

Reproduced with permission from Puri, B.K. 1996: *Statistics for the health sciences*. London: W.B. Saunders.

Frequency distributions

FREQUENCY DISTRIBUTION   This is a systematic way of arranging data, with frequencies being given for categories of a qualitative or quantitative variable. For continuous quantitative variables the categories should be contiguous and mutually exclusive, and are known as **class intervals**.

FREQUENCY TABLE   This is a frequency distribution arranged in the form of a table, with the first column giving contiguous mutually exclusive values (which may be class intervals) of a variable and the adjoining column giving the corresponding frequencies.

RELATIVE FREQUENCY   The relative frequency of a category/class interval/variable is the proportion of the total frequency corresponding to that category/class interval/variable:

relative frequency = (frequency of category)/(total frequency)

CUMULATIVE FREQUENCY   The cumulative frequency of a given value of a variable is the total frequency up to that value.

CUMULATIVE FREQUENCY TABLE   This is a cumulative frequency distribution arranged in the form of a table, with the first column giving contiguous mutually exclusive values (which may be class intervals) of a variable and the adjoining column giving the corresponding cumulative frequencies.

CUMULATIVE RELATIVE FREQUENCY   The cumulative relative frequency of a given value of a variable is the total relative frequency up to that value.

CUMULATIVE RELATIVE FREQUENCY TABLE   This is a cumulative relative frequency distribution arranged in the form of a table, with the first column giving contiguous mutually exclusive values (which may be class intervals) of a variable and the adjoining column giving the corresponding cumulative relative frequencies.

Discrete probability distributions

BERNOULLI TRIAL   This is a trial or experiment having two and only two alternative outcomes.

BERNOULLI DISTRIBUTION   This is the probability distribution for a discrete binary variable (range = 0, 1), which is a special case of the binomial distribution $B(1, p)$, where p is the probability of 'success':

$$\text{mean} = p$$
$$\text{variance} = p(1 - p)$$

BINOMIAL DISTRIBUTION   The binomial distribution, $B(n, p)$, is the probability distribution for a discrete finite variable (range = 0, 1, 2, . . ., n):

$$\text{mean} = np$$
$$\text{variance} = np(1 - p)$$

POISSON DISTRIBUTION   The Poisson distribution, Poisson (μ), is the probability distribution for a discrete infinite variable (range $= 0, 1, 2, \ldots$) where $\mu = np$:

$$\text{mean} = \mu$$
$$\text{variance} = \mu$$

The Poisson distribution can be used in situations in which the following criteria are fulfilled:

- events occur randomly in time or space (length, area or volume)
- the events are independent (that is, the outcome of any given event does not affect the outcome of any other)
- two or more events cannot take place simultaneously
- the mean number of events per given unit of time or space is constant

Continuous probability distributions

NORMAL DISTRIBUTION   The normal distribution, $N(\mu, \sigma^2)$, is the probability distribution for a continuous variable (range $= \mathbb{R}$).

$$\text{mean} = \mu$$
$$\text{variance} = \sigma^2$$

Properties of the normal distribution probability density function curve include:

- it is unimodal
- it is continuous
- it is symmetrical about its mean
- its mean, median and mode are all equal
- the area under the curve is one
- the curve tends to zero as the variable moves in either direction from the mean

The interval one standard deviation either side of the mean of the probability density function of a normal distribution encloses 68.27 per cent of the total area under the curve.

The interval two standard deviations either side of the mean of the probability density function of a normal distribution encloses 95.45 per cent of the total area under the curve.

The interval three standard deviations either side of the mean of the probability density function of a normal distribution encloses 99.73 per cent of the total area under the curve.

If $X \sim N(\mu, \sigma^2)$, then the standard normal variate Z is given by:

$$Z = (X - \mu)/\sigma$$

For $Z \sim N(0, 1)$:

$$\text{mean} = 0$$
$$\text{variance} = 1$$

The cumulative distribution function, $P(Z < z)$, is given by $\Phi(z)$.

For $N(\mu, \sigma^2)$ the two-tailed 5 per cent points are given by:

$$\mu - 1.96\sigma$$
$$\mu + 1.96\sigma$$

t DISTRIBUTION   When $n < 30$, the t distribution, $t(\nu)$ or t_ν, is used in making inferences about the mean of a normal population when its variance is unknown.

The t distribution is symmetrical about the mean but has longer tails than the normal distribution.

v is the number of degrees of freedom, and is given by:

$$v = n - 1$$

For $n \geq 30$, $t(v) \approx N(0, 1)$.

χ^2 DISTRIBUTION   The chi-squared distribution with v degrees of freedom, $\chi^2(v)$, is obtained from the sum of the squares of v independent variables, Z_1 to Z_v, where each $Z \sim N(0, 1)$:

$$\text{If } W = \Sigma Z_i^2, \text{ where } i = 1 \text{ to } v, \text{ and } Z_i \sim N(0, 1)$$
$$\text{then } W \sim \chi^2(v)$$

The chi-squared distribution is asymmetrical.

F DISTRIBUTION   The F distribution is related to the χ^2 distribution and is asymmetrical. A given F distribution is described in terms of v_1 and v_2, each of which gives a number of degrees of freedom. This is usually abbreviated to $F(v_1, v_2)$.

Summary statistics: measures of location

MEASURES OF CENTRAL TENDENCY   The **(arithmetic) mean** (or average) of a sample with n items $(x_1, x_2, x_3, \ldots x_n)$, $\bar{x}$, is given by:

$$\bar{x} = (\Sigma x)/n$$

The population mean, μ, of a population of size N is given by:

$$\mu = (\Sigma x)/N$$

The arithmetic mean is suitable for use with data measured on at least an interval scale. A major disadvantage is that it can be unduly influenced by an extreme value.

The **median** is the middle value of a set of observations ranked in order. If the number of observations is odd:

$$\text{median} = \text{middle value}$$

If the number of observations is even:

$$\text{median} = \text{arithmetic mean of the two middle values}$$

The median is suitable for use with data measured on at least an ordinal scale. It gives a better measure of central tendency than the mean for skewed (asymmetrical) distributions.

The **mode** of a distribution is the value of the observation occurring most frequently. The category/interval occurring most frequently is the modal category. It can be used with all measurement scales.

QUANTILES   Quantiles are cut-off points that split a continuous distribution into equal groups. They include:

- the median: this splits a distribution into two equal parts
- the two tertiles: these split the distribution into three equal parts
- the three quartiles: these split the distribution into four equal parts
- the four quintiles: these split the distribution into five equal parts
- the nine deciles: these split the distribution into 10 equal parts
- the 99 percentiles: these split the distribution into 100 equal parts

The kth quantile of n observations ranked in increasing order from the first to the nth is calculated by interpolating between the two observations adjacent to the qth, where q is given by:

$$q = k(n + 1)/Q$$

where Q is the number of groups into which the quantiles divide the distribution.

Summary statistics: measures of dispersion

RANGE   The range is the difference between the smallest and largest values in a distribution:

$$\text{range} = (\text{largest value}) - (\text{smallest value})$$

It can be used with data that are measured on at least an interval scale.

MEASURES RELATING TO QUANTILES   The most commonly used measures relating to quantiles include:

- the interquartile range = the difference between the third and first quartiles
- the semi-quartile range = half the interquartile range
- the 10 to 90 percentile range = the difference between the 90th and 10th (per)centiles, or equivalently, between the ninth and first deciles
- the interdecile range = the difference between the 90th and 10th (per)centiles, or equivalently, between the ninth and first deciles

The median and interquartile or 10 to 90 percentile range can be more useful summary statistics than the mean and standard deviation for skewed distributions.

STANDARD DEVIATION   The standard deviation of a distribution is based on deviations from the mean and has the same units as the original observations.

For a population of size N and mean μ, the population standard deviation, σ, is given by:

$$\text{population standard deviation, } \sigma = \sqrt{\{[\Sigma(x - \mu)^2]/N\}}$$

For a sample of size n and mean $\bar{x}$, the sample standard deviation, s, is given by:

$$\text{sample standard deviation, } s = \sqrt{\{[\Sigma(x - \bar{x})^2]/(n - 1)\}}$$

The standard deviation can be used for data measured on at least an interval scale.

VARIANCE   The variance is the square of the standard deviation and has units that are the square of those of the observations.

For a population of size N and mean μ, the population variance, σ^2, is given by:

$$\text{population variance, } \sigma^2 = [\Sigma(x - \mu)^2]/N$$

For a sample of size n and mean $\bar{x}$, the sample variance, s^2, is given by:

$$\text{sample variance, } s^2 = [\Sigma(x - \bar{x})^2]/(n - 1)$$

The variance can be used for data measured on at least an interval scale.

Graphs

DEFINITION   The graph of a function f is the set of points $(x, f(x))$.

DRAWING GRAPHS   A properly drawn graph should have the following properties:

- clearly labelled axes
- the independent variable is usually represented on the horizontal axis
- a clear heading/caption or reference in the accompanying text

- the units for both axes are clearly stated
- the scales for both axes are given; these may, for example, be:

  - linear
  - logarithmic
  - broken (which can be represented by a break in the axis)

LINEAR RELATIONSHIP   If the graph of variable y against variable x is a straight line, these variables are related by the equation

$$y = mx + c$$

in which m and c are constants:

- m is the gradient of the line
- c is the intercept of the line on the vertical axis (y-axis)

POWER LAW RELATIONSHIP   If the graph of y against x is a straight line, where

$$y = \log Y$$
$$x = \log X$$

(the logarithm is to any base, so long as it is the same one in both cases)

then variables X and Y are related by the equation

$$Y = CX^m$$

in which m and C are constants such that:

- m is the gradient of the line
- $\log C$ is the intercept of the line on the vertical axis (y-axis)

EXPONENTIAL RELATIONSHIP   If the graph of y against x is a straight line, where

$$y = \ln Y$$
$$x = X$$

($\ln Y$ is the logarithm of Y to base e, that is, $\log_e Y$)

then variables X and Y are related by the equation

$$Y = Ce^{mx}$$

in which m and C are constants such that:

- m is the gradient of the line
- $\ln C$ is the intercept of the line on the vertical axis (y-axis)

This exponential relationship also holds if:

- e is replaced by 10
- $\ln Y$ is replaced by $\log_{10} Y$
- $\ln C$ is replaced by $\log_{10} C$

OTHER RELATIONSHIPS INVOLVING EXPRESSIONS   If the graph of y against x is a straight line, where

$$y = g(Y)$$
$$x = f(X)$$

($f(X)$ is an expression involving X and $g(Y)$ is an expression involving Y)

then variables X and Y are related by the equation

$$g(Y) = m\,f(X) + c$$

in which m and c are constants:

- m is the gradient of the line
- c is the intercept of the line on the vertical axis (y-axis)

Outliers

Outliers are extreme values.

MEASURES OF CENTRAL TENDENCY   Outliers can exert an extreme effect on the arithmetic mean, particularly when the total number of values is small. The median is less affected in such a case and may therefore be preferred.

MEASURES OF DISPERSION   Outliers exert an extreme effect on the range. Measures relating to quantiles are less affected in such a case and may therefore be preferred. Since it takes into account all the values in a distribution, the standard deviation (or variance) may be affected by outliers, although less so than the range.

CORRELATION AND LINEAR REGRESSION   Outliers may exert an extreme effect on the results of correlation and linear regression. In such cases it may be necessary to consider excluding outliers from the calculations.

Stem-and-leaf plots

Stem-and-leaf plots can be used to represent a continuous variable. Their advantage over histograms is that they allow the representation of all the individual data. The stems consist of a vertical column of numbers on the left-hand side of the plot. The leaves are numbers to the right of the stems, which may, for example, represent tenths. All the individual data can then be derived by combining the individual leaves with their corresponding stems, while the shape of the overall plot indicates the shape of the distribution. They are particularly easy to represent in computer printouts. For instance, the distribution 13.5, 13.7, 14.5, 14.6, 14.6, 14.7, 15.2, 15.9, and 16.4 (arbitrary units) may be represented as the following stem-and-leaf plot:

```
13   5 7
14   5 6 6 7
15   2 9
16   4
```

Boxplots (box-and-whisker plots)

Boxplots (box-and-whisker plots) can be used to represent a continuous variable. A boxplot consists of a box whose longer sides are placed vertically, with vertical lines (whiskers) extending vertically. It has the following features:

- the upper boundary of the box is the upper (third) quartile
- the lower boundary of the box is the lower (first) quartile
- the length of the box is the interquartile range
- a thick horizontal line inside the box is the median (second quartile)
- the lower whisker extends to the smallest observation, excluding outliers
- the upper whisker extends to the largest observation, excluding outliers
- outliers are indicated by the symbol O

The above arrangement is sometimes represented horizontally (the whole plot being rotated through $-\pi/2$) if more convenient. Boxplots can be useful for comparing two or more sets of observations diagrammatically, before or in addition to more formal statistical analyses.

Scattergrams (scatter diagrams or dot graphs)

Scattergrams (scatter diagrams or dot graphs) can be used to represent two continuous variables. Two orthogonal axes divide two-dimensional space into a coordinate system, in which each pair of observations is plotted. The two variables can then be compared diagrammatically, before or in addition to more formal statistical analyses.

DESCRIPTIVE AND INFERENTIAL STATISTICS

Descriptive statistics

Descriptive statistics are ways of organizing and describing data. Examples include:

- diagrams
- graphical representations
- numerical representations
- tables

Inferential statistics

Inferential statistics allow conclusions to be inferred from data. An example is inferring a likely range of values for the population mean from the sample mean.

Hypothesis testing: significance tests

A value or range of values for an unknown population parameter is hypothesized. A study/experiment is then carried out and the value of the observed random variable is used to test whether or not the hypothesis should be rejected.

NULL HYPOTHESIS   The initial hypothesis is the null hypothesis, H_0, usually representing no change:

$$H_0: \theta = \theta_0$$

where θ is the unknown parameter and θ_0 is its hypothesized value.

ALTERNATIVE HYPOTHESIS The alternative hypothesis, H_1, may, for example, be one of the following types:

- $H_1: \theta \neq \theta_0$
- $H_1: \theta > \theta_0$
- $H_1: \theta < \theta_0$
- $H_1: \theta = \theta_1$

SIMPLE HYPOTHESIS   A simple hypothesis is one involving a single value for the population parameter.

COMPOSITE HYPOTHESIS   A composite hypothesis is one involving more than one value for the population parameter.

ONE-SIDED SIGNIFICANCE TEST   A one-sided significance test is an hypothesis test involving a composite alternative hypothesis of the following types:

- $H_1: \theta > \theta_0$
- $H_1: \theta < \theta_0$

TWO-SIDED SIGNIFICANCE TEST   A two-sided significance test is an hypothesis test involving a composite alternative hypothesis of the following type:

- $H_1: \theta \neq \theta_0$

CRITICAL REGION   The critical region is the region of the range of the random variable X such that if the observed value x falls in it the null hypothesis, H_0, is rejected.

CRITICAL VALUE   The critical value(s) is (are) the value(s) of the test statistic expected from the null hypothesis, H_0, that define the boundary (boundaries) of the critical region.

SIGNIFICANCE LEVEL   The significance level, α, is the size of the critical region and represents the following probability:

$$\alpha = P(\text{type I error})$$

where a type I error is the error of wrongly rejecting H_0 when it is true.

STEPS IN CARRYING OUT A SIGNIFICANCE/HYPOTHESIS TEST   Hypothesis testing is carried out as follows:

- Formulate H_0
- Formulate H_1
- Specify α
- Decide on the study/experiment to be carried out
- Calculate the test statistic

$$\text{test statistic} = (\text{appropriate statistic} - \text{hypothesized parameter})/ \\ (\text{standard error of statistic})$$

- From the sampling distribution of the test statistic create the test criterion for testing H_0 versus H_1
- Carry out the study/experiment
- Calculate the value of the test statistic from the sample data
- Calculate the value of the difference, d, between the value of the test statistic from the sample and that expected under H_0 (the critical value(s), defining the critical range)
- If $P(d) < \alpha$, the result is statistically significant at the level of α (the 'p value') and H_0 is rejected
- If $P(d) \geq \alpha$, the result is not statistically significant at the level of α and H_0 cannot be rejected
- If H_0 is composite, the hypothesis test is designed so that the critical region size is the maximum value of the probability of rejecting H_0 when it is true

Estimation: confidence intervals

From sample statistics, confidence statements can be made about the corresponding unknown parameters, by constructing confidence intervals. A confidence interval can be two-sided or one-sided; two-sided confidence intervals need not necessarily be symmetrical (central).

If a $100(1 - \alpha)$ per cent confidence interval from a statistic (or statistics) is calculated, this implies that if the study were repeated with other random samples taken from the same parent population and further $100(1 - \alpha)$ per cent confidence intervals similarly individually calculated, the overall proportion of these confidence intervals which included the corresponding population parameter(s) would tend to $100(1 - \alpha)$ per cent.

The two-sided central confidence interval for the unknown parameter θ of a distribution with confidence level $(1 - \alpha)$ can be derived from the random interval of the type:

$$(\theta_-(X), \theta_+(X))$$

By substituting the observation x for X the realization of the random interval,

$$(\theta_-(x),\ \theta_+(x))$$

is the two-sided central confidence interval for θ, in which:

- $\theta_-(x)$ = lower confidence limit (confidence bound) for θ
- $\theta_+(x)$ = upper confidence limit (confidence bound) for θ

Advantages of confidence intervals over *p* values

There has been a recent move away from simply quoting p values in psychiatric research to giving instead, or additionally, the corresponding confidence intervals. Advantages of estimation over hypothesis-testing include:

- Testing the null hypothesis is often inappropriate for psychiatric research; for example they may reverse an investigator's idea (for instance that a new treatment will be more effective than a current one) and substitute instead the notion of no effect or no difference.
- An hypothesis test evaluates the probability of the observed study result, or a more extreme result, occurring if the null hypothesis were in fact true.
- Proper understanding of a study result is obscured in hypothesis-testing by transforming it on to a remote scale constrained from zero to one.
- Obtaining a low p value, particularly $p < 0.05$, is widely interpreted as implying merit and leads to the findings being deemed important and publishable, whereas this status is often denied study results which have not achieved this arbitrary level.
- The p value on its own implies nothing about the magnitude of any difference between treatments.
- The p value on its own implies nothing even about the direction of any difference between treatments.
- This overemphasis on hypothesis-testing and the use of p values to dichotomize results into significant and non-significant has detracted from more useful procedures for interpreting the results of psychiatric research.
- Levels of significance are often quoted alone in the abstracts and texts of published papers without mentioning actual values, proportions, and so on, or their differences.
- Confidence intervals do not carry with them the pseudo-scientific hypothesis-testing language of significance tests.
- Estimation and confidence intervals give a plausible range of values for the unknown parameter.
- Inadequate sample size is indicated by the relatively large width of the corresponding confidence interval.

SPECIFIC TESTS

t-test

The *t*-test is used for testing the null hypothesis that two population means are equal when the variable being investigated has a normal distribution in each population and the population variances are equal; that is, the *t*-test is a parametric test.

INDEPENDENT SAMPLES *t*-TEST   This procedure tests the null hypothesis that the data are a sample from a population in which the mean of a test variable is equal in two independent (unrelated) groups of cases. Assuming equal population variances (which can be checked using Levene's test), the standard error of the difference between two means, $\bar{x}_1$ and $\bar{x}_2$, of two independent samples (taken from the same parent population) of respective sizes n_1 and n_2, and respective standard deviations s_1 and s_2, $(s_1 \approx s_2)$ is given by

$$\text{standard error of difference} = s \sqrt{[1/n_1 + 1/n_2]}$$

where the pooled standard deviation s is given by

$$s = \sqrt{\{[(n_1 - 1)s_1^2 + (n_2 - 1)s_2^2]/(n_1 + n_2 - 2)\}}$$

If the population variances cannot be assumed to be equal, then the standard error is given by

$$\text{standard error of difference} = \sqrt{[s_1^2/n_1 + s_2^2/n_2]}$$

PAIRED SAMPLES t-TEST   This procedure tests the null hypothesis that two population means are equal when the observations for the two groups can be paired in some way. Pairing (a repeated measures or within-subjects design) is used to make the two groups as similar as possible, allowing differences observed between the two groups to be attributed more readily to the variable of interest.

For n pairs the appropriate standard error is given by

$$\text{standard error of differences of paired observations} = s_d/\sqrt{n}$$

where s_d is the standard deviation of the differences of the paired observations.

Chi-squared test

The chi-squared (χ^2) test is a non-parametric test that can be used to compare independent qualitative and discrete quantitative variables presented in the form of contingency tables containing the data frequencies.

NULL HYPOTHESIS   For a given contingency table, under H_0,

$$\text{expected value of a cell} = (\text{row total})(\text{column total})/(\text{sum of cells})$$

CALCULATION OF χ^2   The value of χ^2 for a contingency table is calculated from

$$\chi^2 = \Sigma[(O - E)^2/E]$$

where O = observed value
E = expected value.

In order to use the χ^2 distribution, the number of degrees of freedom of a contingency table, ν, is given by

$$\nu = (r - 1)(k - 1)$$

where r = number of rows
k = number of columns.

2 × 2 CONTINGENCY TABLE   A 2 × 2 contingency table has one degree of freedom:
For a 2 × 2 contingency table the following formula can be used to calculate χ^2:

$$\chi^2 = (az - by)^2(a + b + y + z)/[(a + b)(y + z)(a + y)(b + z)]$$

SMALL EXPECTED VALUES   For a contingency table with more than one degree of freedom, the following criteria (Cochran 1954) should be fulfilled for the test to be valid:

- each expected value ≥ 1
- in at least 80 per cent of cases, expected value > 5

Table 6.2 Observed values in a 2 × 2 contingency table

	—	—	**Total**
—	a	y	$a + y$
—	b	z	$b + z$
Total	$a + b$	$y + z$	$a + b + y + z$

Reproduced with permission from Puri, B.K. 1996: *Statistics for the health sciences*. London: W.B. Saunders.

For a 2 × 2 contingency table all the expected values need to be at least 5 in order to use the above formula; therefore the overall total must be at least 20. If the total is less than 20, Fisher's exact probability test can be used. If $20 \leq$ total < 100, then a better fit with the continuous χ^2 distribution is provided by using Yates' continuity correction:

$$\chi^2_{corrected} = \{|az - by| - \tfrac{1}{2}(a + b + y + z)\}^2(a + b + y + z)/[(a + b)(y + z)(a + y)(b + z)]$$

GOODNESS-OF-FIT The χ^2 test can be used to test how well an observed distribution fits a given distribution, such as the normal distribution. This can be applied to both discrete and continuous data and tests the hypothesis that a sample derives from a particular model.

Fisher's exact probability test
This test determines exact probabilities for 2 × 2 contingency tables. With the nomenclature of Table 6.2, the formula used is:

$$\text{exact probability of table} =$$
$$(a + y)! \, (b + z)! \, (a + b)! \, (y + z)! \, /[(a + b + y + z)! \, a! \, b! \, y! \, z!]$$

In order to test H_0, in addition to calculating the probability of the given table, the probabilities also have to be calculated of more extreme tables occurring by chance.

Mann–Whitney U test
This is a non-parametric alternative to the independent samples t-test. The test statistic, U, is the smaller of U_1 and U_2:

$$U_1 = n_1 n_2 + \tfrac{1}{2} n_1(n_1 + 1) - R_1$$
$$U_2 = n_1 n_2 + \tfrac{1}{2} n_2(n_2 + 1) - R_2$$

where n_1 = number of observations in the first group
n_2 = number of observations in the second group
R_1 = sum of the ranks assigned to the first group
R_2 = sum of the ranks assigned to the second group.
For $n_1 \geq 8$, and $n_2 \geq 8$, $U \approx N(\mu, \sigma^2)$, where

$$\mu = n_1 n_2/2$$
$$\sigma^2 = n_1 n_2 (n_1 + n_2 + 1)/12$$

Confidence interval for the difference between two means
The $100(1 - \alpha)$ per cent confidence interval for the difference between two means is given by

$$\text{difference} - t_{1 - \alpha/2} \text{ (standard error of difference)}$$
$$\text{to} \quad \text{difference} + t_{1 - \alpha/2} \text{ (standard error of difference)}$$

Confidence interval for the difference between two proportions

For large sample sizes and population proportions not too close to 0 or 1, the $100(1 - \alpha)$ per cent confidence interval for the difference between two proportions is given by

$$\text{difference} - z_{1 - \alpha/2} \text{ (standard error of difference)}$$
$$\text{to} \quad \text{difference} + z_{1 - \alpha/2} \text{ (standard error of difference)}$$

where the standard error of the difference is given by

$$\text{standard error of difference} = \sqrt{[\hat{p}_1(1 - \hat{p}_1)/n_1 + \hat{p}_2(1 - \hat{p}_2)/n_2]}$$

where $\hat{p}_1$ = sample estimate of first proportion
$\hat{p}_2$ = sample estimate of second proportion
n_1 = sample size of the first group
n_2 = sample size of the second group.

Confidence interval for the difference between two medians

For the following confidence intervals to be valid, the assumption is made that the two distributions whose possible difference is being estimated have the same shape but may differ in location.

TWO UNPAIRED SAMPLES In order to determine the $100(1 - \alpha)$ per cent confidence interval for the difference between two medians the value of K must first be calculated from

$$K = n_1 n_2/2 - z_{1 - \alpha/2} \sqrt{[n_1 n_2 (n_1 + n_2 + 1)/12]}$$

where n_1 and n_2 are the sample sizes
$n_1 > 25$
$n_2 > 25$
K is rounded up to the nearest integer.

The total number of possible differences $= n_1 n_2$.

The $100(1 - \alpha)$ per cent confidence interval for the median of these differences is from the Kth smallest to the Kth largest of the $n_1 n_2$ differences ($K \in \mathbb{Z}^+$).

If n_1 and/or n_2 is less than or equal to 25, then tables based on the value of the corresponding Mann–Whitney test statistic can be used.

TWO PAIRED SAMPLES In this case the value of K is calculated from

$$K = n(n + 1)/4 - z_{1 - \alpha/2} \sqrt{[n(n + 1)(2n + 1)/24]}$$

where n = the number of paired cases
$n > 50$
K is rounded up to the nearest integer.

The total number of possible means of two differences (including differences with themselves) $= n(n + 1)/2$.

The $100(1 - \alpha)$ per cent confidence interval for the median of these mean differences is from the Kth smallest to the Kth largest of the $n(n + 1)/2$ mean differences ($K \in \mathbb{Z}^+$).

If $n \leq 50$, then tables based on the value of the corresponding Mann–Whitney test statistic can be used.

CLINICAL TRIALS

Definition
Clinical trials are planned experiments carried out on humans to assess the effectiveness of different forms of treatment.

Classification
The following classification of clinical trials is used by the pharmaceutical industry:

- Phase I trial: clinical pharmacology and toxicity
- Phase II trial: initial clinical investigation
- Phase III trial: full-scale treatment evaluation
- Phase IV trial: postmarketing surveillance

Advantages of randomized trials
In a randomized trial all the subjects have the same probability of receiving each of the different forms of treatment being compared. The advantages of such randomization include:

- The effects of concomitant variables are distributed in a random manner between the comparison groups; these variables may be unknown.
- The allocation of subjects is not carried out in a subjective manner influenced by the biases of the investigators.
- Statistical tests used to analyse the results are on a firm foundation as they are based on what is expected to occur in random samples from parent populations having specified characteristics.

The gold standard of clinical trials is the randomized double-blind controlled trial in which:

- allocation of treatments to subjects is randomized
- each subject does not know which treatment they have received
- the investigator(s) do not know the treatment allocation before the end of the trial

Disadvantages of non-randomized trials
Non-randomized trials may have concurrent or historical (that is, non-concurrent) controls. Both types of non-randomized trials have associated disadvantages in comparison with randomized trials.

CONCURRENT CONTROLS   It is not usually possible to confirm that the different treatment groups are comparable. Volunteer bias may also occur, with volunteers faring better than those who refuse to participate in a trial.

HISTORICAL CONTROLS   Here the control group consists of a group previously given an older/alternative treatment. This group is compared with suitable subjects receiving a new treatment being tested. The disadvantages of using historical controls include:

- It cannot be assumed that everything apart from the new treatment being tested has remained unchanged over time.
- The monitoring and care of current subjects receiving the new treatment are likely to be greater than was that of the historical controls.
- The efficacy of the new treatment is likely to be overestimated.
- The findings of such a trial may be not be widely accepted because of the lack of randomization.

MORE COMPLEX METHODS

Factor analysis

Factor analysis is an attempt to express a set of multivariate data as a linear function of unobserved, underlying dimensions, or (common) factors together with error terms (specific factors). The common factors associated with each observed variable have individual loadings.

Principal components analysis

Principal components analysis is used to produce uncorrelated linear combinations of the observed variables of a multivariate dataset. The first component has maximum variance. Successive components account for progressively smaller parts of the total variance. Each component is uncorrelated with preceding components. A plot of the variance of each principal component against the principal component number is known as a scree plot.

Correspondence analysis

A correspondence analysis is similar to a principal components analysis but is applied to contingency tables. It allows a two-dimensional contingency table to be presented as a two-dimensional graph in which one set of coordinates represents the rows of the table and the other set represents the columns. Rather than partitioning the total variance, as in principal components analysis, there is a partition of the value of χ^2 for the contingency table.

Discriminant analysis

This is a method of classification applied to a multivariate dataset. Independent variables used to discriminate among the groups are known as discriminating variables. The discriminant function is a linear function of discriminating variables which maximizes the distance (or separation) between groups.

Cluster analysis

This is also a method of classification applied to a multivariate dataset which derives homogeneous groups or clusters of cases based on their values for the variable set. Hierarchical methods can be applied to the clusters.

Multivariate regression analysis

In this method a linear multivariate regression equation is fitted to a multivariate dataset. The multiple regression coefficient is the maximum correlation between the dependent variable and multiple non-random independent variables, using a least-squares method.

Path analysis

A series of multiple regression analyses are used to allow hypotheses of causality between variables to be modelled and tested. A path diagram allows these variables and their hypothetical relationships to be represented graphically. It shows arrows between the variables, with regression coefficients (known as path coefficients) associated with these arrows. χ^2 tests are used to test the model.

Canonical correlation analysis

This is an extended form of multivariate regression in which the number of dependent variables is no longer confined to one. The maximum correlation between the set of independent variables and the set of dependent variables is known as the canonical correlation and gives information about interrelationships among the variables.

PROBLEMS OF MEASUREMENT IN PSYCHIATRY

Aims of measurement
The main aims of measurement in psychiatry are:

- to help in the diagnostic process or in other forms of categorization
- to measure symptomatology ± its change

Problems of measurement
Problems in measurement in psychiatry include:

- defining caseness
- assessment of behaviour
- assessment of cognitive performance
- assessment of mood
- assessment of delusions and hallucinations
- assessment of personality
- assessment of psychophysiological functioning
- assessing the degree to which an individual suffers from a psychiatric/psychological disorder

Measurement methods
A range of measurement methods can be employed in psychiatric/psychological assessments. Examples include:

- observer rated scales: structured and semistructured standardized psychiatric interview schedules
- screening instruments
- behavioural observation studies
- self-predictions
- self-recording: e.g. diaries
- self-rating scales for the assessment of mood
- self-rating scales for the assessment of personality
- psychophysiological techniques
- naturalistic observations
- psychometric measurements: e.g. of intelligence and personality

Latent traits (constructs)
Psychological concepts such as attitude and intelligence are considered to be latent traits or hypothetical constructs that are believed to exist. Although not directly observable, constructs can be used to explain phenomena which can be observed and to make predictions. In the development and use of psychometric tests, in particular, factor analysis may be used to identify factors, corresponding to latent traits or hypothetical constructs, that may account for correlations observed between the scores on tests or subtests by a large sample of subjects.

Reliability
DEFINITION The reliability of a test or measuring instrument describes the level of agreement between repeated measurements. It can be expressed as the ratio of the variance of the true scores to the variance of the observed scores:

$$\text{reliability} = \sigma_t^2/(\sigma_t^2 + \sigma_e^2)$$

where σ_t^2 = true score variance
σ_e^2 = measurement error variance.

With this definition, the range of values that the reliability can take is given by:

$$0 \leq \text{reliability} \leq 1.$$

A low value, close to zero, implies low reliability, while a high value, close to one, implies high reliability.

INTER-RATER RELIABILITY Inter-rater reliability describes the level of agreement between assessments of the same material made by two or more assessors at roughly the same time.

INTRA-RATER RELIABILITY Intra-rater reliability describes the level of agreement between assessments made by two or more assessors of the same material presented at two or more times.

TEST–RETEST RELIABILITY Test–retest reliability describes the level of agreement between assessments of the same material made under similar circumstances but at two different times.

ALTERNATIVE FORMS RELIABILITY Alternative forms reliability describes the level of agreement between assessments of the same material by two supposedly similar forms of the test or measuring instrument made either at the same time or immediately consecutively.

SPLIT-HALF RELIABILITY Split-half reliability describes the level of agreement between assessments by two halves of a split test or measuring instrument of the same material made under similar circumstances. Since some tests or measuring instruments contain different sections measuring different aspects, in such cases it may be appropriate to create the halves by using alternative questions, thereby maintaining the balance of each half.

Statistical tests of reliability

PERCENTAGE AGREEMENT Measuring the percentage agreement is the simplest but most unsatisfactory method of assessing the reliability, since it does not take into account the agreement between observers owing to chance.

PRODUCT-MOMENT CORRELATION COEFFICIENT The product-moment correlation coefficient, r, may give spuriously high results, particularly if there is chance agreement of many values. It may even give the maximum value of one for the agreement between two raters, even if they do not agree at all, if, for example, one of the raters consistently rates scores on the test or measuring instrument at twice the values rated by the other rater.

KAPPA STATISTIC The kappa statistic, or kappa coefficient, κ, is a measure of agreement in which allowance is made for chance agreement. It is most appropriate when different categories of measurement are being recorded and is calculated from the following formula:

$$\kappa = (P_o - P_c)/(1 - P_c)$$

where P_c = the chance agreement
P_o = observed proportion of agreement.

The range of values that κ can take is:

- $\kappa = 1$: complete agreement
- $0 < \kappa < 1$: observed agreement > chance agreement
- $\kappa = 0$: observed agreement = chance agreement
- $\kappa < 0$: observed agreement < chance agreement

The weighted kappa, κ_w, is a version of κ that takes into account differences in the seriousness of disagreements (represented by the weightings).

INTRA-CLASS CORRELATION COEFFICIENT   The intra-class correlation coefficient, r_i, is more appropriate than κ or r if agreement is being measured for several items that can be regarded as part of a continuum or dimension. For two raters the value of r_i is derived from the corresponding value of r:

$$r_i = \{[\Sigma(s_1^2 + s_2^2) - (s_1 - s_2)^2]r - (\bar{x}_1 - \bar{x}_2)^2 /2\}/\{(s_1^2 + s_2^2) + (\bar{x}_1 - \bar{x}_2)^2/2\}$$

where r = the product-moment correlation coefficient between the scores of the two raters

  s_1 = the standard deviation of the scores for the first rater

  s_2 = the standard deviation of the scores for the second rater

  $\bar{x}_1$ = the mean of the scores for the first rater

  $\bar{x}_2$ = the mean of the scores for the second rater.

It follows that:

$$\text{if } \bar{x}_1 = \bar{x}_2 \text{ and } s_1 = s_2$$
$$\text{then } r_i = r$$
$$\text{else } r_i < r$$

For more than two raters the value of r_i is derived from the corresponding two-way ANOVA for (raters $\times$ subjects):

$$r_i = n_s(s_{ms} - e_{ms})/\{n_s\, s_{ms} + n_r\, r_{ms} + (n_s\, n_r - n_s - n_r)e_{ms}\}$$

where n_r = number of raters

  n_s = number of subjects

  e_{ms} = errors mean square

  r_{ms} = raters mean square

  s_{ms} = subjects mean square.

CRONBACH'S ALPHA   Cronbach's alpha, α, gives a measure of the average correlation between all the items when assessing split-half reliability. It thereby indicates the internal consistency of the test or measuring instrument.

Validity

DEFINITION   The validity of a test or measuring instrument is the term used to describe whether it measures what it purports to measure.

FACE VALIDITY   Face validity is the subjective judgement as to whether a test or measuring instrument appears on the surface to measure the feature in question. In spite of its name it is not strictly a type of validity.

CONTENT VALIDITY   Content validity examines whether the specific measurements aimed for by the test or measuring instrument are assessing the content of the measurement in question.

PREDICTIVE VALIDITY   Predictive validity determines the extent of agreement between a present measurement and one in the future.

CONCURRENT VALIDITY   Concurrent validity compares the measure being assessed with an external valid yardstick atthe same time.

CRITERION VALIDITY   Criterion validity refers to predictive and concurrent validity together.

INCREMENTAL VALIDITY   Incremental validity indicates whether the measurement being assessed is superior to other measurements in approaching true validity.

CROSS-VALIDITY   Cross-validation of a test or measuring instrument is used to determine whether, after having its criterion validity established for one sample, it maintains criterion validity when applied to another sample.

CONVERGENT VALIDITY Convergent validity is established when measures expected to be correlated, since they measure the same phenomena, are indeed found to be associated.

DIVERGENT VALIDITY Divergent validity is established when measures discriminate successfully between other measures of unrelated constructs.

CONSTRUCT VALIDITY Construct validity is determined by establishing both convergent and divergent validity, and is closely connected with the theoretical rationale underpinning the test or measuring instrument. It involves showing the power of the hypothetical construct(s) or latent traits both to explain observations and to make predictions.

Type I error

A type I error is the error of wrongly rejecting H_0 when it is true. As mentioned above, the probability of making a type I error is denoted by α, the significance level:

$$\alpha = P(\text{type I error})$$

Type II error

A type II error is the error of wrongly accepting H_0 when it is false. The probability of making a type II error is denoted by β:

$$\beta = P(\text{type II error})$$

Power

The power of a test is the probability that H_0 is rejected when it is indeed false. It is related to β, the probability of making a type II error, in the following way:

$$\text{power} = 1 - \beta$$

Sensitivity

The sensitivity of a test or measuring instrument is the proportion of positive results/cases correctly identified:

$$\text{sensitivity} = (\text{true positive})/(\text{true positive} + \text{false negative})$$

This ratio needs to be multiplied by 100 if the sensitivity is to be given as a percentage.

Specificity

The specificity of a test or measuring instrument is the proportion of negative results/cases correctly identified:

$$\text{specificity} = (\text{true negative})/(\text{true negative} + \text{false positive})$$

This ratio needs to be multiplied by 100 if the sensitivity is to be given as a percentage.

Predictive values

The predictive value of a positive result from a research measure is the proportion of the positive results that is true positive:

$$\text{predictive value of a positive result} = (\text{true positive})/(\text{true positive} + \text{false positive})$$

The predictive value of a negative result from a research measure is the proportion of the negative results that is true negative:

$$\text{predictive value of a negative result} =$$
$$(\text{true negative})/(\text{true negative} + \text{false negative})$$

Bias
SELECTION BIAS   Selection bias occurs when a characteristic associated with the variable(s) of interest leads to higher or lower participation in the research study, such as an epidemiological cross-sectional survey.

OBSERVER BIAS   In epidemiological studies, observer bias occurs when the researcher has clues about whether the subject is in the case or comparison group, leading to a biased assessment. This is particularly likely in studies involving retrospective assessments.

RECALL BIAS   In epidemiological studies, recall bias occurs when there is a difference in knowledge between the subjects in the case and in the comparison groups, leading to a biased recall. For example, in case-control studies the knowledge on the part of subjects (or, in the case of childhood disorders, their parents) as to whether or not they have a given disorder may bias their recall of exposure to putative risk factors.

INFORMATION BIAS   Information bias includes both observer bias and recall bias.

CONFOUNDING BIAS   In epidemiological studies, confounding bias occurs when the actual, but unexamined, underlying cause of the disorder being researched is associated with both the suspected risk factor and the disorder.

META-ANALYSIS, SURVIVAL ANALYSIS AND LOGISTIC REGRESSION

Meta-analysis
DEFINITION   The term meta-analysis is used to describe the process of evaluating and statistically combining results from two or more existing independent randomized clinical trials addressing similar questions in order to give an overall assessment.

DIFFICULTIES   Difficulties associated with meta-analysis include:

- The existence of publication bias: trials showing a statistically significant difference are more likely to be published than those not finding a statistically significant result.
- Researchers finding 'non-significant' results may be less likely formally to write up their results for publication.
- Arriving at selection criteria to determine which studies to include and which not to include in the meta-analysis.
- The different centres in which the different clinical trials have taken place may differ with respect to important variables in such a way as seriously to question the validity of combining their data.
- If the meta-analysis is of clinical trials carried out on widely differing population groups, to whom can the results of the meta-analysis properly be applied?

Survival analysis
This is a collection of statistical analysis techniques that can be applied to situations in which the time to a given event, such as death, illness onset or recovery, is measured, but not all individuals necessarily have to have reached this event during the overall time interval studied.

SURVIVAL FUNCTION   The survival function, $S(t)$, is given by

$$S(t) = P(t_s > t)$$

where t = time

t_s = survival time.

The survival function is also given by

$$S(t) = 1 - \text{(cumulative distribution function of } t_s)$$

SURVIVAL CURVE   This is a plot of $S(t)$ (on the ordinate) versus t (on the abscissa). Instead of being drawn as continuous curves, sometimes survival curves are drawn in a stepwise fashion, with the steps occurring between estimated cumulative survival probabilities.

HAZARD FUNCTION   This measures the likelihood of an individual experiencing a given event, such as death, the onset of illness, or recovery, as a function of time.

Logistic regression

This is a regression model used to predict the probability of a dichotomous variable, such as better/not better at the end of the treatment period, on the basis of a set of independent variables, x_1 to x_n:

$$P(\text{event}) = 1/(1 + \exp(-(\alpha_0 + \alpha_1 x_1 + \ldots + \alpha_n x_n)))$$

where the coefficients α_0 to α_n are estimated using a maximum likelihood method.

BIBLIOGRAPHY

Altman, D.G. 1991: *Practical statistics for medical research*. London: Chapman & Hall.

Bryman, A. and Cramer, D. 1994: *Quantitative data analysis for social scientists*, revised edn. London: Routledge.

Cochran, W.G. 1954: Some methods for strengthening the common χ^2-test. *Biometrics* 10, 417–51.

Coolican, H. 1994: *Research methods and statistics in psychology*, 2nd edn. London: Hodder & Stoughton.

Dunn, G. and Everitt, B. 1995: *Clinical biostatistics: an introduction to evidence-based medicine*. London: Arnold.

Everitt, B. and Hay, D. 1992: *Talking about statistics: a psychologist's guide to design and analysis*. London: Arnold.

Puri, B.K. 1996: *Statistics for the health sciences*. London: W.B. Saunders.

Puri, B.K. 1996: *Statistics in practice: an illustrated guide to SPSS*. London: Arnold.

7
Social sciences

DESCRIPTIVE TERMS

Social class
A social class is a segment of the population sharing a broadly similar type and level of resources, with a broadly similar style of living and some shared perception of its common condition.

DETERMINANTS The determinants of social class include:

- education
- financial status
- occupation
- type of residence
- geographical area of residence
- leisure activities

OCCUPATIONAL CLASSIFICATION In British psychiatry, the following occupationally based classification given by the Office of Population Censuses and Surveys has traditionally been used:

- social class I: professional, higher managerial, landowners
- social class II: intermediate
- social class III: skilled, manual, clerical
- social class IV: semi-skilled
- social class V: unskilled
- social class 0: unemployed, students

Members of the same household are assigned to the social class of the head of the household.

Socioeconomic status
The socioeconomic status of an individual is their position in the social hierarchy. It is related to social class and may increase, for example through educational achievement, or decrease, for example through unemployment or mental illness.

Relevance to psychiatric disorder and healthcare delivery
PSYCHIATRIC DISORDER The incidence and prevalence of many psychiatric disorders have been found to vary with social class. In particular, the following disorders are more likely to be diagnosed in lower social classes:

- schizophrenia
- alcohol dependence
- organic psychosis
- depressive episodes in women
- parasuicide/deliberate self-harm
- personality disorder

The following disorders are more likely to be diagnosed in upper social classes:

- anorexia nervosa in females
- bulimia nervosa in females
- bipolar mood disorder

RELATIONSHIP BETWEEN SOCIAL CLASS AND PSYCHIATRIC DISORDER   The existence of a relationship between social class and a given psychiatric disorder does not necessarily imply causation, from social class to the disorder. In general, the possible explanations of such a relationship may include:

- downward social drift: e.g. the increased representation of schizophrenia in lower social classes may be partly a result of social drift
- environmental stress: lower social class is associated with adverse life situations, material deprivation and the lower self-esteem that manual jobs entail; women in lower social classes are more likely to experience severe life events and vulnerability factors
- differential labelling: e.g. it may be that some people in Britain of Afro-Caribbean origin are more likely to be detained under mental health legislation and diagnosed as suffering from schizophrenia (although this may in fact reflect genuine differences in prevalence and incidence rates)
- differential treatment: e.g. there is a difference in the type of psychiatric treatment likely to be received by those from different social classes (see below)

HEALTHCARE DELIVERY   Those with a psychiatric disorder who are from lower social classes are more likely to:

- be admitted to hospital as psychiatric inpatients
- remain as psychiatric inpatients for longer
- receive physical treatments e.g. electroconvulsive therapy

Those with a psychiatric disorder who are from upper social classes are more likely to:

- spend a shorter period of time as psychiatric inpatients
- be treated as psychiatric outpatients without inpatient admission
- receive psychological treatments e.g. individual psychotherapy

PATHWAYS TO PSYCHIATRIC CARE   Goldberg and Huxley (1980) described the existence of filters to psychiatric care, each of which depends on:

- social factors: such as age, sex, ethnic background, socioeconomic status
- service organization and provision: e.g. time and location of clinics, length of waiting list
- aspects of the disorder itself: e.g. its severity and chronicity

These filters include:

- the decision to consult the general practitioner
- recognition of the disorder by the general practitioner
- the decision by the general practitioner as to whether or not to refer the patient to a specialist

The Black Report on socioeconomic inequalities in health

According to the Black Report 1980, exploring the difference in health and mortality in Britain between the social classes, compared with those in social class I, individuals in social class V:

- have twice the neonatal mortality
- are twice as likely to die before retirement
- have an increased rate of almost all diseases

EXPLANATIONS   The following explanations for the relationship between social class and illness found in the Black Report on socioeconomic inequalities in health have been suggested:

- artefactual: the health inequalities found are artificial
- natural and social selection: good health is associated with an improvement in social class while poor health is associated with social drift downwards
- materialist/structural: poor health is primarily a function of material deprivation; inequalities in wealth and income distribution is associated with inequalities in health
- cultural/behavioural: certain unhealthy behaviour patterns are more common in lower social classes (e.g. smoking, unhealthy diets), leading to health inequalities

CHANGES AFTER 10 YEARS   A decade after the publication of the Black Report, Smith *et al.* (1990) found:

- social class differences in mortality had widened
- better measures of socioeconomic position showed greater inequalities in mortality
- inequalities in health had been found in all countries that collect relevant data
- measurement artefacts and social selection did not account for mortality differences
- social class differences existed for health during life as well as for the length of life
- trends in income distribution suggested a further likely widening of mortality differences

SOCIAL ROLES OF DOCTORS AND ILLNESS

Social role
The social role of an individual in social life is the pattern of behaviour in given social situations expected of them in relation to their social status. It consists of:

- obligations: behaviours towards others expected of the individual
- rights: behaviours from others expected in return for obligations

Social role of doctors
In the model proposed by Parsons (1951) the role of the doctor includes:

- defining illness
- legitimizing illness
- imposing an illness diagnosis if necessary
- offering appropriate help

Doctors therefore control access to the sick role and they and patients have reciprocal obligations and rights.

Sick role
The sick role was defined by Parsons (1951) as the role given by society to a sick individual, and was considered to carry rights or privileges and obligations.

RIGHTS (PRIVILEGES)   According to Parsons (1951) the sick role carries the following two rights for the sick individual:

- exemption from blame for the illness
- exemption from normal responsibilities while sick, such as the need to go to work

OBLIGATIONS   The sick individual has the following obligations:

- the wish to recover as soon as possible, including seeking appropriate help from the doctor
- cooperation with medical investigations and acceptance of medical advice and treatment

Illness behaviour

Illness behaviour is a set of stages describing the behaviour adopted by sick individuals (Mechanic 1978). It describes the way in which individuals respond to somatic symptoms and signs and the conditions under which they come to view them as abnormal. Illness behaviour therefore involves the manner in which individuals:

- monitor their bodies
- define and interpret their symptoms and signs
- take remedial action
- utilize sources of help

STAGES   Illness behaviour includes the following stages:

- initially well
- symptoms of the illness begin to be experienced
- the opinion of immediate social contacts is sought
- contact is made with a doctor (or doctors)
- the illness is legitimized by the doctor(s)
- the individual adopts the sick role
- on recovery (or death) the dependent stage of the sick role is given up
- a rehabilitation stage is entered if the individual recovers

DETERMINANTS   The determinants of illness behaviour, according to Mechanic (1978), are:

- the visibility, recognizability or perceptual salience of deviant signs and symptoms
- the extent to which symptoms are seen as being serious
- the extent to which symptoms disrupt the family, work, and other social activities
- the frequency of the appearance of deviant signs or symptoms, their persistence, and the frequency of recurrence
- the tolerance threshold of exposed deviant signs and symptoms
- available information, knowledge and cultural understanding of exposed deviant signs and symptoms
- basic needs leading to denial
- the competition between needs and illness responses
- competing interpretations assigned to recognized symptoms
- the availability and physical proximity of treatment resources and the costs in terms of time, money, effort and stigma

FAMILY LIFE IN RELATION TO MAJOR MENTAL ILLNESS

Family life is guided by the explicit and implicit relationship rules that prescribe and limit the behaviour of members of the family and provide expectations within the family with respect to the roles, actions and consequences of individuals.

Elements of family functioning

Elements of family functioning of importance in relation to major mental illness (after Dare 1985) include:

- interactional patterns: family members and relationships, communication patterns, hierarchical structure, control/authority systems, relationship with the outside world
- sociocultural context of the family: socioeconomic status, social mobility, migration status
- location of the family in the lifecycle: number of transitions, adaptation requirements
- intergenerational structure: experiences of parents as children, influences of grandparents and extended family
- significance of symptoms of mental illness for the family
- family problem-solving skills: family style, previous experience

Schizophrenia

Historically, the following types of family dysfunction were at various times believed to be a cause of schizophrenia:

- schizophrenogenic mother
- double-bind
- marital skew and marital schism
- abnormal family communication

These theories are now out of favour, but there is evidence for the more recent theory relating to the effects of expressed emotion with respect to relapse in schizophrenia.

SCHIZOPHRENOGENIC MOTHER This concept was put forward by Fromm-Reichman in 1948. Schizophrenia was said to be a consequence of an inadequate relationship between the future sufferer from schizophrenia, as a child, and their mother. Characteristics of the schizophrenogenic mother were said to include her being:

- rejecting
- aloof
- overly protective
- overtly hostile

DOUBLE-BIND This concept was put forward by Bateson and colleagues in 1956. The parents communicated with the child (the future sufferer from schizophrenia) in abnormal ways leading to feelings of ambivalence and ambiguity, with messages that were typically:

- vague
- ambiguous
- confusing

Schizophrenia developed as a result of exposure to such double-bind situations.

MARITAL SKEW AND MARITAL SCHISM   This concept was put forward by Lidz and colleagues in 1957:

- marital skew: dominant and eccentric mother; passive and dependent father
- marital schism: parental conflict, argument, and hostility leading to divided loyalties to mother and father on the part of the child (the future sufferer from schizophrenia)

ABNORMAL FAMILY COMMUNICATION   This concept was put forward by Wynne and colleagues in 1958 and suggested that disordered communication took place between the parents of those with schizophrenia.

EXPRESSED EMOTION   In an outcome study of 200 patients, mainly with schizophrenia, Brown *et al.* (1958) found that those discharged to their families had a poor outcome, with the highest relapse rate occurring in those families having close and frequent contact with the patients.

Subsequent follow-up studies have confirmed the association of high expressed emotion in families, characterized by the frequent, intense expression of emotion and a pushy and critical attitude by relatives to the patient, with an increased relapse rate in family members with schizophrenia.

In assessing expressed emotion, the five relevant scales of the Camberwell Family Interview (CFI) are:

- critical comments: indicating unambiguous dislike or disapproval
- hostility: expressed towards the person rather than their behaviour
- emotional overinvolvement: exaggerated self-sacrificing or overprotective concern
- warmth: based on sympathy, affection and empathy
- positive remarks: expressing praise or approval of the patient

The first three of these are associated with high expressed emotion and predict relapse (Vaughn and Leff 1976). See Table 7.1.

Mood disorders

EXPRESSED EMOTION   As with schizophrenia, high expressed emotion at home is associated with an increased risk of relapse of depression.

VULNERABILITY FACTORS   Two of the four vulnerability factors found by Brown and Harris (1978) to make women more susceptible to suffer from depression following life events (see below) were:

- the lack of a confiding relationship
- having three or more children under the age of 15 years at home

Table 7.1   Effects of expressed emotion on the relapse rates of treated and untreated patients with schizophrenia in the nine months following discharge

	Relapse rate in nine months following discharge
Antipsychotic medication, low expressed emotion family	12%
Antipsychotic medication, high expressed emotion family, < 35 hours/week face-to-face contact	42%
No antipsychotic medication, high expressed emotion family, > 35 hours/week face-to-face contact	92%

Source: Vaughn and Leff 1976.

Problem drinking and alcohol dependence

Family life often suffers as a result of excessive alcohol consumption, with the breakdown of relationships, marriages and families being common. This may result from the following consequences of excessive alcohol consumption:

- mood changes
- personality deterioration
- verbal abuse
- physical violence
- psychosexual disorders
- pathological jealousy
- associated gambling
- associated abuse of other psychoactive substances

Learning difficulty/mental retardation

Psychological processes that may occur in families with an impaired or diabled member (after Bicknell 1983) include:

- shock → panic → denial
- denial → shopping around
- denial → over-protection/rejection
- grief → projection of grief
- guilt
- anger
- bargaining → late rejection
- acceptance → infantilization
- ego-centred work → 'other'-centred work
- over-identification

LIFE EVENTS

Definition

Life events are sudden changes, which may be positive or negative, in an individual's social life which disrupt its normal course.

Life-change scale

The full Holmes and Rahe Social Readjustment Rating Scale introduced in 1967 consists of a self-report questionnaire containing 43 classes of life event.

Aetiology of psychiatric disorders

In order to demonstrate that life events have an aetiological role in a given psychiatric disorder, the following criteria should be fulfilled:

- the occurrence of life events should correlate with the onset of the disorder
- the life events should precede the onset of the disorder and not the other way round
- a hypothetical construct should exist with confounded variables excluded
- the relationship between life events and the psychiatric disorder should be found to occur in different populations and at different times

Difficulties in the evaluation of life events

Methodological problems in the evaluation of life events include:

Table 7.2 Some life-change values for life events in the Holmes and Rahe Social Readjustment Rating Scale

Life event	Life-change value
Death of spouse	100
Divorce	73
Marital separation	65
Jail term	63
Death of close family member	63
Personal injury or illness	53
Marriage	50
Being sacked from job	47
Retirement	45
Marital reconciliation	45
Pregnancy	40
Birth of child	39
Death of close friend	37
Child leaving home for good	29
Problems with in-laws	29
Problems with boss	23
Change in sleeping habits	16
Change in eating habits	15
Minor legal violation	11

After Holmes and Rahe (1967)

- assessments tend to be retrospective, which can lead to difficulties such as
  - biased recall
  - fall-off in recall with time
  - retrospective contamination
  - effort after meaning
- causation and association need to be separated
- contextual evaluation
- subjective evaluation

A widely used instrument for current research into life events and psychiatric disorder is the Life Events and Difficulties Schedule (LEDS) of Brown and Harris (1978, 1989) which has the following features:

- semistructured interview schedule
- 38 areas probed
- detailed narratives collected about events, including their circumstances
- high reliability
- high validity

Clinical significance

DEPRESSION   Many studies have found a relationship between life events and the onset of depression. In the six to 12 months before the onset, compared with normal controls, patients have a three to five times greater chance of having suffered at least one life event with major negative long-term implications (involving threat or loss). However, most people who experience adverse life events do not develop depression; as mentioned above, Brown and Harris (1978) identified four vulnerability factors that make women more susceptible to suffer from depression following life events:

- the loss of their mother before the age of 11 years
- not working outside the home
- the lack of a confiding relationship
- having three or more children under the age of 15 years at home

SCHIZOPHRENIA   The evidence tends to suggest that independent life events are more likely to occur before relapse rather than before the first onset of schizophrenia (Brown and Birley 1968; Tennant 1985).

ANXIETY   There is some evidence that life events are more likely to occur prior to anxiety (Finlay-Jones and Brown 1981; Miller and Ingham 1985). From their study of life events occurring in the year before the onset of three types of cases of psychiatric disorder of recent onset (depression, anxiety, and mixed depression/anxiety) in young women, and normal controls, Finlay-Jones and Brown (1981) argued that life events involving severe loss were a causal agent in the onset of depression and life events involving severe danger were a causal agent in the onset of anxiety states. Cases of mixed depression/anxiety were more likely to report both a severe loss and a severe danger before onset.

MANIA   In general the results of life-event studies of mania are conflicting.

PARASUICIDE/DELIBERATE SELF-HARM   There is strong evidence that threatening life events are more common before self-poisoning attempts (for example, Morgan *et al.* 1975; Farmer and Creed 1989).

FUNCTIONAL DISORDERS   Threatening life events have been found to be more likely to precede functional disorders presenting physically such as abdominal pain without an organic cause (Creed 1981; Craig and Brown 1984) and menorrhagia (Harris 1989).

RESIDENTIAL INSTITUTIONS

Social institutions
DEFINITION   A social institution is an established and sanctioned form of relationship between social beings.

EXAMPLES   Examples of social institutions include:

- the family
- political parties
- religious groups

Total institutions
DEFINITION   A total institution is an organization in which a large number of like-situated individuals, cut off from the wider social world for an appreciable period of time, together lead an enclosed formally administered round of life (Goffman 1961).

EXAMPLES   Examples of total institutions include:

- older large psychiatric hospitals
- prisons
- monasteries
- large ships

Goffman
From his study of the large St Elizabeth's Hospital, in Washington DC, Goffman (1961) was one of the first to suggest that total institutions may be harmful. Concepts introduced by Goffman include:

- total institution
- binary management: the daily lives of patients were highly regulated by staff who appeared to live in a different world to the patients
- binary living
- batch living: whereas normally life consists of a balance between work, home life, and leisure time, these three distinct entities did not exist in the total institution studied
- institutional perspective: the existence of an institutional perspective leads to the assumption that there exists an overall rational plan
- mortification process: the process whereby an individual becomes an inhabitant of a total institution
- betrayal funnel: the start of the mortification process through which relatives, via doctors, send the individual into a psychiatric hospital
- role-stripping: the patient is processed through the admissions procedure, which would also usually include being physically stripped naked for the purposes of a physical examination
- patient/inmate role: patients or inmates could be considered to be metaphorically baptized into this role through the admissions procedure, which would usually include bathing before being given institutional clothing
- moral career: gradual changes in the perception of patients about themselves and others, occurring as a result of institutionalization

REACTIONS TO THE MORTIFICATION PROCESS   According to Goffman, patients were said to show various possible reactions to the mortification process, including:

- withdrawal
- open rebellion
- colonization: the patient pretends to show acceptance
- conversion
- institutionalization: actual acceptance both outwardly and inwardly

Institutional neurosis
Barton (1959) used the term institutional neurosis to describe a syndrome he considered to be caused by institutions in which the individual shows:

- apathy
- an inability to plan for the future
- submissiveness
- withdrawal
- low self-esteem

Secondary handicap
Wing (1967, 1978) used the term secondary handicap to include both institutional neurosis and similar features occurring in individuals living outside total institutions.

PRIMARY HANDICAP   This may be psychiatric illness, somatic illness, or social difficulties with which the individual has to contend.

SECONDARY HANDICAP   This results from the unfortunate way in which other people may react to the primary handicap, both inside and outside total institutions.

The three mental hospitals study
In the 1960s Wing and Brown (1961, 1970) carried out an important comparative study of three British mental hospitals – Netherne Hospital, South London;

Severalls Hospital, Essex; and Mapperley Hospital, Nottingham. These hospitals were chosen because they had different social conditions but otherwise were similar in that they had patients with schizophrenia who suffered illnesses of similar severity, similar catchment-area populations, and all such patients were accepted for admission. Thus it was hoped to test the hypothesis that social environment could influence schizophrenic symptoms and behaviour. A strong association was found between the poverty of the social environment and the severity of clinical poverty. Clinical poverty consisted of:

- blunted affect
- poverty of speech
- social withdrawal

STIGMA AND PREJUDICE

Stigma
DEFINITION   Stigma is an attribute of an individual which marks them as being unacceptable, inferior or dangerous and 'spoils' identity.

EXAMPLE   Psychiatric disorders are highly stigmatized in societies which value rationality.

ENACTED STIGMA   This is the experience of the discrimination of an individual who bears a stigma.

FELT STIGMA   This is the fear of the discrimination of an individual who bears a stigma.

DEVELOPMENT   Stigma first appears during the psychoanalytic stage of latency, approximately corresponding with Erikson's stage of industry versus inferiority, during which children develop a strong awareness of the ways in which they are similar to and differ from others.

Prejudice
DEFINITION   Prejudice is a preconceived set of beliefs held about others who are 'pre-judged' on this basis. The negative meaning of the term is the one usually used.

EXAMPLE   Racism or racial prejudice is the dogmatic belief that one race is superior to another one, and that there exist identifiable racial characteristics that influence cognition, achievement, behaviour, etc.

DISCRIMINATION   This is the enactment of prejudice. (In the case of racism, the enactment is also termed racialism.)

CAUSES   The causes of prejudice may include:

- the person holding the prejudice is rigid in their beliefs and does not tolerate weaknesses in others; this is sometimes referred to by sociologists as an authoritarian personality
- scapegoating of the victims of the prejudice
- stereotyping of the victims of the prejudice

ETHNIC MINORITIES, ADAPTATION AND MENTAL HEALTH

Prevalence of schizophrenia
In Britain, there is a higher rate of diagnosis of schizophrenia in Afro-Caribbean and Irish populations, compared with the indigenous population, and a lower rate in those of South Asian origin.

Causes of different prevalence rates
Explanations of the different prevalence rates of schizophrenia in ethnic minorities in Britain include:

- Those who migrate from their countries of origin have a greater likelihood of having schizophrenia or a predisposition for schizophrenia (social selection); however, there is a reduced rate in Asians and an increased rate in second generation Afro-Caribbeans.
- Migration is associated with increased stress leading to an increased precipitation of schizophrenia in those with an underlying predisposition; however, there is a reduced rate in Asians and an increased rate in second generation Afro-Caribbeans.
- Discrimination and deprivation lead to an increased rate of schizophrenia, or an increased precipitation of schizophrenia in those with an underlying predisposition (social causation); however, there is a reduced rate in Asians.
- Schizophrenia is over-diagnosed in Afro-Caribbeans.

Depression and anxiety
Those from ethnic minorities may not tell their doctor they feel depressed or anxious. For example:

- Afro-Caribbean men when depressed may instead complain of erectile dysfunction or reduced libido
- South Asians may somatize depression
- South Asians may somatize anxiety

PROFESSIONS

Characteristics of professions
The characteristics of professional status include:

- the possession of practical skills based on theoretical knowledge
- requiring an extended period of formal training and education
- assessments of competence carried out by the profession
- belonging to an organization
- recognition by the state of the professional organization
- adherence to a code of conduct
- providing altruistic service
- the possession of a monopoly of practice in their field

Professional groups involved in patient care
Long-established professions in healthcare services include:

- doctors
- pharmacists
- dentists

Newer 'semi-professions' or 'sub-professions' include:

- psychiatric nurses
- clinical psychologists
- non-medically trained psychotherapists
- occupational therapists

'Semi-professions' or 'sub-professions' may increase their 'professionalization' over time, for instance by increasing the length of training and training requirements. Conversely, professional groups involved in patient care may decrease their 'professionalization' over time, for instance by going on strike even if this adversely affects patient care.

BIBLIOGRAPHY

Barton, W.R. 1959: *Institutional neurosis*. Bristol: Wright.

Bicknell, J. 1983: The psychopathology of handicap. *British Journal of Medical Psychology* 56, 167–78.

Boulton, M. 1998: Sociology. In Puri, B.K. and Tyrer (eds), *Sciences basic to psychiatry*, 2nd edn. Edinburgh: Churchill Livingstone.

Brown, G.W. and Birley, J.L. 1968: Crises and life changes and the onset of schizophrenia *Journal of Health Social Behaviour* 9, 203–14.

Brown, G.W., Carstairs, G.M. and Topping, G.C. 1958: The posthospital adjustment of chronic mental patients. *Lancet* ii, 658–9.

Brown, G.W. and Harris, T.O. (eds) 1978: *Social origins of depression: a study of psychiatric disorder in women*. London: Tavistock.

Brown, G.W. and Harris, T.O. (eds) 1989: *Life events and illness*. New York: Guildford Press.

Craig, T.K.J. and Brown, G.W. 1984: Goal frustration and life events in the etiology of painful gastrointestinal disorder. *Journal of Psychosomatic Research* 28, 411–21.

Creed, F. 1981: Life events and appendicectomy. *Lancet* i, 1381–5.

Creed, F. 1992: Life-events. In Weller, M. and Eysenck, M. (eds), *The scientific basis of psychiatry*, 2nd edn. London: W.B. Saunders.

Dare, C. 1985: Family therapy. In Rutter, M. and Hersov, L. (eds), *Child and adolescent psychiatry: modern approaches*. Oxford: Blackwell Scientific.

Farmer, R. and Creed, F. 1989: Life events and hostility in self-poisoning. *British Journal of Psychiatry* 154, 390–5.

Finlay-Jones, R. and Brown, G.W. 1981: Types of stressful life event and the onset of anxiety and depressive disorders. *Psychological Medicine* 11, 803–15.

Goffman, E. 1961: *Asylums: essays on the social situation of mental patients and other inmates*. New York: Doubleday.

Goldberg, D. and Huxley, P. 1980: *Mental illness in the community: the pathways to psychiatric care*. London: Tavistock Publications.

Harris, T.O. 1989: Disorders of menstruation. In Brown, G.W. and Harris, T.O. (eds), *Life events and illness*. New York: Guildford Press.

Holmes, T.H. and Rahe, R.H. 1967: The social readjustment rating scale. *Journal of Psychosomatic Research* 11, 213–17.

Jones, K. 1993: Social sciences in relation to psychiatry. In Kendall, R.E. and Zealley, A.K. (eds), Edinburgh: Churchill Livingstone.

Mechanic, D. 1978: *Medical sociology*, 2nd edn. Glencoe: Free Press.

Miller, P.M. and Ingham, J.G. 1985: Dimensions of experience and symptomatology. *Journal of Psychosomatic Research* 29, 475–88.

Morgan, H.G., Burns-Cox, C.J., Pocock, H. *et al.* 1975: Deliberate self-harm: clinical and socio-economic characteristics of 368 patients. *British Journal of Psychiatry* 127, 564–74.

Parsons, T. 1951: *The social system*. Glencoe: Free Press.

Scrambler, G. (ed.) 1991: *Sociology as applied to medicine*, 3rd edn, London: Baillière Tindall.

Smith, G.D., Bartley, M., and Blane, D. 1990: The Black report on socioeconomic inequalities in health 10 years on. *British Medical Journal* 301, 373–7.

Tantum, D. and Birchwood, M. (eds) 1994: *Psychiatry and social sciences*. London: Gaskell.

Tennant, C.C. 1985: Stress and schizophrenia: a review. *Integrative Psychiatry* 3, 248–61.

Vaughn, C.E. and Leff, J.P. 1976: The influence of family and social factors on the course of schizophrenic illness. *British Journal of Psychiatry* 129, 125–37.

Wing, J.K. 1967: Social treatment, rehabilitation and management. In Coppen, A. and Walker, A. (eds), *Recent developments in schizophrenia*. British Journal of Psychiatry Special Publication No. 1, London.

Wing, J.K. 1978: *Schizophrenia: towards a new synthesis*. London: Academic Press.

Wing, J.K. and Brown, G.W. 1961: Social treatment of chronic schizophrenia: a comparative survery of three mental hospitals. *Journal of Mental Science* 107, 847–61.

Wing, J.K. and Brown, G.W. 1970: *Institutionalism and schizophrenia: a comparative study of three mental hospitals 1960–1968*. London: Cambridge University Press.

8
Descriptive psychopathology

DISORDERS OF GENERAL BEHAVIOUR

Underactivity

STUPOR   The key features of stupor, when the term is used in its psychiatric sense, include:

- mutism
- immobility
- occasional periods of excitement and overactivity

Stupor is seen in:

- catatonic stupor
- depressive stupor
- manic stupor
- epilepsy
- hysteria

In neurology the term stupor refers to a patient who responds to pain and loud sounds; they may exhibit brief monosyllabic utterances and some spontaneous motor activity takes place.

DEPRESSIVE RETARDATION   This is a lesser form of psychomotor retardation occurring in depression which, in its extreme form, merges with depressive stupor.

OBSESSIONAL SLOWNESS   This may occur secondary to repeated doubts and compulsive rituals.

Overactivity

PSYCHOMOTOR AGITATION   A patient with psychomotor agitation manifests:

- excess overactivity: thus is usually unproductive
- restlessness

HYPERKINESIS   In hyperkinesis, which may be seen in children and adolescents, the following features occur:

- overactivity
- distractibility
- impulsivity
- excitability

SOMNAMBULISM (SLEEP WALKING)   A complex sequence of behaviours is carried out by a person who rises from sleep and is not fully aware of their surroundings.

COMPULSION (COMPULSIVE RITUAL)   This is a repetitive and stereotyped seemingly purposeful behaviour. It is the motor component of an obsessional thought. Examples of compulsions include:

- checking rituals
- cleaning rituals
- counting rituals
- dipsomania: a compulsion to drink alcohol
- dressing rituals
- kleptomania: a compulsion to steal
- nymphomania: a compulsive need in the female to engage in sexual intercourse
- polydipsia: a compulsion to drink water
- satyriasis: a compulsive need in the male to engage in sexual intercourse
- trichotillomania: a compulsion to pull out one's hair

Abnormal posture and movements

Particularly in schizophrenia, but sometimes also in other disorders such as some learning disabilities, the following abnormal movements may occur: ambitendency, echopraxia, mannerisms, negativism, posturing, stereotypies and waxy flexibility.

AMBITENDENCY   The patient makes a series of tentative incomplete movements when expected to carry out a voluntary action.

ECHOPRAXIA   This refers to the automatic imitation by the patient of another person's movements. It occurs even when the patient is asked not to do so.

MANNERISMS   These are repeated involuntary movements that appear to be goal directed.

NEGATIVISM   This is a motiveless resistance to commands and to attempts to be moved.

POSTURING   The patient adopts an inappropriate or bizarre bodily posture continuously for a long time.

STEREOTYPIES   These are repeated regular fixed patterns of movement (or speech) which are not goal directed.

WAXY FLEXIBILITY (*CEREA FLEXIBILITAS*)   There is a feeling of plastic resistance resembling the bending of a soft wax rod as the examiner moves part of the patient's body; that body part then remains 'moulded' by the examiner in the new position.

TICS   These are repeated irregular movements involving a muscle group and may be seen following encephalitis, in Huntington's disease and in Gilles de la Tourette's syndrome, for example.

PARKINSONISM   The features of Parkinsonism include:

- a resting tremor
- cogwheel rigidity
- postural abnormalities
- a festinant gait

DISORDERS OF SPEECH

Disorders of rate, quantity and articulation

DYSARTHRIA   This is difficulty in the articulation of speech.

DYSPROSODY   This is speech with the loss of its normal melody.

LOGORRHOEA (VOLUBILITY)   The speech is fluent and rambling with the use of many words.

MUTISM   This is the complete loss of speech.

POVERTY OF SPEECH   There is a restricted amount of speech. If the patient replies to questions, they may do so with monosyllabic answers.

PRESSURE OF SPEECH   In pressure of speech there is an increase in both the quantity and rate of speech, which is difficult to interrupt.

STAMMERING   The flow of speech is broken by pauses and the repetition of parts of words.

Disorders of the form of speech

CIRCUMSTANTIALITY   Thinking appears slow with the incorporation of unnecessary trivial details. The goal of thought is finally reached, however.

ECHOLALIA   This is the automatic imitation by the patient of another person's speech. It occurs even when the patient does not understand the speech (which may be in another language, for example).

FLIGHT OF IDEAS   The speech consists of a stream of accelerated thoughts with abrupt changes from topic to topic and no central direction. The connections between the thoughts may be based on:

- chance relationships
- clang associations
- distracting stimuli
- verbal associations: e.g. alliteration and assonance

NEOLOGISM   This is a new word constructed by the patient or an everyday word used in a special way by the patient.

PASSING BY THE POINT (*VORBEIGEHEN*)   The answers to questions, although clearly incorrect, demonstrate that the questions are understood. For example, when asked 'What colour is grass?', the patient may reply 'Blue'. It is seen in the Ganser syndrome, first described in criminals awaiting trial.

PERSEVERATION   In perseveration (of both speech and movement) mental operations are continued beyond the point at which they are relevant. Particular types of perseveration of speech are:

- **palilalia**: the patient repeats a word with increasing frequency
- **logoclonia**: the patient repeats the last syllable of the last word

THOUGHT BLOCKING   There is a sudden interruption in the train of thought, before it is completed, leaving a 'blank'. After a period of silence, the patient cannot recall what they had been saying or had been thinking of saying.

DISORDERS (LOOSENING) OF ASSOCIATION (FORMAL THOUGHT DISORDER)   These occur particularly in schizophrenia and may be considered to be a schizophrenic language disorder. Examples include **knight's move thinking**, in which there are odd tangential associations between ideas, leading to disruptions in the smooth continuity of the speech, and **schizophasia**, also called **word salad** or **speech confusion**, in which the speech is an incoherent and incomprehensible mixture of words and phrases. Schneider described the following features of formal thought disorder:

- **derailment**: the thought derails on to a subsidiary thought
- **drivelling**: there is a disordered intermixture of the constituent parts of one complex thought
- **fusion**: heterogeneous elements of thought are interwoven with each other

- **omission**: a thought or part of a thought is senselessly omitted
- **substitution**: a major thought is substituted by a subsidiary thought

DISORDERS OF EMOTION

Disorders of affect

Affect is a pattern of observable behaviours which is the expression of a subjectively experienced feeling state (emotion), and is variable over time, in response to changing emotional states (DSM-IV).

BLUNTED AFFECT   In a patient with a blunted affect the externalized feeling tone is severely reduced.

FLAT AFFECT   This consists of a total or almost total absence of signs of expression of affect.

INAPPROPRIATE AFFECT   This is an affect that is inappropriate to the thought or speech it accompanies.

LABILE AFFECT   A patient with a labile affect has a labile externalized feeling tone which is not related to environmental stimuli.

Disorders of mood

Mood is a pervasive and sustained emotion which, in the extreme, markedly colours the person's perception of the world (DSM-IV).

DYSPHORIA   This is an unpleasant mood.

DEPRESSION   This is a low or depressed mood. It may be accompanied by **anhedonia**, in which the ability to enjoy pleasurable activities is lost. In normal **grief** or mourning, the sadness is appropriate to the loss.

ELATION   This is an elevated mood or exaggerated feeling of wellbeing that is pathological. It is seen in mania.

EUPHORIA   This is a personal and subjective feeling of unconcern and contentment, usually seen after taking opiates or as a late sequel to head injury.

IRRITABILITY   This is a liability to outbursts or a state of reduced control over aggressive impulses towards others. It may be a personality trait or may accompany anxiety. It also occurs in premenstrual syndrome.

APATHY   There is a loss of emotional tone and the ability to feel pleasure, associated with detachment or indifference.

ALEXITHYMIA   This is difficulty in the awareness of or description of one's emotions.

Disorders related to anxiety

ANXIETY   This is a feeling of apprehension, tension or uneasiness caused by the anticipation of an external or internal danger. Types of anxiety include:

- **phobic anxiety**: in which the focus of the anxiety is avoided (phobias are a disorder of thought content)
- **free-floating anxiety**: the anxiety is pervasive and unfocused
- **panic attacks**: anxiety is experienced in acute, episodic, intense attacks and may be accompanied by physiological symptoms

FEAR   This is anxiety caused by a realistic danger that is recognized at a conscious level.

AGITATION   In agitation there is excessive motor activity associated with a feeling of inner tension.

TENSION   In tension there is an unpleasant increase in psychomotor activity.

DISORDERS OF THOUGHT CONTENT

Preoccupations

HYPOCHONDRIASIS   This is a preoccupation with a fear of having a serious illness which is not based on real organic pathology but instead on an unrealistic interpretation of physical signs or sensations as being abnormal.

MONOMANIA   This is a pathological preoccupation with a single object.

EGOMANIA   This is a pathological preoccupation with oneself.

Obsessions

Obsessions are repetitive senseless thoughts which are recognized as irrational by the patient and which are unsuccessfully resisted. Themes include:

- aggression
- dirt and contamination
- fear of causing harm
- religion
- sex

Phobias

A phobia is a persistent irrational fear of an activity, object or situation leading to avoidance. The fear is out of proportion to the real danger and cannot be reasoned away, being out of voluntary control. Some types of phobia are:

- **acrophobia**: fear of heights
- **agoraphobia**: literally a fear of the market place, it is a syndrome with a generalized high anxiety level about, or avoidance of, places or situations from which escape might be difficult, or embarrassing, or in which help may not be available in the event of having a panic attack or panic-like symptoms; objects of fear may include:
  - crowds
  - open and closed spaces
  - shopping
  - social situations
  - travelling by public transport

- **algophobia: fear of pain**
- **claustrophobia**: fear of closed spaces
- **social phobia**: fear of personal interactions in a public setting, such as:
  - public speaking
  - eating in public
  - meeting people

- **specific (simple) phobia**: fear of discrete objects (e.g. snakes) or situations
- **xenophobia**: fear of strangers
- **zoophobia**: fear of animals

PHOBIAS OF INTERNAL STIMULI   These include obsessive phobias and illness phobias, which overlap with hypochondriasis.

ABNORMAL BELIEFS AND INTERPRETATIONS OF EVENTS

Overvalued ideas
An overvalued idea is an unreasonable and sustained intense preoccupation maintained with less than delusional intensity; that is, the patient is able to acknowledge the possibility that the belief may not be true. The idea or belief held is demonstrably false and is not one that is normally held by others of the patient's subculture. There is a marked associated emotional investment.

Delusions
A delusion is a false belief based on incorrect inference about external reality that is firmly sustained despite what almost everyone else believes and despite what constitutes incontrovertible and obvious proof or evidence to the contrary. The belief is not one ordinarily accepted by other members of the person's culture or subculture (e.g. it is not an article of religious faith). When a false belief involves a value judgement, it is regarded as a delusion only when the judgement is so extreme as to defy credibility (DSM-IV).

MOOD CONGRUENT DELUSION   In a mood congruent delusion the content of the delusion is appropriate to the mood of the patient.

MOOD INCONGRUENT DELUSION   In a mood incongruent delusion the content of the delusion is not appropriate to the mood of the patient.

PRIMARY DELUSION   This is a delusion that arises fully formed without any discernible connection with previous events. It may be preceded by a **delusional mood** in which the patient is aware of something strange and threatening happening.

BIZARRE DELUSION   This is a delusion involving a phenomenon that the person's culture would regard as totally implausible.

DELUSIONAL JEALOUSY (PATHOLOGICAL JEALOUSY; OTHELLO SYNDROME; DELUSION OF INFIDELITY)   This is a delusion that one's sexual partner is unfaithful.

DELUSION OF BEING CONTROLLED   This is a delusion in which the feelings, impulses, thoughts, or actions of the patient are experienced as being under the control of some external force rather than under their own control.

DELUSION OF DOUBLES (L'ILLUSION DE SOSIES)   This is a delusion that a person known to the patient has been replaced by a double. It is seen in Capgras' syndrome.

DELUSION OF POVERTY   This is a delusion that one is in poverty.

DELUSION OF REFERENCE   A delusion whose theme is that events, objects, or other persons in one's immediate environment have a particular and unusual significance. These delusions are usually of a negative or pejorative nature, but also may be grandiose in content (DSM-IV). When similar thoughts are held with less than delusional intensity they are **ideas of reference**.

DELUSION OF SELF-ACCUSATION   This is a delusion of one's guilt.

EROTOMANIA (DE CLÉRAMBAULT'S SYNDROME)   This is a delusion that another person, usually of higher status, is deeply in love with the individual.

GRANDIOSE DELUSION   This is a delusion of inflated worth, power, knowledge, identity, or special relationship to a deity or famous person.

PASSIVITY PHENOMENON   This is a delusional belief that an external agency is controlling aspects of the self which are normally entirely under one's own control. Passivity phenomena include:

- **thought alienation**: the patient believes that their thoughts are under the control of an outside agency or that others are participating in their thinking. It includes:

    - **thought insertion**: the delusion that certain of one's thoughts are not one's own, but rather are inserted into one's mind by an external agency
    - **thought withdrawal**: the delusion that one's thoughts are being removed from one's mind by an external agency
    - **thought broadcasting**: the delusion that one's thoughts are being broadcast out loud so that they can be perceived by others

- **made feelings**: the delusional belief that one's own free will has been removed and that an external agency is controlling one's feelings
- **made impulses**: the delusional belief that one's own free will has been removed and that an external agency is controlling one's impulses
- **made actions**: the delusional belief that one's own free will has been removed and that an external agency is controlling one's actions
- **somatic passivity**: the delusional belief that one is a passive recipient of somatic or bodily sensations from an external agency

PERSECUTORY (QUERULANT) DELUSION   A delusion in which the central theme is that one (or someone to whom one is close) is being attacked, harassed, cheated, persecuted, or conspired against (DSM-IV).

SOMATIC DELUSION   A delusion whose main content pertains to the appearance or functioning of one's body (DSM-IV).

Delusional perception
In a delusional perception the patient attaches a new and delusional significance to a familiar real perception without any logical reason.

ABNORMAL EXPERIENCES

Sensory distortions
HYPERAESTHESIAS   These are changes in sensory perception in which there is an increased intensity of sensation. **Hyperacusis** is an increased sensitivity to sounds.

HYPOAESTHESIAS   These are changes in sensory perception in which there is a decreased intensity of sensation. **Hypoacusis** is a decreased sensitivity to sounds.

CHANGES IN QUALITY   Changes in the quality of sensations occur particularly with visual stimuli, giving rise to **visual distortions**. Colourings of visual perceptions include:

- **chloropsia**: green
- **erythropsia**: red
- **xanthopsia**: yellow

DYSMEGALOPSIA   Changes in spatial form include:

- **macropsia**: objects are seen larger or nearer than is actually the case
- **micropsia**: objects are seen smaller or farther away than is actually the case

Sensory deceptions
ILLUSIONS   An illusion is a false perception of a real external stimulus.

HALLUCINATIONS   An hallucination is a false sensory perception in the absence of a real external stimulus. An hallucination is perceived as being located in objective space and as having the same realistic qualities as normal perceptions. It is not subject to conscious manipulation and only indicates a psychotic disturbance when there is also impaired reality testing. Hallucinations can be mood congruent or mood incongruent. Types of hallucination include:

- **auditory**
- **autoscopy (phantom mirror image)**: the patient sees him or herself and knows that it is he or she
- **extracampine**: the hallucination occurs outside the patient's sensory field
- **functional**: the stimulus causing the hallucination is experienced in addition to the hallucination itself
- **gustatory**
- **hallucinosis**: hallucinations (usually auditory) occur in clear consciousness
- **hypnagogic**: the hallucination (usually visual or auditory) occurs while falling asleep
- **hypnopompic**: the hallucination (usually visual or auditory) occurs while waking from sleep
- **olfactory**
- **reflex**: a stimulus in one sensory field leads to an hallucination in another sensory field
- **somatic**: somatic hallucinations include:
    - **tactile (haptic)** hallucinations: superficial and usually involving sensations on or just under the skin in the absence of a real stimulus; these include the sensation of insects crawling under the skin (**formication**)
    - **visceral** hallucinations of deep sensations
- **trailing phenomenon**: moving objects are seen as a series of discrete discontinuous images
- **visual**

PSEUDOHALLUCINATIONS   A pseudohallucination is a form of imagery arising in the subjective inner space of the mind. It lacks the substantiality of normal perceptions and occupies subjective space rather than objective space. It is not subject to conscious manipulation. An **eidetic image** is a vivid and detailed reproduction of a previous perception. In **pareidolia**, vivid imagery occurs without conscious effort while looking at a poorly structured background.

Disorders of self-awareness (ego disorders)
These include disturbances of:

- awareness of self-activity, including:
    - **depersonalization**: one feels that one is altered or not real in some way
    - **derealization**: the surroundings do not seem real
- the immediate awareness of self-unity
- the continuity of self
- the boundaries of the self

COGNITIVE DISORDERS

Disorientation
This is a disturbance of orientation in time, place or person.

Disorders of attention

DISTRACTIBILITY   A distractible subject's attention is drawn too frequently to unimportant or irrelevant external stimuli.

SELECTIVE INATTENTION   In selective inattention anxiety-provoking stimuli are blocked out.

Disorders of memory

AMNESIA   This is the inability to recall past experiences.

HYPERMNESIA   In hypermnesia the degree of retention and recall is exaggerated.

PARAMNESIA   A paramnesia is a distorted recall leading to falsification of memory. Paramnesias include:

- **confabulation**: gaps in memory are unconsciously filled with false memories
- **déjà vu**: the subject feels that the current situation has been seen or experienced before
- **déjà entendu**: the illusion of auditory recognition
- **déjà pensé**: the illusion of recognition of a new thought
- **jamais vu**: the illusion of failure to recognize a familiar situation
- **retrospective falsification**: false details are added to the recollection of an otherwise real memory

Disorders of intelligence

LEARNING DISABILITY (MENTAL RETARDATION)   Learning difficulty or mental retardation is classified by DSM-IV and ICD-10 according to the intelligence quotient (IQ) of the subject:

- $50 \leq IQ \leq 70$ ($50 \leq IQ \leq 69$ in ICD-10): **mild** mental retardation
- $35 \leq IQ \leq 49$: **moderate** mental retardation
- $20 \leq IQ \leq 34$: **severe** mental retardation
- $IQ < 20$: **profound** mental retardation

DEMENTIA   This is a global organic impairment of intellectual functioning without the impairment of consciousness.

PSEUDODEMENTIA   Pseudodementia resembles dementia clinically, but is not organic in origin.

Disorders of consciousness

LEVELS OF CONSCIOUSNESS   The **neurological** terms used to describe progressively more unconscious levels are:

- **somnolence (drowsiness)**: a patient who is drowsy or somnolent can be awoken by mild stimuli and will be able to speak comprehensibly, albeit perhaps for only a little while before falling asleep again
- **stupor**: a stuporose patient responds to pain and loud sounds; brief monosyllabic utterances and some spontaneous motor activity may occur
- **semi-coma**: a **semi-comatose** patient will withdraw from the source of pain but spontaneous motor activity does not take place
- **deep coma**: no response can be elicited from the patient and there is no response to deep pain nor is there any spontaneous movement; tendon, pupillary and corneal reflexes are usually absent
- **death**

CLOUDING OF CONSCIOUSNESS   The patient is drowsy and does not react completely to stimuli. There is disturbance of attention, concentration, memory, orientation and thinking.

DELIRIUM   The patient is bewildered, disoriented and restless. There may be associated fear and hallucinations. Variations include:

- **oneiroid state**: a dreamlike state in a patient who is not asleep
- **torpor**: the patient is drowsy and easily falls asleep
- **twilight state**: a prolonged oneiroid state of disturbed consciousness with hallucinations

FUGUE   This is a state of wandering from the usual surroundings in which there is also loss of memory.

Aphasias

RECEPTIVE (SENSORY) APHASIA (WERNICKE'S FLUENT APHASIA)   Difficulty is experienced in comprehending the meaning of words. Types include:

- **agnosic alexia**: words can be seen but cannot be read
- **pure word deafness**: words that are heard cannot be understood
- **visual asymbolia**: words can be transcribed but cannot be read

INTERMEDIATE APHASIA   Types of intermediate aphasia include:

- **central (syntactical) aphasia**: there is difficulty in arranging words in their proper sequence
- **nominal aphasia**: there is difficulty in naming objects

EXPRESSIVE (MOTOR) APHASIA (BROCA'S NONFLUENT APHASIA)   This refers to difficulty in expressing thoughts in words while comprehension remains.

GLOBAL APHASIA   Both receptive aphasia and expressive aphasia are present at the same time.

JARGON APHASIA   The patient utters incoherent meaningless neologistic speech.

APRAXIAS AND AGNOSIAS

Apraxias

Apraxia is an inability to perform purposive volitional acts, which does not result from paresis, incoordination, sensory loss or involuntary movements. It may be considered to be the motor equivalent of agnosia. Types include:

- **constructional apraxia**: difficulty in constructing objects or copying drawings; it is closely associated with **visuospatial agnosia**, with some authorities treating the two as being essentially the same
- **dressing apraxia**: difficulty in putting on one's clothes correctly
- **ideomotor apraxia**: difficulty in carrying out progressively more difficult tasks, for example involving touching parts of the face with specified fingers
- **ideational apraxia**: difficulty in carrying out a coordinated sequence of actions

Agnosias and disorders of body image

Agnosia is an inability to interpret and recognize the significance of sensory information, which does not result from impairment of the sensory pathways, mental deterioration, disorders of consciousness and attention or, in the case of an object, a lack of familiarity with the object. Types of agnosia and disorders of body image incinclude:

- **visuospatial agnosia**: see **constructional apraxia** above
- **visual (object) agnosia**: a familiar object which can be seen though not

recognized by sight, can be recognized through another modality such as touch or hearing

- **prosopagnosia**: an inability to recognize faces; in the **mirror sign**, which may occur in advanced Alzheimer's disease, a patient may misidentify their own mirrored reflection
- **agnosia for colours**: the patient is unable correctly to name colours, although colour sense is still present
- **simultanagnosia**: the patient is unable to recognize the overall meaning of a picture whereas its individual details are understood
- **agraphognosia** or **agraphaesthesia**: the patient is unable to identify, with closed eyes, the numbers or letters traced on their palm
- **anosognosia**: there is a lack of awareness of disease, particularly of hemiplegia (most often following a right parietal lesion)
- **coenestopathic state**: a localized distortion of body awareness
- **autotopagnosia**: the inability to name, recognize or point on command to parts of the body
- **astereognosia**: objects cannot be recognized by palpation
- **finger agnosia**: the patient is unable to recognize individual fingers, be they their own or those of another person
- **topographical disorientation**: this can be tested by using a locomotor map-reading task in which the patient is asked to trace out a given route by foot
- **distorted awareness of size and shape**: for example, a limb may be felt to be growing larger
- **hemisomatognosis** or **hemidepersonalization**: the patient feels that a limb (which in fact is present) is missing
- **phantom limb**: the continued awareness occurs of the presence of a limb that has been removed
- **reduplication phenomenon**: the patient feels that part or all of their body has been duplicated

BIBLIOGRAPHY

Hamilton, M. (ed.) 1985: *Fish's clinical psychopathology*, 2nd edn. Bristol: Wright.
Institute of Psychiatry 1973: *Notes on eliciting and recording clinical information*. Oxford: Oxford University Press.
Leff, J.P. and Isaacs, A.D. 1990: *Psychiatric examination in clinical practice*, 3rd edn. Oxford: Blackwell Scientific.
Sims, A.C.P. 1985: *Symptoms in the mind*. London: Baillière Tindall.

9
Psychoanalytic theories

SIGMUND FREUD (1856–1939)

Early influences
Those who had an important early influence on Freud, and his pre-psychoanalytic theories, included:

- **Helmholz** and **Brücke**: the physicochemical basis of brain function; concepts of energy and conservation; the Helmholtz School of Medicine
- **Meynert**: neuroanatomy and behaviour
- **Charcot**: hysteria and hypnosis

Freud also gained important ideas from the writings of:

- **Darwin**: the theory of evolution by natural selection
- **Hughlings Jackson**: the relationship of brain structure and function

Protopsychoanalytic phase (1887 to c.1897)
STUDIES ON HYSTERIA   In 1895 Josef Breuer and Sigmund Freud published *Studies on hysteria*. This included the case of Anna O. (Bertha Pappenheim) who had been treated by Breuer for hysterical symptomatology, including limb paralysis, associated with her father's illness. The development of hysteria in general was considered to take the following course:

- the cause consisted of real experiences, which were usually traumatic
- the (traumatic) event(s) gave rise to painful/unpleasant memories and represented ideas incompatible with conscious belief structures
- these memories and ideas were then repressed
- however, the powerful affects associated with them gave rise to somatic hysterical manifestations, sometimes including re-enactments of the (traumatic) event(s)
- in consciousness there remain mnemonic symbolic representations of the event(s)
- bringing the event(s) to consciousness leads to a discharge or release of the associated affects ('psychic pus') and resolution of the hysterical symptomatology (**abreaction**)

TECHNICAL DEVELOPMENT   The techniques employed by Freud progressed gradually through the following major phases:

- the use of **hypnosis**
- the **concentration method**: the patient, lying on a couch with closed eyes, was asked leading questions, and Freud would press his hands on the patient's forehead

- **free association**: the patient, with open eyes but lying on a couch, was encouraged to articulate, without censorship, all thoughts that came to mind

PROJECT FOR A SCIENTIFIC PSYCHOLOGY   This was mostly written by Freud in1895, and published after his death in 1950. It consists essentially of an attempt to link psychological processes with neurophysiology.

Topographical model of the mind
This was set out in Freud's *The interpretation of dreams* (1900) and developed during the following two decades until its eventual replacement by the structural model. In this model the mind is considered to consist of the following three parts:

- the **unconscious**
- the **preconscious**
- the **conscious**

THE UNCONSCIOUS   This contains memories, ideas, and affects that are repressed. Characteristic features include:

- outside awareness
- operating system: **primary process** thinking
- motivating principle: the pleasure principle
- access: access to its repressed contents is difficult, occurring when the censor gives way, for instance by becoming:

  - relaxed, e.g. in dreaming
  - fooled, e.g. in jokes
  - overpowered, e.g. in neurotic symptomatology

- system position:

  - no negation
  - timelessness (reference to time is bound up in unconsciousness)
  - image oriented
  - connotative
  - symbolic
  - non-linear

THE PRECONSCIOUS   This part of the mind develops during childhood and serves to maintain repression and censorship. Characteristic features include:

- outside awareness
- operating system: **secondary process** thinking
- motivating principle: the reality principle
- access: access can occur through focused attention
- system position:

  - bound by time
  - word oriented
  - denotative
  - linear

THE CONSCIOUS   This can be considered to be an attention sensory organ. Characteristic features include:

- within awareness
- operating system: **secondary process** thinking
- motivating principle: the reality principle

- access: easy
- system position:
  - bound by time
  - word oriented
  - declarative
  - linear

CENSORSHIP Freud described the censorship process in the following way:

Let us compare the system of the unconscious to a large entrance hall, in which the mental impulses jostle one another like separate individuals. Adjoining this entrance hall there is a second narrow room, a kind of drawing room, in which consciousness also resides but on the threshold between these two rooms a watchman performs his function; he examines the different mental impulses, acts as a censor, and will not admit them into the drawing room if they displease him. It does not make much difference if the watchman turns away from a particular impulse at the threshold itself or if he pushes it back across the threshold after it has entered the drawing room. If they have already pushed their way forward to the threshold and have been turned back by the watchman then they are inadmissible to the consciousness; we speak of them as *repressed* but even the impulses which the watchman has allowed to cross the threshold are not on that account necessarily conscious as well; they can only become so if they succeed in catching the eye of consciousness. They are therefore justified in calling the second room the system of the *preconscious.*

PRIMARY PROCESS This is the operating system of the unconscious. Its attributes include:

- **displacement**: an apparently insignificant idea is invested with all the psychical depth of meaning and intensity originally attributed to another idea
- **condensation**: all the meanings and several chains of association converge on to a single idea standing at their point of intersection
- **symbolization**: symbols are used rather than words

Characteristics of primary process thinking include (Sklar 1989):

- **timelessness**: the concept of time only develops after a period in the mind of a child in connection to conscious reality, e.g. periodicity or chaos of feeding
- **disregard of reality** of the conscious world
- **psychical reality**: memories of a real event and of imagined experience are not distinguished; abstract symbols are treated concretely
- **absence of contradiction**: opposites have a psychic equivalence
- **absence of negation**

SECONDARY PROCESS This is the operating system of the preconscious and the conscious. Characteristics of secondary process thinking include:

- **time** flows forward linearly
- **reality** is regarded: the content and logical basis of ideas is important
- **verbal word-presentations** are used
- **contradictions** are recognized and should not exist

PLEASURE PRINCIPLE This is the motivating principle of primary process. It is mainly inborn. Pain/'unpleasure' is avoided and pleasure is sought through tension discharge. This leads to:

- wish fulfilment
- the discharge of instinctual drives

REALITY PRINCIPLE   This is the motivating principle of secondary process. It is the result of external reality. It leads to:

- delayed gratification

Dreaming

In his *The interpretation of dreams* (1900), Freud referred to dreams as 'the Royal Road to the Unconscious'.

DREAM COMPOSITION   Dreams were considered to be composed of:

- the **day residue**: memories of the waking hours before the dream that are particularly emotionally charged
- **nocturnal stimuli**: external stimuli, e.g. noise, moisture, touch, and internal stimuli, e.g. pain, and urinary bladder distension
- **unconscious wishes**
- **latent dream**: the day residue, nocturnal stimuli and unconscious wishes

DREAM WORK   This refers to the process whereby the latent dream is converted into the manifest dream. Operations that contribute to dream work can include:

- **displacement**
- **condensation**
- **symbolization**
- **secondary elaboration (secondary revision)**: the process of revising and/or elaborating the dream after awakening in order to make it more consistent with the rules of secondary process

Structural model of the mind

This was set out in Freud's *The ego and the id* (1923) and replaced the topographical model. In this model the mind is considered to consist of the following three parts:

- the **id**
- the **ego**
- the **superego**

ID   Most of the id is unconscious. It contains primordial energy reserves derived from instinctual drives. Its aim is to maximize pleasure by fulfilling these drives.

EGO   According to Freud, the principal characteristics of the ego are as follows:

> In consequence of the preestablished connection between sense and perception and muscular action, the ego has voluntary movement at its command. It has the task of self-preservation. As regards external events, it performs that task by becoming aware of stimuli by storing up experiences about them (in the memory), by avoiding excessively strong stimuli (through adaptation), and finally by learning to bring about expedient changes in the external world to its own advantage (through activity). As regards internal events in relation to the id, it performs that task by gaining control over the demands of the instinct, by deciding whether they are to be allowed satisfaction, by postponing that satisfaction to times and circumstances favourable in the external world, or by suppressing their excitations entirely. It is guided in its activity by consideration of the tension produced by stimuli, whether these tensions are present in it or introduced into it.

Although much of the ego is conscious, most of its activity occurs without consciousness. Owing to its direct access to perception, reality testing takes place in the ego. However, the ego can be said to serve the following 'three harsh masters':

- the superego
- reality
- the id

SUPEREGO The superego is concerned with issues of morality. It develops initially as a result of the imposition of parental restraint. Although more of the superego is conscious than is the case for the id, most of its activity occurs without consciousness.

RELATIONSHIP BETWEEN THE ID, EGO AND SUPEREGO Freud described this relationship in the following way:

> We were justified . . . in dividing the ego from the id . . . [But] the ego is identical with the id, and is merely a specially differentiated part of it . . . . if a real split has occurred between the two, the weakness of the ego becomes apparent. But if the ego remains bound up with the id and indistinguishable from it, then it displays its strength. The same is true of the relation between the ego and the super-ego. In many situations the two are merged; and as a rule we can only distinguish one from the other when there is a tension or conflict between them. In repression the decisive fact is that the ego is an organization and the id is not. The ego is, indeed, the organized portion of the id. We should be quite wrong if we pictured the ego and the id as two opposing camps.

Resistance

This is everything, in words and actions of the analysand, that obstructs them from gaining access to their unconscious. It can be used in psychoanalysis as a means to reach the repressed; indeed the forces at work in resistance and repression are the same.

Transference

Sklar (1989) described the important features of the transference:

> The transference is an unconscious process in which the patient transfers to the therapist feelings, emotions and attitudes that were experienced and/or desired in the patient's childhood, usually in relation to parents and siblings. It can be a passionate demand for love and hate in past relationships between the child and the adult. This is a complex field that includes the unconscious splitting of the therapist into masculine and feminine and locating unconscious affect and thinking of the 'child' part of the patient in relation to the maternal and paternal aspects of the therapist (i.e. Oedipal transference). Furthermore, the direction of such a transference can be both positive and negative. Thus, Freud encountered transference in many variations and certainly also in its hidden form, transformed by resistance. The therapist's transference represents on the one hand the most powerful ally but, on the other, in terms of transference's resistance, a therapeutic difficulty.

Countertransference

Sklar (1989) described the important features of the countertransference:

> The countertransference is the therapist's own feelings, emotions and attitudes to his patient. In the treatment mode, the therapist needs to screen out those that are mediated only by the therapist, and take note of those generated in the therapist from emotional contact with the patient. The latter can be an interesting aspect of the patient, e.g. the therapist may have the feelings of the patient as child in relation to the patient enacting the parent. Thus, in the reverse transference, an aspect of the patient is located in the therapist *as a communication*.

Instinctual drives

Freud used the German word *trieb* to refer to a instinctual drive. Unfortunately, this has often been translated into the word 'instinct', a concept different from a 'drive'. Important instinctual drives identified by Freud were:

- **libido**: sexual 'instinct' and energy of the eros
- **eros**: life preservation 'instinct'
- **thanatos**: death 'instinct'

Psychosexual development
The stages of psychosexual development identified by Freud were:

ORAL PHASE From birth to around 15–18 months of age. Erotogenic pleasure is derived from sucking. In addition to the mother's breast, the infant has a desire to place other objects in their mouth.

ANAL PHASE From around 15–18 months to 30–36 months of age. Erotogenic pleasure is derived from stimulation of the anal mucosa, initially through faecal excretion, and later also through faecal retention.

PHALLIC PHASE From around three years of age to around the end of the fifth year. Boys pass through the Oedipal complex. Girls develop penis envy and pass through the Electra complex.

LATENCY STAGE From around five to six years to the onset of puberty. The sexual drive remains relatively latent during this period.

GENITAL STAGE From the onset of puberty to young adulthood. A strong resurgence in the sexual drive takes place. Successful resolution of conflicts from this and previous psychosexual stages leads to a mature well-integrated adult identity.

CARL JUNG (1875–1961)

Jung founded the psychoanalytic school of **analytic psychology**.

Early influences
Jung was originally an important member of Sigmund Freud's inner circle and indeed at one time his designated successor.

Differences between Jungian and Freudian theory
Jung came to different conclusions to Freud on a number of issues, including the following.

LIBIDO THEORY Jung did not believe that libido was confined to being sexual, but considered the libido as being the unitary force of every manifestation of psychic energy.

NATURE OF THE UNCONSCIOUS Jung believed in the **collective unconscious**, later referred to as the **objective psyche**, which he considered contained latent memories of our cultural, racial and phylogenetic past. In Jungian theory the objective psyche gives rise to consciousness.

CAUSALITY Rather than explaining present events in terms of Freudian psychic determinism, Jungian theory employs:

- **causality**: it offers an explanation in terms of the past
- **teleology**: it offers an explanation in terms of the future potential
- **synchronicity**: it offers an explanation in terms of causation at the boundary of the physical world with the psychical ('mystic') world

DREAMING Jungian theory views the contents of dreams within a phylogenetic framework in which archetypes may be projected on to others.

Archetypes

The archetypes of the objective psyche are energy-field configurations manifesting themselves as representational images having universal symbolic meaning and typical emotional and behavioural patterns. Five important types of archetype are identified in Jungian theory:

ANIMA   The feminine prototype within each person.

ANIMUS   The masculine prototype within each person.

PERSONA   The outward mask covering the individual's personality and allowing social demands to be balanced with internal needs. Both a public and a private persona may be possessed by a person. The persona may be represented in terms of clothing in dreams.

SHADOW   This represents repressed animal instincts arising from phylogenetic development and in dreams manifests itself as another person of the same sex.

SELF   A central archetype holding together conscious and unconscious aspects, including future potential, archetypes and complexes.

Complexes

Complexes surround archetypes and can be defined as feeling-toned ideas. They develop from an interaction of personal experiences and archetypal models.

Mental operations

Jungian theory postulates four operations of the mind.

FEELING   This allows feelings:

- anger and joy
- love and loss
- pleasure and pain

Judgements regarding good and evil also use this operation.

INTUITION   This is perception through unconscious processes.

SENSATION   This allows the acquisition of factual data.

THINKING   This is composed of logic and reasoning. It is verbal and ideational.

Extroversion and introversion

EXTROVERSION   The individual's concerns and mental operations are directed to the objective reality in the external world.

INTROVERSION   The individual's concerns and mental operations are directed to the subjective reality of the inner world.

Individuation

This is the process of personality growth leading to the development of a unique realization of what one intrinsically is.

MELANIE KLEIN (1882–1960)

Background

Klein, who lacked any formal higher education and never developed a full theory of development, was a controversial figure in the British Psycho-Analytical Society. When she began developing her theories, Sigmund Freud viewed her as potentially challenging the work in child analysis of his daughter, Anna Freud.

It is now known that Klein analysed her three children and wrote them up as disguised clinical cases. She proposed that the aim of child psychoanalysis was to 'cure' all children of their 'psychoses'.

Differences between Kleinian and Freudian theory

Among the important differences between the theories of Klein and Freud were the following.

OBJECT RELATIONS   Klein believed that the infant was capable of object relations.

PARANOID–SCHIZOID POSITION   Rejecting the critical importance of autoeroticism for the infant, Klein believed instead that the **paranoid position**, later, under the influence of Fairburn, renamed the **paranoid–schizoid position**, developed as a result of frustration during the first year of life with pleasurable contact with objects such as the **good breast**. The paranoid–schizoid position, characterized by isolation and persecutory fears, developed as a result of the infant viewing the world as **part objects**, using the following defence mechanisms:

- introjection (internalization)
- projective identification
- splitting

Objects viewed by the infant as good are believed to be introjected, while those viewed as bad are split or projected.

AGGRESSION   A strong emphasis was placed on aggression, occurring particularly during the paranoid-schizoid position.

DEPRESSIVE POSITION   This is said to develop by the age of six months when the child no longer views the world in terms of part objects but realizes that objects are whole, and the world is not perfect.

DEVELOPMENT OF THE EGO AND SUPEREGO   The ego and a primitive superego are present, according to Klein, during the first year of life.

Early development

The stages of development during the first year were considered to include, in chronological order:

- **oral frustration**
- **oral envy** (of parental 'oral' sex) and **oral sadism**, leading to Oedipal impulses
- a longing for the **oral incorporation of father's penis**, by **aggressive desires** to bring about the destruction of mother's body (which contains father's penis)
- **castration anxiety** in boys and fear of destruction of her own body in girls
- emergence of the **primitive superego**
- **introjection** of pain-causing objects
- development of a **cruel superego**
- **ejection of the superego**

Analytic play technique

The analysis of children's play was considered to be the homologue, for children, of the free association technique and dream interpretation for adults.

DONALD WINNICOTT (1897–1971)

Background

Winnicott was a British paediatrician who became a psychoanalyst. He was a contemporary of Anna Freud and Melanie Klein, between whom he at one time tried to mediate. He made important contributions to object relations theory and his reputation has grown steadily since his death.

The mother-baby dyad

Winnicott believed it was wrong to consider the baby in isolation, noting that there was:

> no such thing as an infant (apart from the maternal provision).

Countertransference

OBJECTIVE COUNTERTRANSFERENCE   Winnicott broadened the understanding of the countertransference from that of Freud, speaking of the **objective counter-transference**. The objectivity derived from his belief that the countertransference was an understandable and normal reaction to the personality and behaviour of the analysand.

COUNTERTRANSFERENCE HATE

Winnicott normalized the existence of countertransference hate. He gave reasons why a mother hates her infant (male or female) even from the start of their relationship. He then drew an analogy from this mother–infant dyad to the therapist–patient relationship. Winnicott suggested that the countertransference hate should be articulated to the analysand at the end of therapy, but most analysts would tend not to go this far.

Motherhood

GOOD-ENOUGH MOTHER   The good-enough mother is a mother who responds to her baby's communications and meets their needs within an optimal zone of frustration and gratification.

PATHOLOGICAL MOTHER   This is a mother who imposes her own needs over those of her baby, causing her baby to create a **false self** in order to protect their **true self**.

CAPACITY TO BE ALONE

Good parenting by the mother, allowing her child to become increasingly autonomous while at the same time being dependent on her, results in the child being able to be themselves in the presence of their mother, and vice versa. This was termed the **capacity to be alone** in the presence of another.

Transitional object

This is an object, which is neither oneself nor another person (including mother), which is selected by an infant between four and 18 months of age for self-soothing and anxiety-reduction. Examples include a blanket or toy that helps the infant to go to sleep. It helps during the process of separation-individuation. In adults, transitional phenomena that may allow us to cope with loneliness and separation can include music, religion and scientific creativitiy.

Other concepts

Other important concepts associated with Winnicott include:

- the **holding environment**: a therapeutic ambiance or setting allowing the patient to experience safety, and so facilitating psychotherapy
- the **potential space**: an area of experiencing identified as existing between the baby and the object; it subsequently underlies all play, imagination, dreams and the interdependence of transference and countertransference
- the **squiggle game**: a play therapy technique
- **at-one-ment**
- **primary maternal preoccupation**
- **regression to dependence**
- **going on being**

- impingement
- object usage

DEFENCE MECHANISMS

Repression
The basic defence, repression is the pushing away (*Verdrängung*) of unacceptable ideas, affects, emotions, memories and drives, relegating them to the unconscious. When successful no trace remains in consciousness but some affective excitation does remain.

Reaction formation
This is a psychological attitude diametrically opposed to an oppressed wish and constituting a reaction against it. It is often seen in patients with obsessive compulsive disorder.

Isolation
Thoughts/affects/behaviour are isolated so that their links with other thoughts or memories are broken. This is often seen in patients with obsessive compulsive disorder.

Undoing (what has been done)
An attempt is made to negate or atone for forbidden thoughts, affects or memories. This defence mechanism is seen, for example, in the compulsion of magic in patients with obsessive compulsive disorder.

Projection
Unacceptable qualities, feelings, thoughts or wishes are projected on to another person or thing. It is often seen in paranoid patients.

Projective identification
The subject not only sees the other as possessing aspects of the self which have been repressed, but constrains the other to take on those aspsects. It is a primitive form of projection.

Identification
Attributes of others are taken into oneself.

Introjection
In phantasy the subject transposes objects and their qualities from the external world into themselves.

Incorporation
Another's characteristics are taken on.

Turning against the self
An impulse meant to be expressed to another is turned against oneself.

Reversal into the opposite
The polarity of an impulse is reversed in the transition from activity to passivity.

Rationalization
This is an attempt to explain in a logically consistent or ethically acceptable way, ideas, thoughts and feelings whose true motive is not perceived. It operates in everyday life as well as in delusional symptoms.

Sublimation

This is a process that utilizes the force of a sexual instinct in drives, affects and memories in order to motivate creative activities having no apparent connection with sexuality.

Idealization

The object's qualities are elevated to the point of perfection.

Regression

This is a transition, at times of stress and threat, to moods of expression and functioning that are on a lower level of complexity, so that one returns to an earlier level of maturational functioning.

Denial

This is denying the external reality of an unwanted or unpleasant piece of information.

Splitting

This involves dividing 'good' objects, affects and memories from 'bad' ones. It is often seen in patients with borderline personality disorder.

Distortion

This involves reshaping external reality to suit inner needs.

Acting out

This involves expressing unconscious emotional conflicts or feelings directly in actions without being consciously aware of their meaning.

Displacement

Emotions, ideas or wishes are transferred from their original object to a more acceptable substitute.

Intellectualization

Excessive abstract thinking occurs in order to avoid conflicts or disturbing feelings.

BIBLIOGRAPHY

Freud, A. 1936: *The ego and the mechanisms of defence*. London: Hogarth Press.
Freud, S. 1953–1966: *The standard edition of the complete psychological works of Sigmund Freud, vols 1–24*. London: Hogarth Press.
Hall, C.S. 1956: *A primer of Freudian psychology*. London: Allen & Unwin.
Jung, C.G. 1961: *Memories, dreams, reflections*. New York: Random House.
Jung, C.G. 1964: *Man and his symbols*. New York: Doubleday.
Klein, M. 1948: *Contributions to psycho-analysis, 1921–1945*. London: Hogarth Press.
Klein, M. 1949: *The psycho-analysis of children*, 3rd edn. London: Hogarth Press.
Ogden, T.H. 1992: The dialectically constituted/decentred subject of psychoanalysis, II: the contributions of Klein and Winnicott. *International Journal of Psycho-Analysis* 73, 613–26.
Segal, H. 1980: *Melanie Klein*. New York: Viking Press.
Sklar, J. 1989: Dynamic psychopathology. In Puri, B.K. and Sklar, J. *Examination notes for the MRCPsych Part I*. London: Butterworth/Heinemann.

Winnicott, D.W. 1949: Hate in the counter-transference. *International Journal of Psycho-Analysis* 30, 69–74.
Winnicott, D.W. 1958: *Collected papers: through paediatrics to psycho-analysis.* New York: Basic Books.
Winnicott, D.W. 1965: *The maturational processes and the facilitating environment.* New York: International Universities Press.
Winnicott, D.W. 1971: *Playing and reality.* New York: International Universities Press.

10
Neuroanatomy

ORGANIZATION OF THE NERVOUS SYSTEM

Structural organization
The nervous system can be divided structurally into:

- the central nervous system (CNS)
- the peripheral nervous system (PNS)

CENTRAL NERVOUS SYSTEM   The CNS consists of:

- the brain
- the spinal cord

It is well protected by the skull and vertebral column and the meninges (layers of connective tissue membrane):

- the dura mater: outermost layer
- the arachnoid mater: middle layer
- the pia mater: inner layer

Cerebrospinal fluid (CSF) in the subarachnoid space offers further protection of the CNS.

PERIPHERAL NERVOUS SYSTEM   The PNS consists of:

- the cranial nerves
- the spinal nerves
- other neuronal processes and cell bodies lying outside the CNS

It is not as well protected as the CNS.

Functional organization
The nervous system can be divided functionally into:

- the somatic nervous system
- the autonomic nervous system

SOMATIC NERVOUS SYSTEM   This is concerned primarily with the innervation of voluntary structures.

AUTONOMIC NERVOUS SYSTEM   This is concerned primarily with the innervation of involuntary structures. It is subdivided into two parts:

- the sympathetic
- the parasympathetic

Developmental organization
During ontogeny, the midline neural tube differentiates into the following vesicles:

- **prosencephalon**, which differentiates into the

    - **telencephalon**: gives rise to the cerebral hemispheres and contains the

                      pallium
                      rhinencephalon
                      corpus striatum
                      medullary centre

- **diencephalon**: consisting of the
  thalamus
  subthalamus
  hypothalamus
  epithalamus, consisting of the

      habenular nucleus
      pineal gland

- **mesencephalon**, consisting of the

  tectum, consisting of the corpora quadrigemina, made up of the

      superior colliculi
      inferior colliculi

  basis pedunculi
  tegmentum, containing

      the red nucleus
      fibre tracts
      grey matter surrounding the cerebral aqueduct

- **rhombencephalon**, which differentiates into the
  - **metencephalon**: consisting of the

        pons
        oral part of the medulla oblongata
        cerebellum
  - **myelencephalon**: the caudal part of the medulla oblongata

TYPES OF NERVOUS SYSTEM CELL

Neurones

CLASSIFICATION BY MORPHOLOGY   On a morphological basis, neurones can be classified as:

- unipolar: the perikaryon has one neurite
- bipolar: the perikaryon has two neurites
- multipolar: each neurone has one axon and more than one dendrite

CLASSIFICATION BY SIZE   An alternative classification is on the basis of size:

- Golgi type I: long axon
- Golgi type II: short axon terminating near the parent cell
- amacrine: no axon

Neuroglia

RELATIVE NUMBERS   Neuroglia, or interstitial cells, outnumber neurones by a factor of five to 10 times.

CENTRAL NERVOUS SYSTEM   The main types of neuroglia in the CNS are:

- astrocytes

- oligodendrocytes
- microglia
- ependyma

PERIPHERAL NERVOUS SYSTEM   The main types of neuroglia in the PNS are:

- Schwann cells
- satellite cells

ASTROCYTES   There are two types of astrocytes or astroglia:

- fibrous astrocytes
- protoplasmic astrocytes

They are multipolar and their functions include:

- structural support of neurones
- phagocytosis
- forming CNS neuroglial scar tissue
- contributing to the blood–brain barrier

OLIGODENDROCYTES   The functions of oligodendrocytes or oligodendroglia include:

- CNS myelin sheath formation
- phagocytosis

MICROGLIA   These are the smallest neuroglial cells and are most abundant in the grey matter. Their functions include:

- acting as scavenger cells at sites of CNS injury

EPENDYMAL CELLS   They line the cavities of the CNS. Their functions include:

- aiding the flow of CSF (cilial beating)

Types of ependymal cell include:

- choroidal epithelial cells: these cover the surfaces of the choroidal plexi
- ependymocytes: these line the central canal of the spinal cord and ventricles
- tanycytes: these line the floor of the third ventricle over the hypothalamic median eminence

SCHWANN CELLS   In addition to being part of myelinated peripheral nerves, Schwann cells encircle some unmyelinated peripheral nerve axons. Their functions include:

- PNS myelin sheath formation
- neurilemma formation

SATELLITE CELLS   Satellite cells, or capsular cells, are found in:

- sensory ganglia
- autonomic ganglia

Their functions include:

- neuronal support in sensory and autonomic ganglia

FRONTAL LOBES

Frontal operculum
This consists of areas 44, 45 and 47.

BROCA'S AREA   This is the core of the frontal operculum on the dominant (usually left) side, and consists of areas 44 and 45. A lesion in this region can lead to expressive (motor) aphasia (Broca's nonfluent aphasia).

RIGHT SIDE   Lesions in the non-dominant frontal operculum can lead to dysprosody.

Superior mesial region
This contains:

- **supplementary motor area** (SMA, mesial part of area 6)
- **anterior cingulate** cortex (area 24)

Lesions of the left or right superior mesial region can lead to akinetic mutism.

Inferior mesial region
This consists of:

- **orbital cortex** (including areas 11, 12 and 32)
- **basal forebrain**

ORBITAL CORTEX   Lesions of the orbital cortex (either side) can lead to a form of acquired sociopathy.

BASAL FOREBRAIN   This includes the following nuclei:

- diagonal band of Broca
- nucleus accumbens
- septal nuclei
- substantia innominata

Lesions of the basal forebrain (either side) can lead to amnesia (retrograde and anterograde) and confabulation.

Dorsolateral prefrontal cortex
The dorsolateral prefrontal cortex (DLPFC) contains areas 8, 9, 10 and 46. Lesions in this region can lead to abnormalities in cognitive executive functions, impairment of verbal (left) or nonverbal (right) intellectual functions, memory impairments affecting recency and frequency judgements, poor organization, poor planning, poor abstraction, and disturbances in motor programming. Left-sided lesions may cause impaired verbal fluency, while right lesions may cause impaired nonverbal (design) fluency.

TEMPORAL LOBES

Superior temporal gyrus
The posterior part of the superior temporal gyrus, area 22, forms, on the left, Wernicke's area. Lesions in this region can lead to a receptive (sensory) aphasia (Wernicke's fluent aphasia).

Posterior inferolateral region
This consists of:

- posterior portion of the **middle temporal gyrus** (part of area 37)
- posterior portion of the **inferior temporal gyrus** (part of area 37)
- posterior portion of the **fourth temporal gyrus** (part of area 37)

Lesions in this region, and in the adjoining occipitotemporal junction, can lead to prosopagnosia and impaired object recognition.

Anterior inferolateral region
This consists of:

- anterior portion of the **middle temporal gyrus** (part of area 21)
- anterior portion of the **inferior temporal gyrus** (part of area 20)
- anterior portion of the **fourth temporal gyrus** (part of area 20)
- **temporal pole** (area 38)

Lesions in the left side can lead to anomia and defects in accessing the reference lexicon. Lesions in the right side can lead to an inability to name facial expressions. Retrograde anmesia may result from bilateral lesions.

Mesial temporal region
This consists of:

- **parahippocampal gyrus** (areas 27 and 28)
- **amygdala**
- **entorhinal cortex**
- **hippocampus**

Left-sided lesions can lead to anterograde amnesia affecting verbal information, while right-sided lesions can lead to anterograde amnesia affecting nonverbal information. Bilateral lesions can lead to verbal and nonverbal anterograde amnesia.

PARIETAL LOBES

Temporoparietal junction
The posterior part of the inferior parietal lobule together with the posterior part of the superior temporal gyrus (Wernicke's area) form the greater Wernicke's area. Left-sided lesions can lead to a receptive (sensory) aphasia (Wernicke's fluent aphasia), while right-sided lesions can lead to phonagnosia (impairment in the ability to recognize familiar voices) and amusia (impaired ability to recognize and process music).

Inferior parietal lobule
This consists of:

- **angular gyrus** (area 39)
- **supramarginal gyrus** (area 40)

Lesions on the left can lead to conduction aphasia and tactile agnosia. Lesions on the right can lead to anosognosia, neglect, tactile agnosia and anosodiaphoria (impaired concern with respect to neurological deficits).

OCCIPITAL LOBES

The occipital lobe contains:

- **primary visual cortex** (area 17)
- **visual association cortices** (areas 18 and 19)

Lesions of the dorsal region (superior to the calcarine fissure) and adjoining parietal region (areas 7 and 39) can lead to partial (unilateral lesions) or a full-blown (bilateral lesions) Balint's syndrome, consisting of:

- simultanagnosia
- ocular apraxia or psychic gaze paralysis
- optic ataxia

Bilateral dorsal lesions can also lead to astereopsis and impaired visual motion perception. Lesions of the left ventral region (inferior to the calcarine fissure) can lead to contralateral (right) acquired (central) hemiachromatopsia (impaired visual colour perception) and acquired (pure) dyslexia. Lesions of the right ventral region can lead to contralateral (left) acquired (central) hemiachromatopsia and apperceptive visual agnosia. Bilateral lesions can lead to acquired (central) hemiachromatopsia affecting the whole visual field, associative visual agnosia, and prosopagnosia.

BASAL GANGLIA

Components
Authorities differ on the components of the basal ganglia. According to Snell (1987) the basal ganglia consist of the:

- corpus striatum
  - caudate nucleus
  - lentiform nucleus
- amygdala (amygdaloid nucleus)
- claustrum

The lentiform nucleus consists of the:

- globus pallidus
- putamen

Connections of the lentiform nucleus
AFFERENTS   Afferents to the putamen come from the:

- caudate nucleus
- cerebral cortex

Afferents to the globus pallidus come from the:

- caudate nucleus
- putamen
- substantia nigra

EFFERENTS   Efferents from the putamen pass to the:

- globus pallidus

Efferents from the globus pallidus pass to the:

- hypothalamus
- reticular formation
- substantia nigra
- subthalamus
- ventroanterior nucleus of the thalamus
- ventrolateral nucleus of the thalamus

Frontal-subcortical circuits

Alexander *et al.* (1986) have identified five parallel frontal-subcortical circuits which together form one of the main organizational networks of the brain and are central to brain-behaviour relationships. They connect specific regions of the frontal cortex with the basal ganglia and the thalamus in circuits that mediate:

- motor activity
- eye movements
- behaviour

The overall structure of each circuit is as follows:

frontal lobe cortex → caudate nucleus → globus pallidus/substantia nigra → thalamus → frontal lobe cortex

MOTOR CIRCUIT   This circuit originates in SMA and subserves motor function.

OCULOMOTOR CIRCUIT   This circuit originates in the frontal eye fields and subserves eye movements.

DORSOLATERAL PREFRONTAL CIRCUIT   This circuit originates in DLPFC and subserves executive cognitive functions.

LATERAL ORBITOFRONTAL CIRCUIT   This circuit originates in the lateral orbital cortex and subserves personality.

ANTERIOR CINGULATE CIRCUIT   This circuit originates in the anterior cingulate cortex and subserves motivation.

LIMBIC SYSTEM

Limbic lobe

This was described by Broca in 1878 as an arrangement of cortical structures around the diencephalon, forming a border on the medial side of each cerebral hemisphere between the neocortex and the remainder of the brain.

CORTICAL AREAS   Cortical areas of the limbic lobe form the limbic cortex and include the:

- cingulate gyrus
- parahippocampal gyrus
- subcallosal gyrus

NUCLEI   Subcortical nuclei that are part of the limbic lobe include the:

- amygdaloid nucleus
- septal nucleus

Components

There is disagreement as to precisely which structures form part of the modern definition of the limbic system. A good guide is provided by both Snell (1987) and Trimble (1981).

CORTICAL AREAS Cortical areas that are generally considered to be part of the limbic system nowadays include the:

- cingulate gyrus
- gyrus fasciolaris
- hippocampal formation

  - dendate gyrus
  - hippocampus
  - parahippocampal gyrus

- indusium griseum
- olfactory tubercle
- paraterminal gyrus (precommissural septum)
- prepiriform cortex
- secondary olfactory area (entorhinal area)
- subcollosal gyrus
- subiculum

NUCLEI Subcortical nuclear groups that are generally considered to be part of the limbic system nowadays include the:

- amygdala (amygdaloid nucleus)
- anterior thalamic nucleus
- dorsal tegmental nucleus
- epithalamic nucleus
- habenula
- hypothalamic nuclei
- mammillary bodies
- raphe nucleus
- septal nucleus (septal area)
- superior central nucleus
- ventral tegmental area

CONNECTING PATHWAYS Connecting pathways of the limbic system include the:

- anterior commissure
- cingulum
- dorsal longitudinal fasciculus
- fornix
- lateral longitudinal striae
- mammillotegmental tract
- mammillothalamic tract
- medial forebrain bundle
- medial longitudinal striae
- stria terminalis
- stria medullaris thalami

INTERNAL ANATOMY OF THE TEMPORAL LOBES

Hippocampal formation

The hippocampal formation consists of the:

- dendate gyrus
- hippocampus

- parahippocampal gyrus

DENDATE GYRUS   This gyrus lies between the hippocampal fimbria and the parahippocampal gyrus. Anteriorly, it is continuous with the uncus. Posteriorly, it is continuous with the indusium griseum. Histologically, it is made up of the following three layers:

- molecular layer (outer)
- granular layer
- polymorphic layer (inner)

HIPPOCAMPUS   This grey matter structure lies mainly in the floor of the inferior horn of the lateral ventricle. Anteriorly, it forms the pes hippocampus. Posteriorly, it ends inferior to the splenium of the corpus callosum. Axons from each alveus converge medially to form the fimbria and crus of the fornix. Histologically, the hippocampus is made up of the following three layers:

- molecular layer (outer)
- pyramidal layer
- polymorphic layer (inner)

Afferent connections of the hippocampus include fibres that originate from the:

- cingulate gyrus
- dendate gyrus
- hippocampus (the opposite one)
- indusium griseum
- parahippocampal gyrus
- secondary olfactory area (entorhinal area)
- septal nucleus (septal area)

PARAHIPPOCAMPAL GYRUS   This gyrus is separated from the remaining cerebral cortex by the collateral sulcus. Anteriorly, it is continuous with the uncus. The subiculum of the parahippocampal gyrus allows the passage of nerve fibres from the secondary olfactory cortex (entorhinal area) to the dendate gyrus.

Amygdala

The amygdala is also known as the amygdaloid nucleus, body or complex. It is continuous with the tail of the caudate nucleus, lying anterior and superior to the tip of the inferior horn of the lateral ventricle.

AFFERENT CONNECTIONS   Afferent connections received by the amygdala include the:

- amygdala (the opposite one, via the anterior commissure)
- dopaminergic brain stem nuclei
- frontal association area
- lateral olfactory stria
- noradrenergic brain stem nuclei
- septal nucleus (septal area)
- serotonergic brain stem nuclei
- temporal association area
- uncus

EFFERENT CONNECTIONS   Parts of the brain to which efferent connections pass from the amygdala include the:

- hypothalamus (via the stria terminalis)
- septal nucleus (septal area) (via the stria terminalis)
- corpus striatum
- frontal association area
- lateral olfactory stria
- temporal association area
- thalamus

MAJOR WHITE MATTER PATHWAYS

Corpus callosum
This is the largest set of interhemispheric connecting fibres. It lies inferior to the longitudinal fissure and superior to the diencephalon. It connects homologous neocortical areas.

DIVISIONS   The main divisions of the corpus callosum (rostral first) are the:

- rostrum
- genu
- body
- splenium

Fornix
This is the major efferent subcortical white matter tract of the hippocampus. The two crura of the fornix, each formed from axons from the alveus of the hippocampus, converge inferior to the corpus callosum and form the body of the fornix. The body of the fornix is connected anteriorly with the inferior surface of the corpus callosum via the septum pellucidum. The body of the fornix then divides into the two columns of the fornix.

DESTINATION OF FIBRES IN THE FORNIX   The efferent connections of the hippo-campus, via the fornix, include the:

- anterior hypothalamus
- anterior nucleus of the thalamus
- habenular nucleus
- lateral preoptic area
- mammillary body (medial nucleus)
- septal nucleus (septal area)
- tegmentum of the mesencephalon

Papez circuit
This is the concept introduced by Papez, in 1937, of a supposed limbic system reverberating circuit constituting the neuronal mechanism of emotion. It consisted of the:

- hippocampus
- hypothalamus
- anterior nucleus of the thalamus
- cingulate gyrus

The postulated circuit was as follows:

hippocampus → (via the fornix)
→ mammillary bodies of the hypothalamus → (via a synaptic connection)
→ anterior nucleus of the thalamus → (the neuroimpulse then radiates up)

→ cingulate gyrus → (via the cingulum)
→ hippocampus

Arcuate bundle
This is a specific group of association fibres arranged in a curved shape running parallel to the cortical surface which, on the dominant (usually left) side, connects the more rostral Broca's area with Wernicke's area.

Anterior commissure
This small nerve fibre bundle crosses the midline in the lamina terminalis and connects homologous areas of the neocortex and paleocortex. Parts of the limbic system in the two cerebral hemispheres that are connected via the anterior commissure include the:

- amygdala
- hippocampus
- parahippocampal gyrus

CRANIAL NERVES

I: Olfactory nerve
This contains the central processes of the olfactory receptors, which pass from the olfactory mucosa, through the cribriform plate of the ethmoid, to synapse with the olfactory bulb mitral cells. Axons then pass in the olfactory tract to the primary olfactory cortex (also known as the periamygdaloid and prepiriform areas) via the lateral olfactory striae.

II: Optic nerve
This contains retinal ganglion cell axons which pass to the optic chiasma. At the optic chiasma:

- medial retinal fibres, containing temporal visual field information, pass to the contralateral optic tract
- lateral retinal fibres, containing nasal visual field information, pass to the ipsilateral optic tract

Most optic tract fibres synapse in the thalamic lateral geniculate body, while a minority (concerned with pupillary and ocular reflexes) pass directly to the pretectal nucleus and superior colliculi, by-passing the lateral geniculate body. From the lateral geniculate body the optic radiation passes, via the retrolenticular part of the internal capsule, to the visual cortex.

III: Oculomotor nerve
This nerve has two motor nuclei:

- the main oculomotor nucleus (also known as the somatic efferent nucleus): supplies all the extrinsic ocular muscles with the exception of the superior oblique and lateral rectus
- the accessory parasympathetic nucleus (also known as the Edinger–Westphal nucleus): sends preganglionic parasympathetic fibres to the constrictor pupillae and ciliary muscles

IV: Trochlear nerve
This supplies one extrinsic ocular muscle, namely the superior oblique.

V: Trigeminal nerve
This is the largest cranial nerve.
NUCLEI   The trigeminal nerve has four nuclei, the:

- main sensory nucleus
- spinal nucleus
- mesencephalic nucleus
- motor nucleus

SENSORY COMPONENTS   The main divisions and branches of the trigeminal nerve, which together constitute the main sensory innervation of most of the head and face, are as follows:

- ophthalmic nerve or division

    - frontal nerve: innervates, via the supraorbital and supratrochlear branches, the

        upper eyelid
        scalp (anterior to the lamboid suture)

    - lacrimal nerve: innervates the

        lacrimal gland
        lateral conjunctiva
        upper eyelid

    - nasociliary nerve: innervates the

        eyeball
        medial lower eyelid
        nasal skin
        nasal mucosa

- maxillary nerve or division

    - infraorbital nerve: innervates the

        skin of the cheek

    - superior alveolar nerve: innervates the

        upper teeth

    - zygomatic nerve: innervates the

        skin of the temple (via the zygomaticotemporal branch)
        skin of the cheek (via the zygomaticofacial branch)

    Branches from the sphenopalatine ganglion include the

        greater palantine nerve
        lesser palantine nerve
        long sphenopalatine nerve
        nasal branches
        pharyngeal branches
        short sphenopalatine nerve

- mandibular nerve or division

    - auriculotemporal nerve: innervates the

        skin of the temple

auricle division

- buccal nerve: innervates the

  skin of the cheek
  mucous membrane of the cheek

- inferior alveolar nerve: innervates the

  lower teeth
  lower lip
  skin of the chin

- lingual nerve: innervates the

  anterior two-thirds of the tongue
  mucous membrane of the mouth

MOTOR COMPONENT   The motor component of the trigeminal nerve supplies the:

- muscles of mastication
- anterior belly of the digastric
- mylohyoid
- tensor tympani
- tensor veli palatini

VI: Abducent nerve

This supplies one extrinsic ocular muscle, namely the lateral rectus.

VII: Facial nerve

NUCLEI   The facial nerve has three nuclei, the:

- main motor nucleus
- parasympathetic nuclei
- sensory nucleus (the superior part of the tractus solitarius nucleus)

MAIN MOTOR NUCLEUS   This supplies the:

- muscles of facial expression
- auricular muscles
- posterior belly of the digastric
- stapedius
- stylohyoid

Corticonuclear fibres from the contralateral cerebral hemisphere are received by the part of the main motor nucleus supplying the lower face muscles. Cortico-nuclear fibres from both cerebral hemispheres are received by the part of the main motor nucleus supplying the upper face muscles.

PARASYMPATHETIC NUCLEI   These include the:

- lacrimal nucleus: supplies the

  lacrimal gland

- superior salivary nucleus: supplies the

  nasal gland
  palatine gland
  sublingual gland
  submandibular gland

SENSORY NUCLEUS This receives taste fibres, via the geniculate ganglion, from the:

- anterior two-thirds of the tongue
- floor of the mouth
- hard palate
- soft palate

CHORDA TYMPANI This is a branch of the facial nerve given off before it passes through the stylomastoid foramen. The chorda tympani joins the lingual branch of the mandibular division of the trigeminal nerve.

VIII: Vestibulocochlear nerve
This nerve consists of the following two parts, the:

- cochlear nerve: concerned with hearing
- vestibular nerve: concerned with the maintenance of equilibrium

COCHLEAR NERVE Its fibres are the central processes of the cochlear spiral ganglion cells, terminating in the anterior and posterior cochlear nuclei.

VESTIBULAR NERVE Its fibres are the central processes of vestibular ganglion neurones, terminating in the lateral, medial, superior and inferior vestibular nuclei.

IX: Glossopharyngeal nerve
NUCLEI The glossopharyngeal nerve has three nuclei, the:

- main motor nucleus
- parasympathetic nucleus (the inferior salivary nucleus)
- sensory nucleus (part of the tractus solitarius nucleus)

MAIN MOTOR NUCLEUS This supplies the:

- stylopharyngeus

Corticonuclear fibres from both cerebral hemispheres are received by the main motor nucleus.

PARASYMPATHETIC NUCLEUS This receives inputs from the:

- hypothalamus
- olfactory system
- tractus solitarius nucleus
- trigeminal sensory nucleus

Preganglionic fibres reach the otic ganglion via the tympanic plexus and the lesser petrosal nerve. Postganglionic fibres supply the parotid gland by means of the auriculotemporal branch of the mandibular nerve.

SENSORY NUCLEUS This receives taste information from the posterior one third of the tongue.

X: Vagus nerve
NUCLEI The vagus nerve has three nuclei, the:

- main motor nucleus
- parasympathetic nucleus (the dorsal nucleus)
- sensory nucleus (the inferior part of the tractus solitarius nucleus)

MAIN MOTOR NUCLEUS This supplies the:

- intrinsic muscles of the larynx
- constrictor muscles of the pharynx

Corticonuclear fibres from both cerebral hemispheres are received by the main motor nucleus.

PARASYMPATHETIC NUCLEUS   This receives inputs from the:

- hypothalamus
- glossopharyngeal nerve
- heart
- lower respiratory tract
- gastrointestinal tract, as far as the transverse colon

It supplies the:

- involuntary muscle of the heart
- lower respiratory tract
- gastrointestinal tract, as far as the distal one-third of the transverse colon

SENSORY NUCLEUS   This receives taste information from the inferior ganglion of the vagus nerve.

XI: Accessory nerve

This nerve consists of the following two parts, the:

- cranial root
- spinal root

CRANIAL ROOT   This supplies, via the vagus nerve, muscles of the:

- larynx
- pharynx
- soft palate

SPINAL ROOT   This supplies the:

- sternocleidomastoid
- trapezius

XII: Hypoglossal nerve

This supplies the:

- intrinsic muscles of the tongue
- styloglossus
- hyoglossus
- genioglossus

SPINAL CORD

Divisions

From rostral to caudal, the spinal cord is divided into the following five parts:

- cervical: 8 pairs of spinal nerves
- thoracic: 12 pairs of spinal nerves
- lumbar: 5 pairs of spinal nerves
- sacral: 5 pairs of spinal nerves
- coccygeal: 1 pair of spinal nerves

Ascending white column tracts

ANTERIOR   The ascending anterior white column tracts include the:

- anterior spinothalamic tract: carries light touch and pressure sensations

LATERAL   The ascending lateral white column tracts include the:

- anterior and posterior spinocerebellar tracts: carry proprioceptive, pressure and touch sensations
- lateral spinothalamic tract: carries pain and temperature sensations
- spino-olivary tract: carries proprioceptive and cutaneous sensations
- spinotectal tract: involved with spinovisual reflexes

POSTERIOR   The ascending posterior white column tracts include the:

- fasciculus cuneatus: carries discriminative touch and proprioceptive sensations
- fasciculus gracilis: carries vibration sensations

Descending white column tracts
ANTERIOR   The descending anterior white column tracts include the:

- anterior corticospinal tract: involved with voluntary movement
- reticulospinal fibres: involved with motor function
- vestibulospinal tract: involved with muscle tone control
- tectospinal tract: involved with a head-turning reflex and movement of the upper limbs in response to acoustic, cutaneous and visual stimuli

LATERAL   The descending lateral white column tracts include the:

- lateral corticospinal tract: involved with voluntary movement
- rubrospinal tract: involved with muscular activity
- lateral reticulospinal tract: involved with muscular activity
- descending autonomic fibres: involved with visceral function control
- olivospinal tract: possibly involved with muscular activity

MAJOR NEUROCHEMICAL PATHWAYS

Nigrostriatal dopaminergic pathway
The presynaptic components of this pathway are formed by:

- A8 dopaminergic neurones: located in the reticular formation of the mesencephalon
- A9 dopaminergic neurones: located in the pars compacta of the substantia nigra

Their axons pass, via the medial forebrain bundle, to terminate mostly in the:

- caudate nucleus
- putamen
- amygdala

This pathway is concerned with sensorimotor coordination.

Mesolimbic-mesocortical dopaminergic pathway
This pathway originates in:

- A10 dopaminergic neurones: located in the ventral tegmental area of the mesencephalon

Their axons pass, via the medial forebrain bundle, to terminate mostly in the:

- nucleus accumbens
- olfactory tubercle
- bed nucleus of the stria terminalis
- lateral septum
- cingulate cortex
- entorhinal cortex
- medial prefrontal cortex

Ascending noradrenergic pathway from the locus coeruleus

The main noradrenergic nucleus is the locus coeruleus, located in the dorsal pons. At least five noradrenergic tracts arise from it:

- 3 ascend, via the medial forebrain bundle, to supply mainly the

  - ipsilateral cerebral cortex
  - thalamus
  - hypothalamus
  - limbic system
  - olfactory bulb

- the 4th, via the superior cerebellar peduncle, supplies the cerebellar cortex
- the 5th descends in the mesencephalon and spinal cord

Basal forebrain cholinergic pathway

Cholinergic neurons of this pathway originate in the basal forebrain, including:

- Ch4 cholinergic neurones: located in the nucleus basalis of Meynert
- Ch2 and Ch3 cholinergic neurones: located in the diagonal band nucleus (of Broca)
- Ch1 cholinergic neurones: located in the medial septal nucleus

Their main innervation is as follows:

- Ch4: cerebral cortex, amygdala and corpus striatum
- Ch1: hippocampal formation
- Ch2: hippocampal formation
- Ch3: olfactory bulb

(Note that most of the cholinergic innervation of the corpus striatum is intrinsic and not from this pathway.)

Brainstem cholinergic pathway

Cholinergic neurons of this pathway originate in the brainstem, including:

- Ch5 cholinergic neurones: located in the pedunculopontine nucleus
- Ch6 cholinergic neurones: located in the laterodorsal tegmental nucleus

Their (Ch5 and Ch6) main innervation is to the:

- thalamus
- cerebral cortex
- basal forebrain
- corpus striatum
- globus pallidus
- subthalamic nucleus
- substantia nigra

Ch5 neurones are more closely interconnected with extrapyramidal structures, while Ch6 neurones send more projections to nuclei of the limbic system and to the medial prefrontal cortex.

Glutamate system

Neurones using glutamate, an excitatory neurotransmitter, include the:

- cerebral cortical pyramidal cells
- hippocampal pyramidal cells
- primary sensory afferents
- cerebellar granule cells
- cerebellar climbing fibres

The cerebral cortex contains abundant NMDA (*N*-methyl-D-aspartate) receptors, which serve an integral role in corticocortical and corticofugal glutamatergic neurotransmission.

Ascending serotonin system

During embryogenesis, two groups of serotonergic neurones develop:

- a superior group: located at the boundary between the mesencephalon and the pons
- an inferior group: located from the pons caudally to the cervical spinal cord

The superior group gives rise to the superior raphe nuclei and is largely responsible for the origin of ascending serotonergic fibres projecting to the forebrain. The main superior raphe nuclei are the:

- caudal linear nucleus (the most rostral)
- dorsal raphe nucleus
- median raphe nucleus
- supralemniscal nucleus

Ascending fibres pass from the superior raphe nuclei, via pathways such as the dorsal raphe cortical tract (the largest pathway in primates) and the medial forebrain bundle (the largest pathway in the rat), to innervate the forebrain. Particularly important destinations include the:

- suprachiasmatic nucleus
- substantia nigra
- limbic system
- periventricular regions
- primary sensory areas of the cerebral cortex
- association areas of the cerebral cortex

BIBLIOGRAPHY

Alexander, G.E., DeLong, M.R. and Strick, P.L. 1986: Parallel organisation of functionally segregated circuits linking basal ganglia and cortex. *Annual Review of Neuroscience* 9, 357–81.
Heimer, L. 1995: *The human brain and spinal cord*. Berlin: Springer.
Snell, R.S. 1987: *Clinical neuroanatomy for medical students*, 2nd edn. Boston: Little, Brown.
Trimble, M.R. 1981: *Neuropsychiatry*. Chichester: John Wiley.

11
Neuropathology

DEMENTIAS

Alzheimer's disease

MACROSCOPIC NEUROPATHOLOGY   Macroscopic changes in Alzheimer's disease include:

- global brain atrophy
- ventricular enlargement
- sulcal widening

The atrophy is usually most marked in the frontal and temporal lobes.

HISTOPATHOLOGY   Histological changes in the cerebral cortex in Alzheimer's disease include:

- neuronal loss
- shrinking of dendritic branching
- reactive astrocytosis
- neurofibrillary tangles
- neuritic plaques (senile plaques)

There is a positive correlation between the number of neurofibrillary tangles and neuritic plaques, on the one hand, and, on the other, the degree of cognitive impairment. Histological changes seen commonly in the hippocampus include:

- granulovacuolar degeneration
- Hirano bodies
- neurofibrillary tangles
- neuritic plaques (senile plaques)

ULTRASTRUCTURAL PATHOLOGY   Neuritic plaques contain a core made of amyloid. This consists of 8 nm extracellular filaments made up mainly of the β-peptide Aβ or β/A4. Scattered deposits of amyloid β protein in the brain in Alzheimer's disease have been found to localize to activated microglia. Aβ or β/A4 is derived from the β-amyloid precursor protein (APP). The gene for APP is located on the long arm of human chromosome 21 and is a member of a gene family which includes the amyloid precursor-like proteins (APLP) 1 and 2.

NEUROCHEMICAL PATHOLOGY   Neurochemical changes that have been reported in Alzheimer's disease include:

- ↓ acetylcholinesterase
- ↓ choline acetyltransferase
- ↓ GABA
- ↓ noradrenaline

Pick's disease

MACROSCOPIC NEUROPATHOLOGY   Macroscopic changes in Pick's disease include:

- selective asymmetrical atrophy of the anterior temporal lobes and frontal lobes
- knife-blade gyri
- ventricular enlargement

HISTOPATHOLOGY   Histological changes in Pick's disease include:

- Pick's bodies
- neuronal loss
- reactive astrocytosis

These changes may be seen in the:

- cerebral cortex
- basal ganglia
- locus coeruleus
- substantia nigra

ULTRASTRUCTURAL PATHOLOGY   Pick's bodies consist of:

- straight neurofilaments
- paired helical filaments
- endoplasmic reticulum

Multi-infarct dementia
ICD-10 classes multi-infarct dementia under vascular dementia.

MACROSCOPIC NEUROPATHOLOGY   Macroscopic changes in multi-infarct dementia include:

- multiple cerebral infarcts
- local or general brain atrophy
- ventricular enlargement
- arteriosclerotic changes in major arteries

Clinically, the following relationships have been found usually to hold approximately for the total volume of the infarcts:

- 50 ml < volume $\leq$ 100 ml: cognitive impairment
- volume > 100 ml: dementia

HISTOPATHOLOGY   Histological changes include those of infarction and ischaemia.

Lewy body disease
HISTOPATHOLOGY   Histological changes in the brain in dementia caused by Lewy body disease include:

- Lewy bodies
- neuronal loss
- neurofibrillary tangles
- neuritic plaques (senile plaques)

Compared with Parkinson's disease, in which Lewy bodies are also found, in dementia caused by Lewy body disease the density of Lewy bodies is much higher in the:

- cingulate gyrus
- parahippocampal gyrus
- temporal cortex

ULTRASTRUCTURAL PATHOLOGY   Lewy bodies contain:

- protein neurofilaments
- granular material
- dense core vesicles
- microtubule assembly protein
- ubiquitin
- tau protein

Creutzfeldt-Jakob disease

MACROSCOPIC NEUROPATHOLOGY   There may be little or no gross atrophy of the cerebral cortex evident in rapidly developing cases. In those surviving the longest, changes seen may include:

- selective cerebellar atrophy
- generalized cerebral atrophy
- ventricular enlargement

HISTOPATHOLOGY   Histological changes in the brain in dementia caused by Creutzfeldt–Jakob disease include:

- status spongiosus
- neuronal degeneration without inflammation
- astrocytic proliferation

Punch-drunk syndrome

This is also known as post-traumatic dementia or boxing encephalopathy.
MACROSCOPIC NEUROPATHOLOGY   Typical macroscopic changes include:

- cerebral atrophy
- ventricular enlargement
- perforation of the septum pellucidum
- thinning of the corpus callosum

HISTOPATHOLOGY   Histological changes in the brain in punch-drunk syndrome include:

- neuronal loss
- neurofibrillary tangles

CEREBRAL TUMOURS

Types

The main types of cerebral tumours, listed in order of relative frequency, are:

- gliomas
- metastases
- meningeal tumours
- pituitary adenomas
- neurilemmomas
- haemangioblastomas
- medulloblastomas

Gliomas

These are tumours derived from glial cells and their precursors, and include:

- astrocytomas: derived from astrocytes
- oligodendrocytomas: derived from oligodendrocytes

- ependymomas: derived from ependymal cells

Metastases
Cerebral metastases derive particularly from primary neoplasia in the:

- lung
- breast
- kidney
- colon
- ovary
- prostate
- thyroid

Meningeal tumours
These include:

- meningiomas
- meningeal sarcomas: very rare
- primary malignant melanomas derived from pia-arachnoid melanocytes: very rare

Pituitary adenomas
These include, in approximate order of relative frequency (most common first):

- sparsely granulated PRL (prolactin/lactotrophin/mamotrophin) cell adenomas
- oncocytomas
- null cell adenomas
- gonadotroph cell adenomas
- corticotroph cell adenomas
- densely granulated GH (growth hormone/somatotrophin) cell adenomas
- sparsely granulated GH cell adenomas
- mixed (GH cell-PRL cell) adenomas
- silent 'corticotroph' adenomas, subtype 2
- unclassified adenomas
- acidophil stem cell adenomas
- silent 'corticotroph' adenomas, subtype 1
- silent 'corticotroph' adenomas, subtype 3
- mammosomatotroph cell adenomas
- thyrotroph cell adenomas
- densely granulated GH cell adenomas

Neurilemmomas
These are also known as Schwannomas. They are derived from Schwann cells and include acoustic neuromas.

Haemangioblastomas
These are derived from blood vessels.

Medulloblastomas
These cerebellar tumours are embryonal tumours.

SCHIZOPHRENIA

Gross neuropathology
BRAIN MASS There is a slight but significant reduction in brain mass in schizo-

phrenia, compared with controls and allowing for differences in height, body mass, sex and year of birth (Brown *et al.* 1986; Pakkenberg 1987; Bruton *et al.* 1990).

BRAIN LENGTH   Bruton *et al.* (1990) found a significant reduction in the maximum anteroposterior length of formalin fixed cerebral hemispheres in schizophrenia, compared with age- and sex-matched normal controls. Both hemispheres were shorter in schizophrenia compared with the controls.

CEREBRAL VOLUME   In the postmortem brains of patients with schizophrenia, compared with age- and sex-matched controls, Pakkenberg (1987) found a significant reduction in the volumes of the:

- cerebral hemispheres
- cerebral cortex
- central grey matter

The volumes of the white matter did not differ significantly.

HIPPOCAMPUS AND PARAHIPPOCAMPAL GYRUS   Altshuler *et al.* (1990) studied the area and shape of the anterior hippocampus and parahippocampal gyrus in postmortem brains from schizophrenic, nonschizophrenic suicide, and nonpsychiatric controls. No significant differences were found in hippocampal area, but the parahippocampal gyrus was significantly smaller in the schizophrenic group compared with the control group.

Bogerts *et al.* (1990) also studied the postmortem brains of schizophrenic patients and control subjects. Compared with the controls, in the schizophrenic group the hippocampal formation was significantly smaller in the right and left hemispheres. The reduction in hippocampal volume in the male schizophrenics was greater than in the female schizophrenics.

VENTRICULAR VOLUME   Ventricular enlargement has been found in a number of postmortem studies of schizophrenic brains (e.g. Brown *et al.* 1986; Pakkenberg 1987; Bruton *et al.* 1990). The ventricular enlargement particularly affects the temporal horn (Crow *et al.* 1989), indicating temporal lobe neuropathology.

TEMPORAL LOBE   The major of postmortem studies have found a reduction in temporal lobe volume in schizophrenia. While the grey matter is reduced in volume, particularly at the level of the amygdala and anterior hippocampus, the volume of the white matter tends not to be reduced.

Morphometric studies

TEMPORAL LOBE   Pyramidal cell disorientation in the hippocampus has been reported by Kovelman and Scheibel (1984) and by Conrad *et al.* (1991), although this failed to be found by Altshuler *et al.* (1987).

Jeste and Lohr (1989) found that schizophrenic patients had a significantly lower pyramidal cell density than normal controls in the left CA4 hippocampal region.

Cytoarchitectural abnormalities have been reported in the entorhinal cortex in schizophrenia (Arnold *et al.* 1991). These changes, which suggest disturbed development, included:

- aberrant invaginations of the surface
- disruption of cortical layers
- heterotopic displacement of neurons
- paucity of neurons in superficial layers

Arnold *et al.* (1995) found that schizophrenic postmortem brains had a smaller neurone size in the hippocampal regions of:

- the subiculum
- CA1
- layer II of the entorhinal cortex

It is of note that the subiculum, CA1, and the entorhinal cortex are the major subfields of the hippocampal region that maintain the afferent and efferent connections of the hippocampus with widespread cortical and subcortical targets. It was therefore concluded that the smaller size of neurones in these subfields may reflect the presence of structural or functional impairments that disrupt these connections, which in turn could have behavioural sequelae. Reduced hippocampal mossy cell fibre staining has also been reported by Goldsmith and Joyce (1995).

Akbarian et al. (1993a) found a distorted distribution of nicotinamide-adenine dinucleotide phosphate-diaphorase (NADPH-d) neurones in the the the hippocampal formation and in the neocortex of the lateral temporal lobe, consistent with anomalous cortical development in the lateral temporal lobe.

OTHER CORTICAL AREAS Compared with control brains, Benes et al. (1986) found significantly lower neuronal density in the following cortical regions in schizophrenic brains:

- prefrontal cortex: layer VI
- anterior cingulate cortex: layer V
- primary motor cortex: layer III

The glial density also tended to be lower throughout most layers of all three above regions. However, there were no differences in the neurone:glia ratios or neuronal size between the two groups. These results suggest the occurrence of a dysplastic process rather than degeneration in schizophrenia.

Benes et al. (1987) confirmed the presence of greater numbers of long, vertical, associative axons in the anterior cingulate cortex of schizophrenic patients relative to control subjects. On the basis of this finding they suggested that there might be an increase of associative inputs into the anterior cingulate cortex in schizophrenia.

Akbarian et al. (1993b) found a distorted distribution of NADPH-d neurones in the dorsolateral prefrontal area of schizophrenic postmortem brains, consistent with anomalous cortical development in this region.

Akbarian et al. (1995) have also found that the prefrontal cortex of schizophrenics shows reduced expression for glutamic acid decarboxylase (GAD) in the absence of significant cell loss, suggesting an activity-dependent down-regulation of neurotransmitter gene expression.

OTHER BRAIN REGIONS The results of studies of the corpus callosum and cerebellum have yielded inconsistent results.

Synaptic pathology

SYNAPTIC VESICLES Soustek (1989) found clusters of large numbers of synaptic vesicles in presynaptic knobs in the cerebral cortex of schizophrenic postmortem brains but not in brains from control subjects.

SYNAPTOPHYSIN Synaptophysin is a presynaptic vesicle protein the distribution and abundance of which provides a synaptic marker which can be reliably measured in postmortem brain. Eastwood et al. (1995b) found that in schizophrenic brains, compared with controls, synaptophysin mRNA was reduced bilaterally in:

- CA4
- CA3
- the subiculum
- the parahippocampal gyrus

(The effect of antipsychotic medication was discounted as a separate rat study showed no effect of haloperidol treatment on hippocampal synaptophysin mRNA.)

Furthermore, Eastwood and Harrison (1995) found decreased synaptophysin in the medial temporal lobe in schizophrenia, compared with controls, using immunoautoradiography. Significant reductions were found in the:

- dentate gyrus
- subiculum
- parahippocampal gyrus

Gliosis

Almost all recent quantitative studies investigating the regions of greatest structural differences in schizophrenic patients have not shown significant gliosis (e.g. Jellinger 1985; Roberts et al. 1987; Bruton et al. 1990). This negative finding is consistent with either of the following possibilities:

- the structural change in schizophrenic brains results from an embryonic insult prior to the third trimester (since the developing brain does not show reactive gliosis until approximately the third trimester)
- a neuropathological process occurs at or after the third trimester but does not usually initiate a glial reaction

AUTISM

Histological changes

Bauman and Kemper (1985) studied the brain of a 29-year-old autistic man and found, compared with the brain of an age- and sex-matched normal control, abnormalities in the:

- hippocampus
- subiculum
- entorhinal cortex
- septal nuclei
- mammillary body
- amygdala (selected nuclei)
- neocerebellar cortex
- roof nuclei of the cerebellum
- inferior olivary nucleus

Neuropathological studies suggest that the microscropic neuroanatomical abnormalities in autism begin early in gestation, probably in the second trimester (Bauman 1991)

Cerebellar pathology

Both neuropathological and structural neuroimaging studies have indicated that hypoplastia of the cerebellar vermis as well as hypoplasia of the cerebellar hemispheres occurs in some subjects with autism.

REDUCED PURKINJE CELL COUNT   Ritvo et al. (1986) compared the cerebellums of four autistic subjects with those of three comparison subjects without central nervous system pathology and one with phenytoin toxicity. Total Purkinje cell counts were found to be significantly lower in the cerebellar hemisphere and vermis of each autistic subject than in the comparison subjects.

NEOCEREBELLAR ABNORMALITY In their study of subjects with autism, Courchesne *et al.* (1988) measured the size of the cerebellar vermis using magnetic resonance imaging and compared these with its size in controls. The neocerebellar vermal lobules VI and VII were found to be significantly smaller in autism. This appeared to be a result of developmental hypoplasia rather than shrinkage or deterioration after full development had been achieved. In contrast, the adjacent vermal lobules I to V, which are ontogenetically, developmentally, and anatomically distinct from lobules VI and VII, were found to be of normal size. Maldevelopment of the vermal neocerebellum had occurred in both retarded and nonretarded patients with autism. The authors suggested that this localized maldevelopment might serve as a temporal marker to identify the events that damage the brain in autism, as well as other neural structures that might be concomitantly damaged. They concluded that the neocerebellar abnormality may:

- directly impair cognitive functions that may be attributable to the neocerebellum
- indirectly affect, through its connections to the brainstem, hypothalamus, and thalamus, the development and functioning of one or more systems involved in cognitive, sensory, autonomic, and motor activities
- occur concomitantly with damage to other neural sites, the dysfunction of which directly underlies the cognitive deficits in autism

MOVEMENT DISORDERS

Parkinson's disease

Idiopathic Parkinson's disease is characterized by a loss of dopaminergic neurones in the substantia nigra.

MACROSCOPIC NEUROPATHOLOGY Macroscopic changes in idiopathic Parkinson's disease include:

- depigmentation of the substantia nigra: particularly the zona compacta
- depigmentation of the locus coeruleus

Diffuse cortical atrophy may take place.

HISTOPATHOLOGY Histological changes in idiopathic Parkinson's disease include:

- neuronal loss
- reactive astrocytosis
- the presence of Lewy bodies in the

  - substantia nigra
  - dorsal motor nucleus of the vagus
  - hypothalamus
  - nucleus basalis of Meynert
  - locus coeruleus
  - Edinger–Westphal nucleus
  - raphe nuclei

- cerebral cortex
- olfactory bulb

- the presence of melanin-containing macrophages

NEUROCHEMICAL PATHOLOGY   Neurochemical changes in idiopathic Parkinson's disease include reduced inhibitory dopaminergic action of the nigrostriatal pathway on striatal cholinergic neurones.

Huntington's disease

Huntington's disease results from a mutation of the protein huntingtin and is characterized by a selective loss of discrete neuronal populations in the brain with progressive degeneration of efferent neurones of the neostriatum and sparing of dopaminergic afferents, resulting in progressive atrophy of the neostriatum.

MACROSCOPIC NEUROPATHOLOGY   Macroscopic changes in Huntington's disease include:

- small brain with reduced mass
- marked atrophy of the corpus striatum: particularly the caudate nucleus
- marked atrophy of the cerebral cortex: particularly the frontal lobe gyri (the parietal lobe is less often affected)
- dilatation of the lateral and third ventricles

HISTOPATHOLOGY   Histological changes in Huntington's disease include:

- neuronal loss in the cerebral cortex: particularly the frontal cortex
- neuronal loss in the corpus striatum: particularly neurones using as neuro-transmitters

    - GABA and enkephalin
    - GABA and substance P

- astrocytosis in affected regions

In the affected regions there is relative sparing of the following neuronal populations:

- diaphorase-positive neurones containing nitric oxide synthase (NOS)
- large cholinesterase-positive neurones

NEUROCHEMICAL PATHOLOGY   Neurochemical changes that have been reported in Huntington's disease include:

- ↓ GABA
- ↓ glutamic acid decarboxylase
- ↓ acetylcholine
- ↓ substance P
- ↑ somatostatin
- ↓ corticotrophin-releasing factor (CRF)
- dopamine hypersensitivity

Tardive dyskinesia

Tardive dyskinesia is a syndrome of potentially irreversible involuntary hyperkinetic dyskinesias that may occur during long-term treatment with antipsychotic (neuroleptic) medication. The most important hypotheses concerning the neurochemical pathology of tardive dyskinesia are:

- dopamine hypersensitivity
- free radical induced neurotoxicity

- GABA insufficiency
- noradrenergic dysfunction

DOPAMINE HYPERSENSITIVITY HYPOTHESIS According to this hypothesis the following sequence of events takes place:

> long-term treatment with antipsychotic (neuroleptic) medication
> → chronic dopamine receptor blockade
> → dopamine D2 receptor hypersensitivity in the nigrostriatal pathway
> → tardive dyskinesia

Evidence in favour of this hypothesis includes:

- studies of denervation-induced hypersensitivity in muscles
- animal experiments in which, following the discontinuation of antipsychotic drugs, acute dopamine agonist challenges → ↑ oral stereotyped behaviour
- animal experiments in which repeated antipsychotic treatment may → ↑ brain dopamine D2 receptors

Problems with the hypothesis include:

- differences in the chronology of the onset of symptoms between humans and animal models
- only limited support for dopamine hypersensitivity from postantipsychotic dopamine turnover experiments in monkeys
- postmortem human brain tissue studies have not shown significant differences in D2 receptor binding between schizophrenic patients with tardive dyskinesia and schizophrenic patients without tardive dyskinesia
- blood biochemical assays have not shown consistent significant differences between patients with tardive dyskinesia and patients without tardive dyskinesia with respect to

  - prolactin
  - somatotrophin

- no consistent significant differences have been shown between patients with tardive dyskinesia and patients without tardive dyskinesia with respect to

  - plasma homovanillic acid
  - urinary homovanillic acid
  - CSF homovanillic acid

- dopamine agonists do not strikingly exacerbate tardive dyskinesia
- dopamine antagonist antipsychotics may sometimes worsen tardive dyskinesia

A modification of this hypothesis includes a role for dopamine D1 receptors, but many of the above problems also apply again. Moreover, postmortem human brain tissue studies have not shown significant differences in D1 receptor binding between schizophrenic patients with tardive dyskinesia and schizophrenic patients without tardive dyskinesia.

FREE RADICAL INDUCED NEUROTOXICITY According to this hypothesis the following sequence of events takes place:

> long-term treatment with antipsychotic (neuroleptic) medication
> → ↑catecholamine turnover
> → free radical byproducts

$\rightarrow$ membrane lipid peroxidation in the basal ganglia (the basal ganglia have a high oxidative metabolism)

$\rightarrow$ tardive dyskinesia

Evidence in favour of this hypothesis includes:

- α-tocopherol (vitamin E) is of benefit in rodent models of antipsychotic induced dyskinesiaa
- some studies have shown $\uparrow$ blood or CSF levels of lipid peroxidation byproducts in patients with tardive dyskinesia compared with those without tardive dyskinesia

Problems with the hypothesis include:

- vitamin E treatment of tardive dyskinesia in general does not lead to major clinical improvement

GABA INSUFFICIENCY   According to one version of this hypothesis the following sequence of events takes place:

long-term treatment with antipsychotic (neuroleptic) medication
$\rightarrow$ destruction of GABAergic neurones in the striatum
$\rightarrow$ $\downarrow$ feedback inhibition
$\rightarrow$ tardive dyskinesia

According to another version, the sequence of events is:

long-term treatment with antipsychotic (neuroleptic) medication
$\rightarrow$ $\downarrow$ GABAergic neuronal activity in the pars reticulata of the substantia nigra
$\rightarrow$ $\downarrow$ inhibition of involuntary movements

$\rightarrow$ tardive dyskinesia

Evidence in favour of these hypotheses includes:

- it has been shown that striatonigral GABAergic neurones feed back on dopaminergic nigrostriatal neurones to reduce their activity
- antipsychotic-treated dyskinetic monkeys have been found to have a decrease in glutamic acid decarboxylase, compared with similarly treated monkeys without tardive dyskinesia, in the

  - substantia nigra
  - globus pallidus
  - subthalamic nucleus

- patients with tardive dyskinesia have been found on postmortem to have a significant decrease in glutamic acid decarboxylase activity, compared with patients without tardive dyskinesia, in the subthalamic nucleus
- the following GABAergic agonists have generally shown promise as potential therapeutic agents

  - benzodiazepines
  - baclofen
  - gamma-vinyl GABA

Problems with the hypothesis include:

- rodent models of tardive dyskinesia do not show consistent GABA function changes with antipsychotic treatment

- it has not so far proved possible effectively to treat tardive dyskinesia with GABAergic drugs

NORADRENERGIC DYSFUNCTION According to this hypothesis noradrenergic overactivity contributes to the pathophysiology of tardive dyskinesia. Evidence in favour of this hypotheses includes:

- patients with tardive dyskinesia have been found to have significantly greater dopamine β-hydroxylase activity than those without tardive dyskinesia
- platelet ^{3}H-dihydroergocryptine-α2 adrenergic receptor binding and CSF noradrenaline have been found to be significantly correlated with the severity of tardive dyskinesia

Problems with the hypothesis include:

- it has not so far proved possible effectively to treat tardive dyskinesia with noradrenergic drugs

BIBLIOGRAPHY

Akbarian, S., Vinuela, A., Kim, J.J., Potkin, S.G., Bunney, W.E. Jr and Jones, E.G. 1993a: Distorted distribution of nicotinamide-adenine dinucleotide phosphate-diaphorase neurons in temporal lobe of schizophrenics implies anomalous cortical development. *Archives of General Psychiatry* 50, 178–87.

Akbarian, S., Bunney, W.E. Jr, Potkin, S.G., *et al.* 1993b: Altered distribution of nicotinamide-adenine dinucleotide phosphate-diaphorase cells in frontal lobe of schizophrenics implies disturbances of cortical development. *Archives of General Psychiatry* 50, 169–77.

Akbarian, S., Kim, J.J., Potkin, S.G., *et al.* 1995: Gene expression for glutamic acid decarboxylase is reduced without loss of neurons in prefrontal cortex of schizophrenics. *Archives of General Psychiatry* 52, 258–66.

Altshuler, L.L., Casanova, M.F., Goldberg, T.E. and Kleinman, J.E. 1990: The hippocampus and parahippocampus in schizophrenia, suicide, and control brains. *Archives of General Psychiatry* 47, 1029–34.

Altshuler, L.L., Conrad, A., Kovelman, J.A. and Scheibel, A. 1987: Hippocampal pyramidal cell orientation in schizophrenia. A controlled neurohistologic study of the Yakovlev collection. *Archives of General Psychiatry* 44, 1094–8.

Arnold, S.E., Hyman, B.T., Van Hoesen, G.W. and Damasio, A.R. 1991: Some cytoarchitectural abnormalities of the entorhinal cortex in schizophrenia. *Archives of General Psychiatry* 48, 625–32.

Arnold, S.E., Franz, B.R., Gur, R.C., *et al.* 1995: Smaller neuron size in schizophrenia in hippocampal subfields that mediate cortical-hippocampal interactions. *American Journal of Psychiatry* 152, 738–48.

Bauman, M.L. 1991: Microscopic neuroanatomic abnormalities in autism. *Pediatrics* 87, 791–6.

Bauman, M. and Kemper, T.L. 1985: Histoanatomic observations of brain in early infantile autism. *Neurology* 35, 866–74.

Benes, F.M., Davidson, J. and Bird, E.D. 1986: Quantitative cytoarchitectural studies of the cerebral cortex of schizophrenics. *Archives of General Psychiatry* 43, 31–5.

Benes, F.M., Majocha, R., Bird, E.D. and Marotta, C.A. 1987: Increased vertical axon numbers in cingulate cortex of schizophrenics. *Archives of General Psychiatry* 44, 1017–21.

Bogerts, B., Falkai, P., Haupts, M., *et al.* 1990: Post-mortem volume measurements of limbic system and basal ganglia structures in chronic schizophrenics. Initial results from a new brain collection. *Schizophrenia Research* 3, 295–301.

Brown, R., Colter, N., Corsellis, J.A., *et al.* 1986: Postmortem evidence of structural brain changes in schizophrenia. Differences in brain weight, temporal horn area, and parahippocampal gyrus compared with affective disorder. *Archives of General Psychiatry* 43, 36–42.

Bruton, C.J., Crow, T.J., Frith, C.D., Johnstone, E.C., Owens, D.G. and Roberts, G.W.

1990: Schizophrenia and the brain: a prospective clinico-neuropathological study. *Psychological Medicine* 20, 285–304.

Conrad, A.J., Abebe, T., Austin, R., Forsythe, S. and Scheibel, A.B. 1991: Hippocampal pyramidal cell disarray in schizophrenia as a bilateral phenomenon. *Archives of General Psychiatry* 48, 413–17.

Courchesne, E., Yeung Courchesne, R., Press, G.A., Hesselink, J.R. and Jerningan, T.L. 1988: Hypoplasia of cerebellar vermal lobules VI and VII in autism. *New England Journal of Medicine* 318, 1349–54.

Crow, T.J., Ball, J., Bloom, S.R., *et al.* 1989: Schizophrenia as an anomaly of development of cerebral asymmetry. A postmortem study and a proposal concerning the genetic basis of the disease. *Archives of General Psychiatry* 46, 1145–50.

Eastwood, S.L. and Harrison, P.J. 1995: Decreased synaptophysin in the medial temporal lobe in schizophrenia demonstrated using immunoautoradiography. *Neuroscience* 69, 339–43.

Eastwood, S.L., Burnet, P.W. and Harrison, P.J. 1995: Altered synaptophysin expression as a marker of synaptic pathology in schizophrenia. *Neuroscience* 66, 309–19.

Goldsmith, S.K. and Joyce, J.N. 1995: Alterations in hippocampal mossy fiber pathway in schizophrenia and Alzheimer's disease. *Biological Psychiatry* 37, 122–6.

Jellinger, K. 1985: Neuromorphological background of pathochemical studies in major psychoses. In: Beckman, H. (ed.) *Pathochemical markers in major psychoses.* Heidelberg: Springer Verlag, 1–23.

Jeste, D.V. and Lohr, J.B. 1989: Hippocampal pathologic findings in schizophrenia. A morphometric study. *Archives of General Psychiatry* 46, 1019–24.

Kovelman, J.A. and Scheibel, A.B. 1984: A neurohistological correlate of schizophrenia. *Biological Psychiatry* 19, 1601–21.

Pakkenberg, B. 1987: Post-mortem study of chronic schizophrenic brains. *British Journal of Psychiatry* 151, 744–52.

Ritvo, E.R., Freeman, B.J., Scheibel, A.B., *et al.* 1986: Lower Purkinje cell counts in the cerebella of four autistic subjects: initial findings of the UCLA-NSAC autopsy research report. *American Journal of Psychiatry* 143, 862–66.

Roberts, G.W., Colter, N., Lofthouse, R., Johnstone, E.C. and Crow, T.J. 1987: Is there gliosis in schizophrenia? Investigation of the temporal lobe. *Biological Psychiatry* 22, 1459–68.

Soustek, Z. 1989: Ultrastructure of cortical synapses in the brain of schizophrenics. *Zentralblatt für Allgemeine Pathologic und Pathologische Anatomie* 135, 25–32.

12
Neuroimaging
techniques

X-RAY

BASIS   Radiography utilizes X-rays.

TYPE OF IMAGING   X-ray radiography is a form of structural imaging.

NEUROPSYCHIATRIC APPLICATIONS   The main use nowadays of skull radiography is:

■   assessment of trauma

It may also be useful in the detection of intracranial expanding lesions.

CT

CT is X-ray computerized tomography or computed tomography. It was previously known as computerized axial tomography, or CAT.

BASIS   The basis of CT is as follows:

X-ray beams are passed through a given tissue plane in different directions
   → scintillation counters record the emerging X-rays
   → computer reconstruction of emerging X-ray data
   → radiodensity maps

This procedure is repeated for successive adjacent planes, thereby building up an image of, for example, the whole brain.

TYPE OF IMAGING   CT is a form of structural imaging.

NEUROPSYCHIATRIC APPLICATIONS   Where available, CT and MRI have largely replaced skull radiography. Its clinical uses include the detection of:

■   shifts of intracranial structures
■   intracranial expanding lesions
■   cerebral infarction
■   cerebral oedema
■   cerebral atrophy and ventricular dilatation
■   atrophy of other structures
■   demyelination changes and other causes of radiodensity change

It is also widely used in neuropsychiatric research.

PET

PET is positron emission tomography.

BASIS   The basis of PET neuroimaging is as follows:

a positron-emitting radioisotope or radiolabelled ligand is introduced into the cerebral circulation; routes commonly used are

- intravenous administration (the radioactive substance is in solution)
- by inhalation (the radioactive substance is in gaseous form)
  - → blood flow ± cerebral tissue binding in the brain
  - → emission of positrons
  - → positron-electron interactions
  - → dual γ photon emissions
  - → detection of γ photons
  - → computer reconstruction of emerging γ photon data
  - → slice images of the distribution of the radioisotopes in the brain

The positron-emitting radioisotopes used can be produced in small cyclotrons.

TYPE OF IMAGING   PET is a form of functional imaging.

NEUROPSYCHIATRIC APPLICATIONS   PET neuroimaging can give information about:

- metabolic changes
- regional cerebral blood flow (rCBF)
- ligand binding

Clinical applications of PET include:

- cerebrovascular disease
- Alzheimer's disease
- epilepsy, prior to neurosurgery
- head injury

PET is likely to be increasingly replaced by functional magnetic resonance imaging (fMRI), since the latter does not require the use of radioactive isotopes.

SPECT

SPECT is single-photon emission computerized tomography. It is also known as SPET or single-photon emission tomography.

BASIS   The basis of SPECT neuroimaging is as follows:

a radioisotope or radiolabelled ligand is introduced into the cerebral circulation; routes commonly used are

- intravenous administration (the radioactive substance is in solution)
- by inhalation (the radioactive substance is in gaseous form)
  - → blood flow ± cerebral tissue binding in the brain
  - → single γ photon emissions
  - → detection of γ photons
  - → computer reconstruction of emerging γ photon data
  - → slice images of the distribution of the radioisotopes in the brain

TYPE OF IMAGING   SPECT is a form of functional imaging.

NEUROPSYCHIATRIC APPLICATIONS   SPECT neuroimaging can give information about:

- regional cerebral blood flow (rCBF)
- ligand binding

It is also of use in conditions in which the onset of the symptomatology being studied (e.g. epileptic seizures, auditory hallucinations) may occur at a time when the patient is not in or near a scanner; a suitable radioligand (e.g. 99m-technetium hexamethylpropylene amine oxime (HMPAO)) can be administered at the material time and the patient scanned afterwards.

Clinical applications of SPECT include:

- Alzheimer's disease

The resolution of SPECT is generally poorer than that of PET, and both are likely to be increasingly replaced by fMRI.

MRI

MRI is magnetic resonance imaging. It was previously referred to as NMR or nuclear magnetic resonance; NMR is now taken to include MRI, MRS (magnetic resonance spectroscopy) and fMRI.

BASIS   The basis of MRI is as follows:

the patient is placed in a strong static magnetic field → alignment of proton spin axes
→ pulses of radiofrequency waves at specified frequencies are administered
→ this additional energy is absorbed
→ some protons jump to a higher quantum level
→ radiowaves are emitted when these protons return to the lower quantum level
→ the radio-frequency (rf) wave frequencies are measured
→ precession in each voxel is determined and T1 (longitudinal relaxation time) and T2 (transverse relaxation time) calculated
→ proton density, T1, T2 pixel intensities
→ anatomical magnetic resonance images

In some circumstances it may be useful to administer a paramagnetic contrast-enhancing agent such as gadolinium DTPA.

TYPE OF IMAGING   MRI is a form of structural imaging.

NEUROPSYCHIATRIC APPLICATIONS   MRI is useful in most clinical and research studies requiring high resolution neuroanatomical imaging.

BIBLIOGRAPHY

Bydder, G.M. 1983: Clinical aspects of NMR imaging. In Steiner, R. (ed.) *Recent advances in radiology and medical imaging.* Edinburgh: Churchill Livingstone.

Costa, D.C. and Ell, P.J. 1991: *Brain blood flow in neurology and psychiatry.* Edinburgh: Churchill Livingstone.

Costa, D.C., Morgan, G.F. and Lassen, N.A. 1993: *New trends in nuclear neurology and psychiatry.* London: John Libbey.

Gadian, D.G. 1995: *NMR and its applications to living systems,* 2nd edn. Oxford: Oxford University Press.

Ketonen, L.M. and Berg, M.J. 1996: *Clinical neuroradiology.* London: Arnold.

13
Neurophysiology

PHYSIOLOGY OF NEURONES, SYNAPSES AND RECEPTORS

Neurones

RESTING MEMBRANE ION PERMEABILITIES   The comparative permeabilities to different ions of the resting neuronal membrane is as follows:

- K^+ (potassium ions): relatively permeable
- Na^+ (sodium ions): relatively impermeable
- Cl^- (chloride ions): freely permeable
- organic anions: relatively impermeable

RESTING MEMBRANE POTENTIAL   There is a negative resting membrane potential of around -70 mV. It is maintained by the sodium pump, which actively transports Na^+ out of the cell and K^+ into the cell. Energy for this process is provided by ATP.

CHANGES IN MEMBRANE ION PERMEABILITIES   The neuronal membrane ion permeabilities may change in response to stimulation:

- depolarization: the membrane potential increases, that is it becomes less negative; this increases the probability of an action potential being generated
- hyperpolarization: the membrane potential decreases, that is it becomes more negative; this decreases the probability of an action potential being generated

ACTION POTENTIAL   Neuronal stimulation leads to local depolarization.

If (degree of depolarization) > (a critical threshold) → nerve impulse or action potential

During an action potential the membrane potential rapidly becomes positive, before returning to become negative. This is caused by an increase first in Na^+ permeability, allowing the inflow of Na^+, and then in K^+ permeability (with a rapid reduction in Na^+ permeability at the same time), causing an outflow of K^+ and thereby restoring the negative membrane potential. The sodium pump then restores the original ionic concentrations.

PROPAGATION OF ACTION POTENTIAL   An action potential is propagated by the depolarization spreading laterally to adjacent parts of the neurone.

ALL-OR-NONE PHENOMENON   The passage of an action potential along a neurone is an all-or-none phenomenon.

ABSOLUTE REFRACTORY PERIOD   This is the period during which the active part of the neuronal membrane has a reversed polarity so that conduction or initiation of another action potential is not possible in it.

RELATIVE REFRACTORY PERIOD   This is the period of repolarization after an action potential, during which hyperpolarization occurs, making it more difficult for stimulation to allow the membrane potential to reach the critical threshold.

CONDUCTION IN UNMYELINATED FIBRES   The greater the diameter of the fibre the faster is the rate of transmission.

CONDUCTION IN MYELINATED FIBRES   The action potential appears to jump from one node of Ranvier to the next, skipping the intervening myelinated parts. This rapid form of conduction is known as saltatory conduction.

Synapses

SYNAPTIC CLEFT   This is the gap at a synapse between the membrane of a presynaptic fibre and that of the postsynaptic fibre.

LOCATION   Synapses may be found between

- two neurones
- motoneurones and muscle cells
- sensory neurones and sensory receptors

TYPES   There are two types of synapse:

- chemical: the commoner type, in which a chemical neurotransmitter is stored in presynaptic vesicles
- electrical: faster than chemical synapses, with direct membrane-to-membrane connection via gap junctions

SYNAPTIC TRANSMISSION   At chemical synapses the following events take place during synaptic transmission:

arrival of action potential at presynaptic membrane
$\rightarrow$ influx of Ca^{2+} (calcium ions)
$\rightarrow$ presynaptic vesicles fuse to the presynaptic membrane
$\rightarrow$ release of neurotransmitter into the synaptic cleft
$\rightarrow$ passage of neurotransmitter across the synaptic cleft
$\rightarrow$ binding of neurotransmitter to postsynaptic receptors
$\rightarrow$ ion permeability changes in postsynaptic membrane
$\rightarrow$ postsynaptic depolarization or hyperpolarization (depending on the type of neurotransmitter)

EXCITATORY POSTSYNAPTIC POTENTIALS   Excitatory postsynaptic potentials, or EPSPs, occur in the postsynaptic membrane (because of depolarization) following the release of an excitatory neurotransmitter from the presynaptic neurone at central excitatory synapses.

INHIBITORY POSTSYNAPTIC POTENTIALS   Inhibitory postsynaptic potentials, or IPSPs, occur in the postsynaptic membrane (because of hyperpolarization) following the release of an inhibitory neurotransmitter from the presynaptic neurone at central inhibitory synapses.

SUMMATION   One EPSP on its own is not usually sufficient to initiate an action potential. However, temporal and/or spatial summation may all decrease the degree of depolarization to reach the critical threshold. IPSPs, on summating with EPSPs, counter the effect of the latter.

Receptors

SENSORY RECEPTORS   The main types of sensory receptor in humans are:

- mechanoreceptors
- thermoreceptors
- light receptors
- nociceptors
- chemoreceptors

ADAPTATION   In response to a continuous prolonged appropriate stimulus, most sensory receptors exhibit adaptation:

Table 13.1 The anterior pituitary hormones and their corresponding hypothalamic releasing factors (hormones) and release-inhibiting factors (hormones)

Anterior pituitary hormone	Hypothalamic releasing factor (hormone) and/or release-inhibiting factor (hormone)
Corticotropin (adrenocorticotrophic hormone, ACTH)	Corticotropin releasing factor (hormone) (CRF or CRH)
Follicle stimulating hormone (FSH)	Gonadotropin releasing factor (hormone) (GnRF or GnRH)
Luteinizing hormone (LH)	Gonadotropin releasing factor (hormone) (GnRF or GnRH)
Melanocyte stimulating hormone (MSH)	MSH release inhibitory factor (MIH)
Prolactin	Prolactin releasing factor (PRF) Prolactin release inhibitory factor (PIF) (dopamine)
Somatotropin (growth hormone, GH)	Growth hormone releasing factor (hormone) (GRF or GRH; somatocrinin) Growth hormone release inhibitory factor (somatostatin)
Thyrotropin (thyroid stimulating hormone, TSH)	Thyrotropin releasing factor (hormone) (TRF or TRH)

- phasic receptors: the receptor firing stops
- tonic receptors: the receptor firing frequency falls to a low maintained level

PITUITARY HORMONES

Anterior pituitary hormones

Posterior pituitary hormones
The hypothalamus is responsible for the neurosecretion of the two posterior pituitary hormones:

- arginine vasopressin (argipressin or antidiuretic hormone; AVP or ADH)
- oxytocin

AROUSAL AND SLEEP

Sleep architecture
REM AND NON-REM SLEEP   Sleep is divided into the following two phases:

- rapid eye movement (REM) sleep: during which the eyes undergo rapid movements and there is a high level of brain activity
- non-REM sleep: during which there is reduced neuronal activity

STAGES OF SLEEP   The following stages normally occur during normal non-REM sleep:

- stage 0: quiet wakefulness and shut eyes; EEG: alpha activity
- stage 1: falling asleep; EEG: low amplitude, ↓ alpha activity, low-voltage theta activity
- stage 2: light sleep; EEG: 2 to 7 Hz, occasional sleep spindles and K complexes
- stage 3: deep sleep; ↑ delta activity (20 to 50 per cent)
- stage 4: deep sleep; ↑ ↑ delta activity (> 50 per cent)

Stage 3 + stage 4 = slow-wave sleep (SWS)

Physiological correlates of sleep

REM SLEEP   Features of REM sleep include:

- ↑ recall of dreaming if awoken during REM sleep
- ↑ complexity of dreams
- ↑ sympathetic activity
- transient runs of conjugate ocular movements
- maximal loss of muscle tone
- ↑ heart rate
- ↑ systolic blood pressure
- ↑ respiratory rate
- ↑ cerebral blood flow
- occasional myoclonic jerks
- penile erection or vaginal blood flow
- ↑ protein synthesis (rat brain)

NON-REM SLEEP   Features of non-REM sleep include:

- ↓ recall of dreaming if awoken during REM sleep
- ↓ complexity of dreams
- ↑ parasympathetic activity
- upward ocular deviation with few or no movements
- abolition of tendon reflexes
- ↓ heart rate
- ↓ systolic blood pressure
- ↓ respiratory rate
- ↓ cerebral blood flow
- penis not usually erect

Causes of the sleeping–waking cycle

There are two main theories accounting for the sleeping–waking cycle, the:

- monoaminergic (or biochemical, two-stage, Jouvet's) model
- cellular (or Hobson's) model

MONOAMINERGIC MODEL   In this model:

- non-REM sleep is associated with serotonergic neuronal activity: raphe complex
- REM sleep is associated with noradrenergic neuronal activity: locus coeruleus

CELLULAR MODEL   In this model three groups of central neurones are of importance. These groups, and their corresponding neurotransmitters, are the:

- pontine gigantocellular tegmental fields (nucleus reticularis pontis caudalis): acetylcholine
- dorsal raphe nuclei: serotonin
- locus coeruleus: noradrenaline

THE EEG

Recording techniques

CONVENTIONAL The conventional EEG (electroencephalogram) recording involves placing electrodes on the scalp, and is therefore non-invasive. The positions of the electrodes is usually according to the International 10–20 System, which entails measurements from the following scalp landmarks:

- the nasion
- the inion
- the right auricular depression
- the left auricular depression

In this system, proportions of scalp distances are 10 per cent or 20 per cent, and midline electrodes are denoted by the subscript z.

In ambulatory electroencephalography the output is stored on a suitable portable recorder.

SPECIALIZED Specialized recording techniques include:

- nasopharyngeal leads: electrodes are positioned in the superior part of the nasopharynx; they can be used to obtain recordings from the inferior and medial temporal lobe
- sphenoidal electrodes: electrodes are inserted between the mandibular coronoid notch and the zygoma; they can be used to obtain recordings from the inferior temporal lobe
- electrocorticography: electrodes are placed directly on the surface of the brain
- depth electroencephalography: electrodes are placed inside the brain

Normal EEG rhythms

CLASSIFICATION ACCORDING TO FREQUENCY BAND Normal EEG rhythms are classified according to frequency as follows:

- delta: frequency < 4 Hz
- theta: 4 Hz ≤ frequency < 8 Hz
- alpha: 8 Hz ≤ frequency < 13 Hz
- beta: frequency ≥ 13 Hz

LAMBDA ACTIVITY Lambda activity occurs over the occipital region in subjects with their eyes open. It is related to ocular movements during visual attention.

MU ACTIVITY Mu activity occurs over the motor cortex. It is related to motor activity and is abolished by movement of the contralateral limb.

Spikes and waves

SPIKES Spikes are transient high peaks that last less than 80 ms.

SHARP WAVES Sharp waves are conspicuous sharply defined wave formations that rise rapidly, fall more slowly, and last more than 80 ms.

The effect of drugs

ANTIDEPRESSANTS In general, antidepressants cause:

- ↑ delta activity

ANTIPSYCHOTICS In general, antipsychotic drugs cause:

- ↓ beta activity
- ↑ low-frequency delta activity and/or ↑ theta activity

ANXIOLYTICS   In general, anxiolytics, including barbiturates and benzodiazepines, cause:

- ↑ beta activity
- ↓ alpha activity (sometimes)

LITHIUM   The therapeutic levels of lithium lead to only small EEG effects which are likely to be missed on visual analysis of routine recordings.

BIBLIOGRAPHY

Carpenter, R.H.S. 1996: *Neurophysiology*, 3rd edn. London: Arnold.
Emslie-Smith, D., Paterson, C.R., Scratcherd, T. and Read, N.W. (eds) 1988: *Textbook of physiology*, 11th edn. Edinburgh: Churchill Livingstone.
Guyton, A.C. and Hall, J.E. 1995: *Textbook of medical physiology*, 9th edn. Philadelphia: W.B. Saunders.

14
Neurochemistry

TRANSMITTER SYNTHESIS, STORAGE AND RELEASE

Transmitter synthesis
The synthesis of the neurotransmitters noradrenaline, serotonin, dopamine, GABA, and acetylcholine is considered later in this chapter.

Transmitter storage
The transmitter at a synaptic cleft is stored in presynaptic vesicles. Each vesicle contains one quantum, usually corresponding to several thousand molecules, of transmitter.

Transmitter release
Transmitter release from synaptic vesicles takes place by exocytosis in a process controlled by Ca^{2+} influx. Because the number of vesicles released is an integer, transmitter release is essentially quantal in nature. The Ca^{2+} enters via voltage-dependent ion channels. Importantly, Na^+ influx and/or K^+ efflux are not needed for transmitter release. Ca^{2+} influences or regulates:

- the probability of vesicular transmitter release
- vesicular fusion
- the transport of synaptic vesicles to the presynaptic active zone of exocytosis
- post-tetanic potentiation
- tonic depolarization of the presynaptic neurone

RECEPTORS

Structure
In general, the receptors to which neurotransmitters bind are proteins located on the external surface of cell membranes. Until the 1980s receptors were classified and identified pharmacologically but not according to their structures. Since 1983, however, when the primary amino acid sequence of a receptor subunit of the nicotinic acetylcholine receptor was discovered, the DNA of an increasing number of receptor proteins has been sequenced, and hence their amino acid sequences discovered. This has led to a further clarification of receptor classification. It has also become evident that, as expected, for receptors of classical neurotransmitters the amino acids forming the binding site are on or close to the extracellular side of the receptor.

Function
The main function of a receptor is the molecular recognition of a signalling molecule, which inthe case of neurotransmission is a neurotransmitter, leading in turn to signal transduction. A receptor generally responds to neurotransmitter binding in one of two ways:

- neurotransmitter binding $\rightarrow$ opening of transmembrane ion channel
- receptor-neurotransmitter $\rightarrow$ second messenger system activation/inhibition

G PROTEINS   G proteins (named after their ability to bind guanosine triphosphate (GTP) and guanosine diphosphate (GDP)) are often involved in transmembrane signalling, linking receptors to intracellular effector systems. For neurotransmitter binding, the following types of G protein may be involved:

- Gs
- Gi
- Go
- Gq

SECOND MESSENGERS   Two of the most important second-messenger systems are:

- receptor-neurotransmitter complex $\rightarrow$ G protein binding to receptor-neurotransmitter complex $\rightarrow$ adenylate cyclase activation (or inhibition) $\rightarrow$ cyclic AMP (cAMP)
- neurotransmitter binding $\rightarrow$ hydrolysis of phosphatidylinositol biphosphate (a membrane phospholipid) $\rightarrow$ diacylglycerol and IP_3 (inositol triphosphate); diacylglycerol activates protein kinase C, while IP_3 causes endoplasmic reticulum calcium release, in turn activating calmodulin-dependent protein kinase

Adrenoceptors

The adrenergic receptors are coupled to G proteins, via which they produce their physiological effects. At the time of writing, the main adrenergic receptors and their main effectors (via G protein α subunits) are believed to be:

- $\alpha_{1A} \rightarrow \uparrow Ca^{2+}$ (via Gi/Go)
- $\alpha_{1B} \rightarrow \uparrow IP_3$ (via Gq)
- $\alpha_{1C} \rightarrow \uparrow IP_3$ (via Gq)
- $\alpha_{1D} \rightarrow \uparrow IP_3$ (via Gq)
- α_{2A} (human)/α_{2D} (probably rat homologue) $\rightarrow \downarrow$ adenylyl cyclase, $\uparrow K^+$, $\downarrow Ca^{2+}$ (via Gi)
- $\alpha_{2B} \rightarrow \downarrow$ adenylate cyclase (via Gi)
- $\alpha_{2C} \rightarrow \downarrow$ adenylate cyclase (via Go)
- $\beta_1 \rightarrow \uparrow$ adenylate cyclase (via Gs)
- $\beta_2 \rightarrow \uparrow$ adenylate cyclase (via Gs)

The excitatory α_1 adrenoceptors are postsynaptic, while the inhibitory α_2 adrenoceptors are found as both presynaptic and postsynaptic receptors.

Serotonergic receptors

The main serotonergic receptors, grouped according to their relative homologies, and their signalling systems, believed to exist at the time of writing, are as follows:

$$5-HT_{1A} \rightarrow \downarrow \text{adenylate cyclase}$$
$$5-HT_{1B} \rightarrow \downarrow \text{adenylate cyclase}$$
$$5-HT_{1D\alpha} \rightarrow \downarrow \text{adenylate cyclase}$$
$$5-HT_{1D\beta} \rightarrow \downarrow \text{adenylate cyclase}$$
$$5-HT_{1E} \rightarrow \downarrow \text{adenylate cyclase}$$

$$5-HT_{2A} \rightarrow \uparrow IP_3$$
$$5-HT_{2B} \rightarrow \uparrow IP_3$$
$$5-HT_{2C} \rightarrow \uparrow IP_3$$

$5\text{-}HT_3$ – ion channel

$5\text{-}HT_{5A}$ – signalling system not known at the time of writing
$5\text{-}HT_{5B}$ – signalling system not known at the time of writing

$5\text{-}HT_6 \rightarrow \uparrow$ adenylate cyclase
$5\text{-}HT_7 \rightarrow \uparrow$ adenylate cyclase

Dopaminergic receptors

The dopaminergic receptors are coupled to G proteins, via which they produce their physiological effects. At the time of writing, the main dopaminergic receptors and their main effectors (via G protein α subunits) are believed to be:

$D_1 \rightarrow \uparrow$ adenylate cyclase (via Gs)
$D_2 \rightarrow \downarrow$ adenylate cyclase, $\uparrow K^+$, $\downarrow Ca^{2+}$ (via Gi/Go)
$D_3 \rightarrow \downarrow$ adenylate cyclase, $\uparrow K^+$, $\downarrow Ca^{2+}$ (via Gi/Go)
$D_4 \rightarrow \downarrow$ adenylate cyclase, $\uparrow K^+$, $\downarrow Ca^{2+}$ (via Gi/Go)
$D_5 \rightarrow \uparrow$ adenylate cyclase (via Gs)

GABA receptors

The GABA receptor superfamilies may be large, with multiple types of GABA subunits having been cloned. In general, there are two main types of receptor, the main effects of which are:

$GABA_A \rightarrow \uparrow Cl^-$ (via a receptor-gated ion channel)
$GABA_B \rightarrow \uparrow K^+ \pm Ca^{2+}$ effects (via G protein coupling)

Cholinergic receptors

Cholinergic receptors transduce signals via coupling with G proteins. At the time of writing, the following types are recognized:

- nicotinic
- M1 (muscarinic)
- M2 (muscarinic)
- M3 (muscarinic)
- M4 (muscarinic)
- M5 (muscarinic)

Glutamate receptors

The types of glutamate receptor recognized are:

- NMDA (N-methyl-D-aspartate) receptors
- AMPA (α-amino-3-hydroxy-5-methyl-4-isoxazole propionic acid) receptors
- KA (kainic acid) receptors
- mGluRs (metabotropic glutamate receptors) (= *trans*-ACPD receptors)

The first three classes are ionotropic glutamate receptors that are coupled directly to cation-specific ion channels.

NMDA RECEPTORS   At the time of writing the NMDA receptor subtype is believed to include two families of subunits:

- NMDAR1 (= NR1)
- NMDAR2 (= NR2)

In turn, the following splice variants of NMDAR1 have been recognized:

- NMDAR1A (= NR1a)
- NMDAR1B (= NR1b)

- NMDAR1C (= NR1c)
- NMDAR1D (= NR1d)
- NMDAR1E (= NR1e)
- NMDAR1F (= NR1f)
- NMDAR1G (= NR1g)

Variants of NMDAR2 are modulatory subunits that form heteromeric channels but not homomeric channels.

AMPA RECEPTORS AMPA receptors can be formed from one or any two of:

- GluR1
- GluR2
- GluR3
- GluR4

KA RECEPTORS KA receptors include:

- GluR5
- GluR6
- GluR7
- KA1
- KA2

MGLURS The mGluRs are coupled to G proteins, unlike the other classes of glutamate receptor. At the time of writing, the following subtypes have been cloned:

- mGluR1
- mGluR2
- mGluR3
- mGluR4
- mGluR5
- mGluR6

These have been categorized into the following subgroups:

- subgroup I = mGluR1 and mGluR5
- subgroup II = mGluR2 and mGluR3
- subgroup III = mGluR4 and mGluR6

The effector system for subgroup I involves stimulation of phospholipase C, while that for both subgroup II and subgroup III involves inhibition of adenylate cyclase.

CLASSICAL NEUROTRANSMITTERS

Noradrenaline
BIOSYNTHESIS The primary biosynthetic pathway is:

> tyrosine
> $\rightarrow$ DOPA (3,4-dihydroxyphenylalanine)
> $\rightarrow$ dopamine
> $\rightarrow$ noradrenaline

The corresponding enzymes are:

- tyrosine hydroxylase (acts on tyrosine)
- aromatic amino acid decarboxylase = DOPA decarboxylase (acts on DOPA)
- dopamine-β-hydroxylase (acts on dopamine)

METABOLISM   The metabolic degradation of noradrenaline may begin with the action of either catechol-O-methyltransferase (COMT) or monoamine oxidase (MAO). The catabolic pathway starting with the action of COMT is as follows:

> noradrenaline
> → normetanephrine
> → 3-methoxy-4-hydroxyphenylglycolaldehyde
> → VMA (vanillyl mandelic acid) = 3-methoxy-4-hydroxymandelic acid

The corresponding enzymes are:

- COMT (acts on noradrenaline)
- MAO (acts on normetanephrine)
- aldehyde dehydrogenase (acts on 3-methoxy-4-hydroxyphenylglycolaldehyde)

The catabolic pathway starting with the action of MAO has two major branches. The first branch is as follows:

> noradrenaline
> → 3,4-dihydroxyphenylglycolaldehyde
> → 3,4-dihydroxymandelic acid
> → VMA (vanillyl mandelic acid) = 3-methoxy-4-hydroxymandelic acid

The corresponding enzymes are:

- MAO (acts on noradrenaline)
- aldehyde dehydrogenase (acts on 3,4-dihydroxyphenylglycolaldehyde)
- COMT (acts on 3,4-dihydroxymandelic acid)

The second branch is as follows:

> noradrenaline
> → 3,4-dihydroxyphenylglycolaldehyde
> → 3,4-dihydroxyphenylglycol
> → MHPG (3-methoxy-4-hydroxyphenylglycol)

The corresponding enzymes are:

- MAO (acts on noradrenaline)
- aldehyde reductase (acts on 3,4-dihydroxyphenylglycolaldehyde)
- COMT (acts on 3,4-dihydroxyphenylglycol)

RE-UPTAKE   Following its release into the synaptic cleft, the main method of inactivation of noradrenaline is by means of re-uptake by presynaptic neurones.

Serotonin
BIOSYNTHESIS   The primary biosynthetic pathway is:

> tryptophan
> → 5-hydroxytryptophan
> → serotonin

The corresponding enzymes are:

- tryptophan hydroxylase (acts on tryptophan)
- 5-hydroxytryptophan decarboxylase = amino acid decarboxylase (acts on 5-hydroxytryptophan)

METABOLISM   The metabolic degradation of serotonin is as follows:

> serotonin
> → 5-HIAA (5-hydroxyindoleacetic acid)

The enzyme catalysing this is:

- MAO_A (MAO type A)

Dopamine
BIOSYNTHESIS   The primary biosynthetic pathway is:

> tyrosine
> → DOPA (3,4-dihydroxyphenylalanine)
> → dopamine

The corresponding enzymes are:

- tyrosine hydroxylase (acts on tyrosine)
- aromatic amino acid decarboxylase = DOPA decarboxylase (acts on DOPA)

METABOLISM   The metabolic degradation of dopamine may begin with the action of either COMT or MAO. The catabolic pathway starting with the action of COMT is as follows:

> dopamine
> → 3-methoxytyramine
> → 3-methoxy-4-hydroxyphenylacetaldehyde
> → HVA (homovanillic acid)

The corresponding enzymes are:

- COMT (acts on dopamine)
- MAO (acts on 3-methoxytyramine)
- aldehyde dehydrogenase (acts on 3-methoxy-4-hydroxyphenylacetaldehyde)

(A less important pathway allows 3-methoxy-4-hydroxyphenylacetaldehyde to be metabolized to 3-methoxy-4-hydroxyphenylethanol via the action of aldehyde reductase.)

The catabolic pathway starting with the action of MAO is as follows:

> dopamine
> → 3,4-dihydroxyphenylacetaldehyde
> → DOPAC (dihydroxyphenylacetic acid)
> → HVA

The corresponding enzymes are:

- MAO (acts on dopamine)
- aldehyde dehydrogenase (acts on 3,4-dihydroxyphenylacetaldehyde)
- COMT (acts on DOPAC)

RE-UPTAKE   Following its release into the synaptic cleft, the main method of inactivation of dopamine is by means of re-uptake by presynaptic neurones.

GABA

BIOSYNTHESIS   GABA is derived from glutamic acid via the action of GAD (glutamic acid decarboxylase).

METABOLISM   The metabolic breakdown of GABA to glutamic acid and succinic semialdehyde involves the action of GABA transaminase (GABA-T).

Acetylcholine

BIOSYNTHESIS   Acetylcholine is derived from acetyl CoA and choline, in a reaction catalyzed by choline acetyltransferase.

METABOLISM   After release into the synaptic cleft, acetylcholine is hydrolyzed by cholinesterase into choline and ethanoic (acetic) acid.

NEUROPEPTIDES

Some neurotransmitters consist of small proteins, or peptides. In this section, the following neuropeptide transmitters are considered: CRH, CCK and the endogenous opioid peptides.

Corticotrophin releasing hormone

The cell bodies responsible for secreting corticotrophin releasing factor or hormone (CRF or CRH) are located in the hypothalamic paraventricular nucleus. CRH is secreted from the hypothalamus into the hypothalamopituitary portal system and in turn regulates the release of POMC (pro-opiomelanocortin) derived peptides, including corticotropin, from the adenohypophysis.

Cholecystokinin

Cholecystokinin (CCK), first located as gastrointestinal and pancreatic hormone, occurs in high concentrations in the central nervous system, particularly in the cerebral cortex, hypothalamus, and limbic system. From a neuropsychiatric viewpoint, important cholecystokinin-like peptide fragments in the brain include CCK-tetrapeptide (CCK-4) and octapeptide (CCK-8).

Endogenous opioids

Endogenous opioids isolated from the central nervous system are derived from peptide precursor molecules:

- POMC → corticotropin, β-lipotropin
- proenkephalin → met-enkephalin, leu-enkephalin
- prodynorphin → dynorphin A, dynorphin B, α-neoendorphin

The enkephalins met-enkephalin and leu-enkephalin are each pentapeptides.

BIBLIOGRAPHY

Carpenter, R.H.S. 1996: *Neurophysiology*, 3rd edn. London: Arnold.
Guyton, A.C. and Hall, J.E. 1995: *Textbook of medical physiology*, 9th edn. Philadelphia: W.B. Saunders.
Stryer, L. 1995: *Biochemistry*, 4th edn. New York: R.H. Freeman.

15
General principles of psychopharmacology

HISTORICAL OVERVIEW

Antidepressants
TRICYCLIC ANTIDEPRESSANTS AND MAOIs Tricyclic antidepressants and mono-amine oxidase inhibitors (MAOIs) were introduced between 1955 and 1958:

- MAOIs: this arose from the observation of elevated mood in patients with tuberculosis being treated with the MAOI iproniazid, and less toxic MAOIs were subsequently developed; Kline was one of the first to report the value of MAOI treatment in depression
- tricyclic antidepressants: Kuhn observed the antidepressant action of imipramine, while studying chlorpromazine-like agents

SSRIs The selective serotonin re-uptake inhibitors (SSRIs) were introduced in the late 1980s.

Lithium
In 1886 Lange proposed the use of lithium for treating excited states. Lithium was introduced by Cade in 1949. Following his finding from animal experiments that lithium caused lethargy, Cade observed (in 1948) that it led to clinical improvement in a patient with mania.

Antipsychotics
RESERPINE Reserpine was introduced by Sen and Bose in 1931; in 1953 Kline confirmed that it was a treatment for schizophrenia.

TYPICAL ANTIPSYCHOTICS Important dates in the introduction of typical antipsychotics in psychiatric treatment in the twentieth century include:

- 1950: chlorpromazine synthesized by Charpentier, who was attempting to synthesize an antihistaminergic agent for anaesthetic use; Laborit then reported that chlorpromazine could induce an artificial hibernation
- the efficacy of chlorpromazine in the treatment of psychosis was reported by Paraire and Sigwald in 1951, and by Delay and Deniker in 1952
- 1958: haloperidol was synthesized by Janssen

CLOZAPINE Important dates in the introduction and, after 1988, the reintroduction of the atypical antipsychotic clozapine include:

- 1958: clozapine synthesized as an imipramine analogue; its actions appeared to be closer to chlorpromazine than to imipramine
- 1961–62: first clinical trial in schizophrenia (University Psychiatric Clinic, Bern) gave disappointing results; low doses of clozapine were used
- 1966: Gross and Langner reported good results in chronic schizophrenia
- 1975 and thereafter: clozapine was withdrawn from general clinical use in some countries owing to cases of fatal agranulocytosis (including eight such deaths in Finland in 1975)
- 1988: Kane and colleagues reported positive results from their multicentre double-blind study of clozapine versus chlorpromazine in treatment-resistant schizophrenia; subsequent studies showed that social functioning also improved in response to clozapine

Anxiolytics

BARBITURATES   The first barbiturate, barbituric acid (malonylurea), was synthesized in 1864. The barbiturates were introduced in 1903.

BENZODIAZEPINES   The benzodiazepine chlordiazepoxide was synthesized in the late 1950s by Sternbach (working for Roche) and introduced in 1960.

CLASSIFICATION

The examples given in each class of drug are not meant to be exhaustive.

Antipsychotics (neuroleptics)

TYPICAL ANTIPSYCHOTICS   In the following classification, note that the piperidine group of phenothiazines includes thioridazine, which is classed here as an atypical antipsychotic.

- phenothiazines: aliphatic

    - chlorpromazine
    - methotrimeprazine
    - promazine

- phenothiazines: piperazines

    - fluphenazine
    - trifluoperazine
    - perphenazine
    - prochlorperazine

- phenothiazines: piperidines
    - pipothiazine palmitate
    - pericyazine
- butyrophenones

    - haloperidol
    - droperidol
    - benperidol
    - trifluperidol

- thioxanthenes

    - flupenthixol
    - zuclopenthixol

- diphenylbutylpiperidines

    - pimozide
    - fluspirilene

- loxapine

ATYPICAL ANTIPSYCHOTICS   The atypical antipsychotics include:

- clozapine
- risperidone
- sulpiride (a substituted benzamide)
- thioridazine
- olanzapine
- sertindole
- zotepine (being tested at the time of writing)
- amperozide (being tested at the time of writing)

Antimuscarinics (anticholinergics)

Antimuscarinic (anticholinergic) drugs used in the treatment of Parkinsonism resulting from pharmacotherapy with antipsychotics include:

- procyclidine
- benzhexol
- benztropine
- orphenadrine
- biperiden
- methixene

Prophylaxis of bipolar mood disorder

The drugs most commonly used in the prophylaxis of bipolar mood disorder are:

- lithium
- carbamazepine

Antidepressants

TRICYCLIC ANTIDEPRESSANTS   Tricyclic antidepressants include:

- dibenzocycloheptanes

    - amitriptyline
    - butriptyline
    - nortriptyline
    - protriptyline

- iminodibenzyls

    - clomipramine
    - desipramine
    - imipramine
    - trimipramine

- others

    - dothiepin
    - doxepin
    - iprindole
    - lofepramine

TRICYCLIC-RELATED ANTIDEPRESSANTS   Tricyclic-related antidepressants include:

- trazodone
- viloxazine

MAOIs   Monoamine oxidase inhibitors include:

- hydrazine compounds

  - phenelzine
  - isocarboxazid

- non-hydrazine compounds

  - tranylcypromine

TETRACYCLIC ANTIDEPRESSANTS   Tetracyclic antidepressants include:

- maprotiline
- mianserin

SSRIs   Selective serotonin re-uptake inhibitors include:

- fluvoxamine
- fluoxetine
- sertraline
- paroxetine
- citalopram
- nefazodone

RIMAs   Reversible inhibitors of monoamine oxidase-A (RIMAs) include:

- moclobemide

At the time of writing, the following RIMAs are being tested:

- brofaromine
- cimoxatone
- toloxatone

SNRIs   At the time of writing there is one serotonin noradrenaline re-uptake inhibitor (SNRI) in clinical use:

- venlafaxine

Benzodiazepines

Long-acting benzodiazepines include:

- alprazolam
- bromazepam
- chlordiazepoxide
- clobazam
- clorazepate
- diazepam
- flunitrazepam
- flurazepam
- medazepam
- nitrazepam

Short-acting benzodiazepines include:

- loprazolam
- lorazepam

- lormetazepam
- oxazepam
- temazepam

Other anxiolytics
Non-benzodiazepine anxiolytics in clinical use include:

- azaspirodecanediones: buspirone
- β-adrenoceptor blocking drugs: e.g. propranolol

Drugs used in alcohol dependence
The following drugs are used in alcohol dependence:

- benzodiazepines
- chlormethiazole
- disulfiram
- acamprosate

Drugs used in opioid dependence
The following drugs are used in opioid dependence:

- methadone
- lofexidine
- naltrexone

Antiandrogens
At the time of writing, there is one antiandrogen used for psychiatric reasons:

- cyproterone acetate

OPTIMIZING PATIENT COMPLIANCE

Factors that can help optimize patient compliance include:

- patient education
- setting reasonable expectations
- ↓ number of tablets to be taken
- ↓ dosage frequency
- labelling medicine containers clearly
- parenteral/depot administration
- using alternative medication if there are troublesome side-effects
- involving family members

It is particularly important to avoid polypharmacy, if possible, and to prescribe a simple, straightforward drug regime for elderly patients. Containers used by the elderly should take into account the possibility that the patient may have arthritis, and may also be designed to allow the pharmacist to place the appropriate medication for each intake in clearly labelled boxes.

PLACEBO EFFECT

Definition
A placebo refers to any therapy or component of therapy that is deliberately used for its nonspecific, psychological, or psychophysiological effect, or its

presumed specific effect, but that is without specific activity for the condition being treated.

Mechanisms of the placebo effect

White *et al.* (1985) have proposed the following biopsychosocial model for the mechanisms of the placebo effect:

- homoestatic mechanisms

    - central nervous system function
    - autonomic nervous system function
    - peripheral nervous system function
    - endocrine function
    - immune function

- classical conditioning
- operant conditioning
- cognitive–affective–behavioural self-control
- hypnosis
- the doctor's attitude
- the patient's expectations
- transitional object phenomena

Pill factors

The strength of the placebo effect varies with the physical form of the medication, including the size, type, colour and number of pills (Buckalew and Coffield, 1982; Blackwell *et al.* 1972). For example, the relative placebo effect for the following physical forms has been found to be stronger:

- multiple pills > single pills
- larger pills > smaller pills
- capsules > tablets

Again, examples of the relative potency of medication varying with pill colour include (Schapira *et al.* 1970):

- anxiety symptoms responded better to green tablets
- depressive symptoms responded better to yellow tablets

Controlling for the placebo effect

The above factors can be taken into account in clinical practice. In clinical trials it is important to control for the placebo effect, and this is achieved in the randomized double-blind placebo-controlled design (see Chapter 6 on principles of evaluation and psychometrics).

PRESCRIBING FOR PSYCHIATRIC PATIENTS

Prescribing for psychiatric patients includes taking into consideration the following factors (Cookson *et al.* 1993):

- the symptoms to be targeted in the short and long term
- age
- physical health
- circumstances
- drugs already being taken, including home remedies
- the effectiveness, or otherwise, of previous drug treatments

- personality
- lifestyle
- social setting
- the choice of actual drugs

    - dose size
    - dose schedule

- when to review outcome and who should help report it
- the role of the community psychiatry nurse and the GP in providing medication and monitoring progress

BIBLIOGRAPHY

Blackwell, B., Bloomfield, S.S. and Buncher, C.R. 1972: Demonstration to medical students of placebo responses and nondrug factors. *Lancet* i, 1279–82.

Buckalew, L.W. and Coffield, K.E. 1982: An investigation of drug expectancy as a function of capsule color and size and preparation form. *Journal of Clinical Psychopharmacology.* 2, 245–8.

Cookson, J., Crammer, J. and Heine, B. 1993: *The use of drugs in psychiatry.* 4th edn. London: Gaskell.

Schapira, K., McClelland, H.A., Griffiths, N.R. *et al.* 1970: Study of the effects of tablet colour in the treatment of anxiety states. *British Medical Journal* ii, 446–9.

Silverstone, T. and Turner, P. 1995: *Drug treatment in Psychiatry*, 5th edn. London: Routledge.

White, L., Tursky, B. and Schwartz, G. (eds) 1985: *Placebo: theory, research, and mechanisms.* New York: Guildford Press, 431–47.

16
Pharmacokinetics

ABSORPTION

Routes of administration

ENTERAL ADMINISTRATION   Enteral administration routes employ the gastrointestinal tract, from which the drug is absorbed into the circulation. They include administration via the following routes:

- oral
- buccal
- sublingual
- rectal

PARENTERAL ADMINISTRATION   This includes administration via the following routes:

- intramuscular
- intravenous
- subcutaneous
- inhalational
- topical

Rate of absorption
The rate of absorption of a drug from its site of administration depends on the following factors:

- the form of the drug
- the solubility of the drug, which is influenced by factors such as

    - the pK_a of the drug
    - particle size
    - the ambient pH

- the rate of blood flow through the tissue in which the drug is sited

Oral administration

MECHANISMS OF ABSORPTION   The main mechanisms of absorption of drugs from the gastrointestinal tract are:

- passive diffusion
- pore filtration
- active transport

SITE OF ABSORPTION   The main site of absorption of most psychotropic drugs (which tend to be lipophilic at a physiological pH) from the gastrointestinal tract is the small intestine.

FACTORS INFLUENCING ABSORPTION   Factors influencing the absorption of drugs from the gastrointestinal tract include:

- gastric emptying
- gastric pH
- intestinal motility
- presence/absence of food: the presence of food delays gastric emptying
- intestinal microflora
- area of absorption
- blood flow

The antimuscarinic actions of some psychotropic medication leads to delayed gastric emptying.

Rectal administration

ADVANTAGES   The advantages of rectal administration over the oral route include:

- it can be used if the patient cannot swallow: e.g. because of vomiting
- gastric factors are by-passed
- it can be used for drugs that are irritant to the stomach
- ↓ first-pass metabolism
- it can be useful in uncooperative patients
- it can be used to administer diazepam during an epileptic seizure, for example in a patient with a learning difficulty

DISADVANTAGES   The disadvantages of rectal administration include:

- embarrassment
- the presence of a variable amount of faecal matter → unpredictable rate of absorption
- local inflammation may occur following frequent use of this route

Intramuscular administration

FACTORS INFLUENCING ABSORPTION   The rate of absorption of drugs administered intramuscularly is increased in the following circumstances:

- lipid-soluble drugs
- drugs with a low relative molecular mass
- ↑ muscle blood flow: e.g. after physical exercise or during emotional excitement

DISADVANTAGES   The disadvantages of intramuscular administration include:

- pain
- usually unacceptable for self-administration
- risk of damage to structures such as nerves
- some drugs, e.g. paraldehyde, may cause sterile abscess formation
- ↓ muscle blood flow (e.g. in cardiac failure) → ↓ absorption
- tissue binding or precipitation from solution after intramuscular administration (e.g. for chlordiazepoxide, diazepam, phenytoin) → ↓ absorption
- this route should not be used if the patient is receiving anticoagulant therapy
- ↑ creatine phosphokinase occurs, which may interfere with diagnostic cardiac enzyme assays

Intravenous administration

ADVANTAGES   The advantages of intravenous administration include:

- rapid intravenous administration → rapid action; useful in emergency situations

- drug dose can be titrated against patient response
- large volumes can be administered slowly
- this route can be used for drugs that cannot be absorbed by other routes
- first-pass metabolism is by-passed

DISADVANTAGES   The disadvantages of intravenous administration include:

- adverse effects may occur rapidly
- dangerously high blood levels may be achieved
- it is difficult to recall the drug once administered
- risk of sepsis
- risk of thrombosis
- risk of air embolism
- risk of injection into tissues surrounding the vein, which may lead to necrosis
- risk of injection into an artery, which may lead to spasm
- cannot be used with insoluble drugs

DISTRIBUTION

The rate and degree of distribution of psychotropic drugs between the lipid, protein and water components of the body are influenced by the:

- lipid solubility of the drug
- plasma protein binding
- volume of distribution
- blood–brain barrier
- placenta

Lipid solubility
Increased lipid solubility is associated with increased volume of distribution. This is the case for most psychotropic drugs at physiological pH.

Plasma protein binding
Drugs circulate around the body partly bound to plasma proteins and partly free in the water phase of plasma. This plasma protein binding, which is reversible and competitive, acts as a reservoir for the drug. The main plasma binding protein for acidic drugs is albumin, while basic drugs, including many psychotropic drugs, can also bind to other plasma proteins such as lipoprotein and α_1-acid glycoprotein. The extent of plasma protein binding varies with a number of factors:

- plasma drug concentration
- plasma protein concentration: ↓ in

    - hepatic disease
    - renal disease
    - cardiac failure
    - malnutrition
    - carcinoma
    - surgery
    - burns

- drug interactions

    - displacement
    - plasma protein tertiary structure change

- concentration of physiological substances: e.g. urea, bilirubin and free fatty acid

Volume of distribution

This is a theoretical concept relating the mass of a drug in the body to the blood or plasma concentration:

volume of distribution = (mass of a drug in the body at a given time)/(the concentration of the drug at that time in the blood or the plasma)

A higher volume of distribution in general corresponds to a shorter duration of drug action.

Factors that may influence the volume of distribution include:

- drug lipid solubility: $\uparrow$ lipid solubility (e.g. most psychotropic drugs) $\leftrightarrow$ $\uparrow$ volume of distribution
- adipose tissue: e.g. some psychotropic drugs $\rightarrow$ weight gain $\rightarrow$ $\uparrow$ adipose tissue $\rightarrow$ $\uparrow$ volume of distribution
- age: $\uparrow$ age $\rightarrow$ $\downarrow$ proportion of lean tissue $\rightarrow$ $\uparrow$ volume of distribution
- sex
- physical disease

Blood–brain barrier and brain distribution

COMPONENTS   Components of the blood–brain barrier include:

- tight junctions between adjacent cerebral capillary endothelial cells
- cerebral capillary basement membrane
- gliovascular membrane

DRUG LIPID SOLUBILITY   A high rate of penetration of the blood–brain barrier occurs for non-polar highly lipid soluble drugs, since the brain is a highly lipid organ. Most psychotropic drugs, being highly lipid soluble, can therefore easily cross the blood-brain barrier.

INFECTION   Infection may alter the normal functioning of the blood–brain barrier.

RECEPTORS   The existence of specific brain receptors for many psychotropic drugs leads to psychotropic drug protein binding in the brain, thereby forming a central nervous system reservoir. This does not occur in the CSF, with its very low protein concentration.

ACTIVE TRANSPORT   Active transport mechanisms are used to cross the blood–brain barrier by some physiological substances and drugs, e.g. levodopa.

DIFFUSION   Some small molecules diffuse readily into the brain and CSF from the cerebral circulation, e.g. lithium ions.

Placenta

Drugs may transfer into the fetal circulation from the maternal circulation across the placenta by means of:

- passive diffusion
- active transport
- pinocytosis

Since drugs may cause teratogenesis during the first trimester, they should be avoided during this time if at all possible.

METABOLISM

While some highly water-soluble drugs, e.g. lithium, are excreted unchanged by the kidneys, others, such as most highly lipid-soluble psychotropic drugs, first undergo metabolism (biotransformation) to reduce their lipid solubility and make them more water-soluble, prior to renal excretion. Metabolism sometimes results in the production of pharmacologically active metabolites, e.g. amitriptyline → nortriptyline. Sites of metabolism include the:

- liver: this is the most important site of metabolism
- kidney
- adrenal (suprarenal) cortex
- gastrointestinal tract
- lung
- placenta
- skin
- lymphocytes

Hepatic phase I metabolism (biotransformation)
This leads to a change in the drug molecular structure by the following non-synthetic reactions:

- oxidation: the most common
- hydrolysis
- reduction

The most important type of oxidation reaction is that carried out by microsomal mixed-function oxidases, involving the cytochrome P450 isoenzymes.

Hepatic phase II metabolism (biotransformation)
This is a synthetic reaction involving conjugation between a parent drug/drug metabolite/endogenous substance and a polar endogenous molecule/group. Examples of the latter include:

- glucuronic acid
- sulphate
- acetate
- glutathione
- glycine
- glutamine

The resulting water-soluble conjugate can be excreted by the kidney if the relative molecular mass < approximately 300. If the relative molecular mass > approximately 300, the conjugate can be excreted in the bile.

First-pass effect
The first-pass effect (first-pass metabolism or presystemic elimination) is the metabolism undergone by an orally absorbed drug during its passage from the hepatic portal system through the liver before entering the systemic circulation. It varies between individuals and may be reduced by, for example, hepatic disease, food or drugs that increase hepatic blood flow.

ELIMINATION

Elimination (excretion) of drugs and drug metabolites can take place by means of the:

- kidney: the most important organ for such elimination
- bile and faeces
- lung
- saliva
- sweat
- sebum
- milk

With the exception of pulmonary excretion, in general water-soluble polar drugs and drug metabolites are eliminated more readily by excretory organs than are highly lipid-soluble non-polar ones.

BIBLIOGRAPHY

Cookson, J., Crammer, J. and Heine, B. 1993: *The use of drugs in psychiatry*, 4th edn. London: Gaskell.
King, D.J. 1995: *Seminars in clinical psychopharmacology*. London: Gaskell.
Silverstone, R. and Turner, P. 1995: *Drug treatment in psychiatry*, 5th edn. London: Routledge.

17
Pharmacodynamics

ANTIPSYCHOTICS

Typical antipsychotics
Many of the actions of chlorpromazine, the archetypal antipsychotic, are believed to result from antagonist action to the following neurotransmitters:

- dopamine
- acetylcholine: muscarinic receptors
- adrenaline/noradrenaline
- histamine

Many of these actions also occur, to varying extents, with other typical antipsychotics.

ANTIDOPAMINERGIC ACTION   In general, typical antipsychotics are postulated to act clinically by causing the postsynaptic blockade of dopamine D2 receptors; their antagonism at these receptors is related to their clinical antipsychotic potencies. It is the antidopaminergic action on the mesolimbic-mesocortical pathway which is believed to be the effect required for this clinical action.

   The antidopaminergic action on the tuberoinfundibular pathway causes hormonal side-effects. Hyperprolactinaemia, resulting from the fact that dopamine is a prolactin-inhibitory factor, causes:

- galactorrhoea
- gynaecomastia
- menstrual disturbances
- ↓ sperm count
- ↓ libido

The antidopaminergic action on the nigrostriatal pathway causes extrapyramidal symptoms:

- parkinsonism
- dystonias
- akathisia
- tardive dyskinesia

ANTIMUSCARINIC ACTION   The central antimuscarinic (anticholinergic) actions may cause:

- convulsions
- pyrexia

Peripheral antimuscarinic symptoms include:

- a dry mouth
- blurred vision
- urinary retention

- constipation
- nasal congestion

ANTIADRENERGIC ACTION   Antiadrenergic actions may cause:

- postural hypotension
- ejaculatory failure

ANTIHISTAMINIC ACTION   Antihistaminic effects include:

- drowsiness

Atypical antipsychotics
The atypical antipsychotics have a greater action than do typical antipsychotics on receptors other than dopamine D2 receptors. For example, clozapine, the archetypal atypical antipsychotic, has a higher potency of action than do typical antipsychotics on the following receptors:

- $5-HT_2$
- D4
- D1
- muscarinic
- α-adrenergic

DRUGS USED IN THE TREATMENT OF AFFECTIVE DISORDER

Lithium
Lithium ions, Li^+, are monovalent cations that cause a number of effects, some of which may account for its therapeutic actions, including:

- $\uparrow$ intracellular Na^+
- $\downarrow$ Na,K-ATPase pump activity
- $\uparrow$ intracellular Ca^{2+} in erythrocytes in mania and depression
- $\uparrow$ erythrocyte choline
- $\uparrow$ erythrocyte phospholipid catabolism (via phospholipase D)
- $\downarrow$ Ca^{2+} in platelets in bipolar disorder

- $\uparrow$ serotonergic neurotransmission
- $\downarrow$ central $5-HT_1$ and $5-HT_2$ receptor density (demonstrated in the hippocampus)
- $\uparrow$ dopamine turnover in hypothalamic-tuberoinfundibular dopaminergic neurones
- $\downarrow$ central dopamine synthesis (dose-dependent)
- normalization of low plasma and CSF levels of GABA in bipolar disorder
- $\uparrow$ GABAergic neurotransmission
- $\downarrow$ low affinity GABA receptors in the corpus striatum and hypothalamus (chronic lithium administration)
- $\uparrow$ met-enkephalin and leu-enkephalin in the basal ganglia and nucleus accumbens
- $\uparrow$ dynorphin in the corpus striatum

Tricyclic antidepressants
The most important postulated modes of action in the brain of tricyclic antidepressants in achieving therapeutic effects are:

- inhibition of re-uptake of noradrenaline
- inhibition of re-uptake of serotonin

For this reason, tricyclic antidepressants are also known as monoamine re-uptake inhibitors, or MARIs. Peripherally, most tricyclic antidepressants also have an antimuscarinic action, which gives rise to peripheral antimuscarinic side-effects such:

- dry mouth
- blurred vision
- urinary retention
- constipation

Postural hypotension occurs as a result of the antiadrenergic action.

SSRIs

The most important postulated mode of action in the brain of SSRIs (selective serotonin re-uptake inhibitors) in achieving therapeutic effects is the:

- inhibition of re-uptake of serotonin

Their relatively selective action on serotonin re-uptake means that SSRIs are less likely than tricyclic antidepressants to cause antimuscarinic side-effects. They are, however, more likely to cause gastrointestinal side-effects such as nausea and vomiting.

MAOIs

The most important postulated mode of action in the brain of MAOIs (mono-amine oxidase inhibitors) in achieving therapeutic effects is the:

- irreversible inhibition of MAO-A and MAO-B

In the central nervous system, MAO-A (monoamine oxidase type A) acts on:

- noradrenaline
- serotonin
- dopamine
- tyramine

In the central nervous system, MAO-B (monoamine oxidase type B) acts on:

- dopamine
- tyramine
- phenylethylamine
- benzylamine

The inhibition of peripheral pressor amines, particularly dietary tryramine, by MAOIs can lead to a hypertensive crisis when foodstuffs rich in tyramine are eaten (see Chapter 18 on adverse drug reactions).

RIMAs

The most important postulated mode of action in the brain of RIMAs (reversible inhibitors of monoamine oxidase-A) in achieving therapeutic effects is the:

- reversible inhibition of MAO-A

SNRIs

The most important postulated modes of action in the brain of SNRIs (serotonin noradrenaline re-uptake inhibitors) in achieving therapeutic effects are the:

- inhibition of re-uptake of noradrenaline
- inhibition of re-uptake of serotonin

ANXIOLYTICS AND HYPNOTICS

Benzodiazepines
The most important postulated mode of action in the brain of benzodiazepines in achieving central therapeutic effects is:

- binding to $GABA_A$ receptors

Buspirone
The most important postulated mode of action in the brain of the azaspiro-decanedione buspirone in achieving central therapeutic effects is:

- partial agonism at $5\text{-}HT_{1A}$ receptors

β-adrenoceptor blocking drugs
The most important postulated mode of action of the β-adrenoceptor blocking drugs in achieving anxiolytic effects is:

- antagonism at peripheral β-adrenoceptors

Zopiclone
The cyclopyrrolone zopiclone is believed to achieve a central hypnotic effect by acting on the same receptors as do benzodiazepines.

Zolpidem
The imidazopyridine zolpidem in believed to achieve a central hypnotic effect by acting on the same receptors as do benzodiazepines.

ANTI-EPILEPTIC AGENTS

Carbamazepine
Carbamazepine, which has a tricyclic antidepressant-like structure, may achieve its anticonvulsant effect on the basis of the following actions:

- binding to and inactivation of voltage dependent Na^+ channels
- $\uparrow K^+$ conductance
- partial agonism at the adenosine A_1 subclass of P_1 purinoceptors

Sodium valproate
Sodium valproate may achieve its anticonvulsant effect on the basis of the following actions:

- $\uparrow$ GABA

    - $\downarrow$ GABA breakdown
    - $\uparrow$ GABA release
    - $\downarrow$ GABA turnover
    - $\uparrow$ GABA-B receptor density
    - $\uparrow$ neuronal responsiveness to GABA

- $\downarrow Na^+$ influx
- $\uparrow K^+$ conductance

Phenytoin

The mechanism of anticonvulsant action of phenytoin is unknown, but may involve:

- membrane stabilization
    - Na^+ channel binding
    - Ca^{2+} channel binding
- benzodiazepine receptor binding
- GABA receptor function modulation

Phenobarbitone

The actions of phenobarbitone may be similar to those given above for phenytoin.

Gabapentin

Gabapentin is believed to achieve its anticonvulsant effect by means of the following action:

- binding to a unique cerebral receptor site

Vigabatrin

Vigabatrin is believed to achieve its anticonvulsant effect by means of the following action:

- inhibition of GABA transaminase → ↑ GABA release

Lamotrigine

Lamotrigine is believed to achieve its anticonvulsant effect by means of the following action:

- inhibition of glutamate release

NEUROCHEMICAL EFFECTS OF ECT

Noradrenaline

ECT probably leads to increased noradrenergic function. In particular, ECT acutely causes:

- ↑ cerebral noradrenaline activity
- ↑ cerebral tyrosine hydroxylase activity
- ↑ plasma catecholamines, particularly adrenaline

Chronic ECS (electroconvulsive shock) leads to:

- ↓ β-adrenergic receptor density

The last effect may be a result of receptor down-regulation.

Serotonin

ECT probably leads to increased serotonergic function. In particular, ECT acutely causes:

- ↑ cerebral serotonin concentration

Chronic ECS leads to:

- ↑ 5-HT$_2$ receptor density

Dopamine

ECT probably leads to increased dopaminergic function. In particular, ECT acutely causes:

- ↑ cerebral dopamine concentration
- ↑ cerebral concentration of dopamine metabolites
- ↑ behavioural responsiveness to dopamine agonists

In rat substantia nigra, repeated electroconvulsive shocks lead to:

- ↑ dopamine D_1 receptor density
- ↑ second-messenger potentiation at dopamine D_1 receptors

GABA

ECT may cause a functional increase in GABAergic activity.

Acetylcholine

ECT probably leads to decreased central cholinergic function. In particular, ECT acutely causes:

- ↓ cerebral acetylcholine concentration
- ↑ cerebral acetyltransferase activity
- ↑ cerebral acetylcholinesterase activity
- ↑ CSF acetylcholine concentration

Chronic ECS leads to:

- ↓ muscarinic cholinergic receptor density in the cerebral cortex
- ↓ muscarinic cholinergic receptor density in the hippocampus
- ↓ second messenger response in the hippocampus

Endogenous opioids

Chronic ECS leads to:

- ↑ cerebral met-enkephalin concentration and synthesis
- ↑ cerebral β-endorphin concentration and synthesis
- changes in opioid ligand binding

Adenosine

Chronic ECS leads to:

- ↑ cerebral adenosine A_1 purinoceptor density

BIBLIOGRAPHY

Bloom, F.E. and Kupfer, D.J. (eds) 1995: *Psychopharmacology: the fourth generation of progress.* New York: Ravens Press.

Cookson, J., Crammer, J. and Heine, B. 1993: *The use of drugs in psychiatry,* 4th edn. London: Gaskell.

King, D.J. 1995: *Seminars in clinical psychopharmacology.* London: Gaskell.

Silverstone, T. and Turner, P. 1995: *Drug treatment in psychiatry,* 5th edn. London: Routledge.

18

Adverse drug reactions

TYPES OF ADVERSE DRUG REACTIONS

Classification
Adverse drug reactions may be classified as:

- intolerance
- idiosyncratic reactions
- allergic reactions
- drug interactions

Causal relationship
The following criteria have been suggested as making it more likely that a causal connection exists between a drug and an alleged effect (Edwards 1995):

- there is a close temporal relationship between the effect and the taking of the drug, or toxic levels of the drug or its active metabolites in body fluids have been demonstrated
- the effect differs from manifestations of the disorder being treated
- no other substances are being taken or withdrawn when the effect occurs
- the reaction disappears when the treatment is stopped
- the effect reappears with a rechallenge test

Intolerance
In drug intolerance the adverse reactions are consistent with the known pharmacological actions of the drug. These adverse drug reactions may be dose-related.

Idiosyncratic reactions
Idiosyncratic adverse drug reactions are reactions which are not characteristic or predictable and which are associated with an individual human difference not present in members of the general population.

Allergic reactions
Allergic reactions to drugs involve the body's immune system, with the drug interacting with a protein to form an immunogen which causes sensitization and the induction of an immune response. Criteria suggesting an allergic reaction include:

- a different time-course from that of the pharmacodynamic action, for example:
  - delayed onset of the adverse drug reaction
  - the adverse drug reaction manifests only following repeated drug exposure
- there may be no dose-related effect, with subtherapeutically small doses leading to sensitization or allergic reactions

- a hypersensitivity reaction occurs, which is unrelated to the pharmacological actions of the drug

Types of allergic reaction to drugs include:

- anaphylactic shock: type I hypersensitivity reaction
- haematological reactions: type II, III or IV hypersensitivity reaction; for example
  - haemolytic anaemia
  - agranulocytosis
  - thrombocytopenia
- allergic liver damage: type II $\pm$ III hypersensitivity reaction
- skin rashes: type IV hypersensitivity reaction
- generalized autoimmune (systemic lupus erythematosus-like) disease: type IV hypersensitivity reaction

Drug interactions

Adverse drug reactions may result from interactions between different drugs. These may result from:

- pharmacokinetic interactions
- pharmacodynamic interactions

PHARMACOKINETIC INTERACTIONS   Pharmacokinetic interactions between drugs include:

- precipitation or inactivation following the mixing of drugs
- chelation
- changes in gastrointestinal tract motility
- changes in gastrointestinal tract pH
- drug displacement from binding sites
- enzyme induction
- enzyme inhibition
- competition for renal tubular transport
- changes in urinary pH $\rightarrow$ changes in drug excretion

PHARMACODYNAMIC INTERACTIONS   Pharmacodynamic interactions between drugs include:

- inhibition of drug uptake
- inhibition of drug transport
- interaction at receptors
- synergism
- changes in fluid and electrolyte balance

PSYCHOTROPIC MEDICATION

Typical antipsychotics

In the previous chapter, the major categories of adverse drug reactions are given that are believed to be caused by antagonist action to the following neurotransmitters:

- dopamine
- acetylcholine: muscarinic receptors

- adrenaline/noradrenaline
- histamine

Other important adverse drug reactions include:

- photosensitization
- hypothermia or pyrexia
- allergic (sensitivity) reactions
- neuroleptic malignant syndrome

PHOTOSENSITIZATION　Photosensitization is more common with chlorpromazine than with other typical antipsychotics.

HYPOTHERMIA OR PYREXIA　Interference with temperature regulation is a dose-related side-effect.

ALLERGIC (SENSITIVITY) REACTIONS　Sensitivity reactions include:

- agranulocytosis
- leucopenia
- leucocytosis
- haemolytic anaemia

NEUROLEPTIC MALIGNANT SYNDROME　Neuroleptic malignant syndrome is characterized by:

- hyperthermia
- fluctuating level of consciousness
- muscular rigidity
- autonomic dysfunction

    - tachycardia
    - labile blood pressure
    - pallor
    - sweating
    - urinary incontinence

Laboratory investigations commonly, but not invariably, demonstrate:

- ↑ creatinine phosphokinase
- ↑ white blood count
- abnormal liver function tests

Neuroleptic malignant syndrome requires urgent medical treatment.

CHRONIC PHARMACOTHERAPY　Long-term high-dose pharmacotherapy may cause ocular and skin changes, such as:

- opacity of the lens
- opacity of the cornea
- purplish pigmentation of the skin
- purplish pigmentation of the conjunctiva
- purplish pigmentation of the cornea
- purplish pigmentation of the retina

Atypical antipsychotics

Clozapine may cause neutropenia and potentially fatal agranulocytosis, because of which regular haematological monitoring is required. Other side-effects of clozapine include hypersalivation and side-effects common to chlorpromazine, including extrapyramidal symptoms.

Antimuscarinic drugs

Antimuscarinic drugs used in parkinsonism may give rise to the following side-effects:

- antimuscarinic side-effects (see previous chapter)
- worsening of tardive dyskinesia
- gastrointestinal tract disturbances
- hypersensitivity

Lithium

RENAL FUNCTION   Since lithium ions are excreted mainly by the kidneys, renal function must be checked before commencing pharmacotherapy with lithium.

PLASMA LEVELS   The therapeutic index of lithium is low and therefore regular plasma lithium level monitoring is required. (Therapeutic index = [toxic dose]/[therapeutic dose].) The dose is adjusted to achieve a lithium level of 0.4 to 1.0 mmol L^{-1} for prophylactic purposes, with lower levels being used in the elderly.

SIDE-EFFECTS   Side-effects of lithium therapy include:

- fatigue
- drowsiness
- dry mouth
- a metallic taste
- polydipsia
- polyuria
- nausea
- vomiting
- weight gain
- diarrhoea
- fine tremor
- muscle weakness
- oedema

Oedema should not be treated with diuretics since thiazide and loop diuretics reduce lithium excretion and can thereby cause lithium intoxication.

INTOXICATION   Signs of lithium intoxication include:

- mild drowsiness and sluggishness → giddiness and ataxia
- lack of coordination
- blurred vision
- tinnitus
- anorexia
- dysarthria
- vomiting
- diarrhoea
- coarse tremor
- muscle weakness

SEVERE OVERDOSAGE   At lithium plasma levels of greater than 2 mmol L^{-1} the following effects can occur:

- hyperreflexia and hyperextension of the limbs
- toxic psychoses
- convulsions
- syncope
- oliguria

- circulatory failure
- coma
- death

CHRONIC THERAPY   Long-term treatment with lithium may give rise to:

- thyroid function disturbances

    - goitre
    - hypothyroidism

- memory impairment
- nephrotoxicity
- cardiovascular changes

    - T-wave flattening on the ECG
    - arrhythmias

Thyroid function tests are usually carried out routinely every six months in order to check for lithium-induced disturbances.

Carbamazepine

Since carbamazepine may lower the white blood count, regular monitoring of plasma carbamazepine levels should be carried out.

Tricyclic antidepressants

The psychopharmacological basis of important side-effects of tricyclic antidepressants is as follows:

- blockade of ACh muscarinic receptors
- blockade of histamine H_1 receptors
- blockade of α_1-adrenoceptors
- blockade of 5–$HT_{2/1c}$ serotonergic receptors
- membrane stabilization

BLOCKADE OF MUSCARINIC RECEPTORS   This leads to antimuscarinic side-effects (see previous chapter).

BLOCKADE OF HISTAMINE H_1 RECEPTORS   This can lead to:

- weight gain
- drowsiness

BLOCKADE OF α_1-ADRENOCEPTORS   This can lead to:

- drowsiness
- postural hypotension
- sexual dysfunction
- cognitive impairment

BLOCKADE OF 5–$HT_{2/1c}$ RECEPTORS   This can lead to:

- weight gain

MEMBRANE STABILIZATION   Membrane stabilization can lead to:

- cardiotoxicity
- ↓ seizure threshold

CARDIOVASCULAR SIDE-EFFECTS   These include:

- ECG changes

- arrhythmias
- postural hypotension
- tachycardia
- syncope

ALLERGIC AND HAEMATOLOGICAL REACTIONS   These include:

- agranulocytosis
- leucopenia
- eosinophilia
- thrombocytopenia
- skin rash
- photosensitization
- facial oedema
- allergic cholestatic jaundice

ENDOCRINE SIDE-EFFECTS   These include:

- testicular enlargement
- gynaecomastia
- galactorrhoea

OTHERS   Other side-effects include:

- tremor
- black tongue
- paralytic ileus
- sweating
- hyponatraemia: particularly in the elderly
- neuroleptic malignant syndrome: very rare with tricyclic antidepressants
- abnormal liver function tests
- movement disorders
- pyrexia
- (hypo)mania
- blood glucose changes

SSRIs

Important side-effects that may occur with SSRIs include:

- dose-related gastrointestinal side-effects

    - nausea
    - vomiting
    - diarrhoea

- headache
- restlessness
- sleep disturbance
- anxiety
- delayed orgasm

MAOIs

DANGEROUS FOOD INTERACTIONS   As mentioned in the previous chapter, the inhibition of peripheral pressor amines, particularly dietary tryramine, by MAOIs can lead to a hypertensive crisis when foodstuffs rich in tyramine are eaten. Foods that should therefore be avoided when on treatment with MAOIs include:

- cheese: except cottage cheese and cream cheese
- meat extracts and yeast extracts
- alcohol: particularly chianti, fortified wines and beer
- non-fresh fish
- non-fresh meat
- non-fresh poultry
- offal
- avocado
- banana skins
- broad-bean pods
- caviar
- herring: pickled or smoked

DANGEROUS DRUG INTERACTIONS Medicines that should be avoided by patients taking MAOIs include:

- indirectly acting sympathomimetic amines, e.g.

  - amphetamine
  - fenfluramine
  - ephedrine
  - phenylpropanolamine

- cough mixtures containing sympathomimetics
- nasal decongestants containing sympathomimetics
- L-dopa
- pethidine
- tricyclic antidepressants

OTHER SIDE-EFFECTS Other side-effects of MAOIs include:

- antimuscarinic actions
- hepatotoxicity
- appetite stimulation
- weight gain
- tranylcypromine may cause dependency

Benzodiazepines

An important side-effect of benzodiazepines is psychomotor impairment. If benzodiazepines are taken regularly for four weeks or more, dependence may develop, so that the sudden cessation of intake may then lead to a withdrawal syndrome whose main features include:

- anxiety symptoms

  - palpitations
  - tremor
  - panic
  - dizziness
  - nausea
  - sweating
  - other somatic symptoms

- low mood
- abnormal experiences

  - depersonalization

- derealization
- hypersensitivity to sensations in all modalities
- distorted perception of space
- tinnitus
- formication
- a strange taste

- influenza-like symptoms
- psychiatric/neurological symptoms

  - epileptic seizures
  - confusional states
  - psychotic episodes

- insomnia
- loss of appetite
- weight loss

Buspirone
The main side-effects of buspirone are:

- dizziness
- headache
- excitement
- nausea

Disulfiram
If alcohol is drunk while disulfiram is being taken regularly, acetaldehyde accumulates. Thus, ingesting even small amounts of alcohol then causes unpleasant systemic reactions, including:

- facial flushing
- headache
- palpitations
- tachycardia
- nausea
- vomiting

The ingestion of large amounts of alcohol while being treated with disulfiram can lead to:

- air hunger
- arrhythmias
- severe hypotension

Cyproterone acetate
The side-effects of this antiandrogen agent in males include:

- the inhibition of spermatogenesis
- tiredness
- gynaecomastia
- weight gain
- the improvement of existing acne vulgaris
- ↑ scalp hair growth
- female pattern of pubic hair growth

Liver function tests should be carried out regularly because of a theoretical risk to the liver. Dyspnoea may result from high-dose treatment.

OFFICIAL GUIDANCE

The official guidance in Britain on the use of antipsychotic drugs and benzodiazepines is given in this section. The BNF is the abbreviation for the latest *British National Formulary*, a six-monthly publication of the British Medical Association and the Royal Pharmaceutical Society of Great Britain.

Antipsychotic doses above the BNF upper limit
The Royal College of Psychiatrists has published advice on the use of antipsychotic doses above the BNF upper limit. This advice is reproduced in the BNF:
   Unless otherwise stated, doses in the BNF are licensed doses: any higher dose is therefore *unlicensed*.

1   Consider alternative approaches including adjuvant therapy and newer or atypical neuroleptics such as clozapine.
2   Bear in mind risk factors, including obesity: particular caution is indicated in older patients especially those over 70.
3   Consider potential for drug interactions [published in an appendix to the BNF].
4   Carry out ECG to exclude untoward abnormalities such as prolonged QT interval; repeat ECG periodically and reduce dose if prolonged QT interval or other adverse abnormality develops.
5   Increase dose slowly and not more often than once weekly.
6   Carry out regular pulse, blood pressure, and temperature checks; ensure that the patient maintains adequate fluid intake.
7   Consider high-dose therapy to be for a limited period and review regularly; abandon if there is no improvement after three months (return to standard dosage).

Important: When prescribing an antipsychotic for administration on an emergency basis it must be borne in mind that the intramuscular dose should be *lower* than the corresponding oral dose (owing to the absence of first-pass effect), particularly if the patient is very active (increased blood flow to muscle considerably increases the rate of absorption). The prescription should specify the dose in the context of *each route* and should *not* imply that the same dose can be given by mouth or by intramuscular injection. The dose should be reviewed *daily*.

Benzodiazepines
In Britain, the Committee on Safety of Medicines has issued the following advice with respect to the presciption of benzodiazepines:

1   Benzodiazepines are indicated for the short-term relief (two to four weeks only) of anxiety that is severe, disabling or subjecting the individual to unacceptable distress, occurring alone or in association with insomnia or short-term psychosomatic, organic or psychotic illness.
2   The use of benzodiazepines to treat short-term 'mild' anxiety is inappropriate and unsuitable.
3   Benzodiazepines should be used to treat insomnia only when it is severe, disabling or subjecting the individual to extreme distress.

Prevention of adverse drug reactions
The BNF gives the following advice for preventing adverse drug reactions:

1   Never use any drug unless there is a good indication. If the patient is pregnant do not use a drug unless the need for it is imperative.
2   It is very important to recognize allergy and idiosyncrasy as causes of adverse drug reactions. Ask if the patient had previous reactions.

3   Ask if the patient is already taking other drugs *including self-medication*; remember that interactions may occur.
4   Age and hepatic or renal disease may alter the metabolism or excretion of drugs, so that much smaller doses may need to be prescribed. Pharmacogenetic factors may also be responsible for variations in the rate of metabolism, notably of isoniazid and the tricyclic antidepressants.
5   Prescribe as few drugs as possible and give very clear instructions to the elderly or any patient likely to misunderstand complicated instructions.
6   When possible use a familiar drug. With a new drug be particularly alert for adverse reactions or unexpected events.
7   If serious adverse reactions are liable to occur warn the patient.

REPORTING

Britain
In Britain, the CSM holds an information database for adverse drug reactions. Doctors practising in Britain are asked to report adverse drug reactions to:

> CSM
> Freepost
> London SW8 5BR
> Tel: 0171–627 3291

Yellow prepaid lettercards for reporting are available from the above address, by dialling a 24-hour Freefone service (dial 100 and ask for 'CSM Freefone'), and in the BNF.

ADROIT
ADROIT (Adverse Drug Reactions On-line Information Tracking) is an online service used in Britain to monitor adverse drug reactions.

Newer drugs
In the BNF these are indicated by the symbol ▼. The BNF advises that doctors are asked to report all suspected reactions.

Established drugs
The BNF advises that doctors are asked to report all serious suspected reactions. These include those that are fatal, life-threatening, disabling, incapacitating, or which result in or prolong hospitalization.

BIBLIOGRAPHY

Bloom, F.E., and Kupfer, D.J. (eds) 1995: *Psychopharmacology: the fourth generation of progress.* New York: Raven Press.
British Medical Association and Royal Pharmaceutical Society of Great Britain. *British national formulary.* London: British Medical Association and Royal Pharmaceutical Society of Great Britain.
Cookson, J., Crammer, J. and Heine, B. 1993: *The use of drugs in psychiatry,* 4th edn. London: Gaskell.
Edwards, J.G. 1995: Adverse reactions to and interactions with psychotropic drugs: mechanisms, methods of assessment, and medicolegal considerations. In: King, D.J. (ed.) *Seminars in clinical psychopharmacology.* London: Gaskell Press, 480–513.

19
Genetics

BASIC CONCEPTS

Chromosomes

NUMBER   In normal humans the genome is distributed on 46 chromosomes in each somatic cell nucleus:

- one pair of sex chromosomes
- 44 autosomes = 22 pairs of chromosomes

SEX CHROMOSOMES   The sex chromosomes are the X and Y chromosomes:

- normal females: XX
- normal males: XY

KARYOTYPE   This is an arrangement of the chromosomal make-up of somatic cells which can be produced by carrying out the following procedures in turn:

- arrest cell division at an appropriate stage
- disperse the chromosomes
- fix the chromosomes
- stain the chromosomes
- photograph the chromosomes
- identify the chromosomes
- arrange the chromosomes

CENTROMERE   This is the somewhat constricted region of each chromosome that is particularly evident during mitosis and meiosis.

METACENTRIC CHROMOSOMES   These are chromosomes with a centrally or almost centrally positioned centromere.

ACROCENTRIC CHROMOSOMES   These are chromosomes in which the centromere is very near to one end.

CHROMOSOMAL MAP   The system agreed at the International Paris Conference in 1971 is as follows:

- 1st position: a number (1 to 22) or letter (X or Y) that identifies the chromosome
- 2nd position: p (short arm of chromosome) or q (long arm of chromosome)
- 3rd position (region): a digit corresponding to a stretch of the chromosome lying between two relatively distinct morphological landmarks
- 4th position (band): a digit corresponding to a band derived from the staining properties of the chromosome

Cell division

MITOSIS   This is the process of nuclear division allowing many somatic cells to undergo cell division via the following stages:

- interphase
- prophase
- metaphase
- anaphase
- telophase

MEIOSIS   This process involves two stages of cell division and occurs in gametogenesis via the following stages:

- interphase
- prophase I
- metaphase I
- anaphase I
- telophase I
- prophase II
- metaphase II
- anaphase II
- telophase II

Chromosomal division takes place once during meiosis, so that the resulting gametes are haploid. Recombination takes place during prophase I.

Gene structure

Genes, the biological units of heredity, consist of codons grouped into exons with intervening nucleotide sequences known as introns. The introns do not code for amino acids. Genes also contain nucleotide sequences at their beginning and end that allow transcription to take place accurately. Thus, starting from the 5′ end (upstream), a typical eukaryotic gene contains the following:

- upstream site regulating transcription
- promoter (TATA)
- transcription initiation site
- 5′ noncoding region
- exons
- introns
- 3′ noncoding region, containing a poly A addition site

Transcription

This is the step in gene expression in which information from the DNA molecule is transcribed on to a primary RNA transcript. This is followed by splicing and nuclear transport, so that the information (minus that from introns) then exists in the cytoplasm of the cell on mRNA (messenger RNA).

Translation

Following transcription, splicing and nuclear transport, translation is the process in gene expression whereby mRNA acts as a template allowing the genetic code to be deciphered to allow the formation of a peptide chain. This process involves tRNA molecules.

Patterns of inheritance

In this section, R and S are dominant alleles, and r and s the corresponding recessive alleles.

LAW OF UNIFORMITY   Consider two homozygous parents with genotypes RR and rr, respectively. Mating (×) results in the next (F1) generation having the genotype shown:

Parents: RR × rr
F1:   Rr

MENDEL'S FIRST LAW   This is also known as the law of segregation.

Parents: Rr × Rr
F1:   RR: Rr: rr = 1:2:1

MENDEL'S SECOND LAW   This is also known as the law of independent assortment.

Parents: RRSS × rrss
F1:   RrSs
F2:   independent assortment of different alleles → RRSS, RRSs, . . ., rrss

AUTOSOMAL DOMINANT INHERITANCE   Autosomal dominant disorders result from the presence of an abnormal dominant allele causing the individual to manifest the abnormal phenotypic trait. Features of autosomal dominant transmission include:

- the phenotypic trait is present in all individuals carrying the dominant allele
- the phenotypic trait does not skip generations: vertical transmission takes place
- males and females are affected
- male to male transmission can take place
- transmission is not solely dependent on parental consanguineous matings
- if one parent is homozgyous for the abnormal dominant allele, all the members of F1 will manifest the abnormal phenotypic trait

Variable expressivity can cause clinical features of autosomal dominant disorders to vary between affected individuals. This, together with reduced penetrance, may give the appearance that the disorder has skipped a generation. The sudden appearance of an autosomal dominant disorder may occur as a result of a new dominant mutation.

AUTOSOMAL RECESSIVE INHERITANCE   Autosomal recessive disorders result from the presence of two abnormal recessive alleles causing the individual to manifest the abnormal phenotypic trait. Features of autosomal recessive transmission include:

- heterozygous individuals are generally carriers who do not manifest the abnormal phenotypic trait
- the rarer the disorder the more likely it is that the parents are consanguineous
- the disorder tends to miss generations but the affected individuals in a family tend to be found among siblings: horizontal transmission takes place

X-LINKED RECESSIVE INHERITANCE   In X-linked recessive disorders a recessive abnormal allele is carried on the X chromosome. All male (XY) offspring inheriting this allele manifest the abnormal phenotypic trait. Other features of X-linked recessive transmission include:

- male-to-male transmission does not take place
- female heterozygotes are carriers

X-LINKED DOMINANT INHERITANCE   In X-linked dominant disorders a dominant abnormal allele is carried on the X chromosome. If an affected male mates with an unaffected female, all the daughters and none of the sons are affected. If an unaffected male mates with an affected heterozygous female, half the daughters and half the sons, on average, are affected. Again, male-to-male transmission does not take place.

ANTICIPATION   This refers to the occurrence of an autonomic dominant disorder at earlier ages of onset or with greater severity in the succeeding generations. In Huntington's disease it has been shown to be caused by expansions of unstable triplet repeat sequences.

MOSAICISM   Abnormalities in mitosis can give rise to an abnormal cell line. Such mosaicism may affect somatic cells (somatic mosaicism) or germ cells (gonadal mosaicism).

UNIPARENTAL DISOMY   This refers to the phenomenon in which an individual inherits both homologues of a chromosome pair from the same parent.

GENOMIC IMPRINTING   This refers to the phenomenon in which an allele is differentially expressed depending on whether it is maternally or paternally derived.

MITOCHONDRIAL INHERITANCE   Since mtDNA (mitochondrial DNA) is essentially maternally inherited, mitochondrial inheritance may explain some cases of disorders that affect both male and females but that are transmitted through females only and not through males.

TRADITIONAL TECHNIQUES

Family studies
METHODOLOGY   The rates of illness in the first and second degree relatives of probands are compared with the corresponding rates in the general population. First degree relatives have, on average, 50 per cent of the genome in common with the proband, and include the biological:

- father
- mother
- brothers
- sisters
- children

Second degree relatives have, on average, 25 per cent of the genome in common with the proband, and include the biological:

- grandfathers
- grandmothers
- uncles
- aunts
- nephews
- nieces
- grandsons
- grandaughters

DIFFICULTIES   Difficulties (and possible solutions) with family studies applied to psychiatric disorders include:

- psychiatric disorders need to be considered longitudinally: lifetime expectancy rates or morbid risks can be used
- at the time of the study some relatives may not have reached an age range during which the disorder manifests itself: Weinberg's age correction method can be used

- genetic factors are not separated well from environmental factors: twin and adoption studies can be used

Twin studies

METHODOLOGY   The rates of illness in cotwins of monozygotic and dizygotic probands are compared. Monozygotic twins share 100 per cent of the genome, whereas dizygotic twins share, on average, 50 per cent of their genome. The rate of concurrence of a disorder in the cotwin of a proband is the concordance rate:

- pairwise rate (as a percentage) = 100(number of concordant pairs of twins)/ (total number of twin pairs) per cent
- probandwise rate (as a percentage) = 100(number of cotwins of probands in whom the disorder is concurrent)/(total number of cotwins) per cent

DIFFICULTIES   Difficulties (and possible solutions) with twin studies applied to psychiatric disorders include:

- pairwise and probandwise concordance rates usually give different results: take care to note the method used to determine the concordance rate
- zygosity was determined less accurately in older twin studies: use modern more accurate methods
- diagnostic variability occurred in older twin studies: use more detailed modern diagnostic criteria
- sampling bias may occur: use twin registers
- twins are at greater risk of central nervous system abnormalities resulting from birth injury or congenital abnormalities (risk to monozygotic twins > risk to dizygotic twins), which may introduce errors if central nervous system abnormalities contribute to the disorder being studied
- assortative mating may lead to a relative increase in the rate of illness in dizygotic twins compared with monozygotic twins
- age correction techniques may introduce errors: do not use age correction techniques
- the environment does not necessarily affect twins equally: use adoption studies

Adoption studies

METHODOLOGY   Individuals are studied who have been brought up by unrelated adoptive parents from an early age, instead of by their biological parents. Types of adoption studies include:

- adoptee studies
- adoptee family studies
- cross-fostering studies
- adoption studies involving monozygotic twins

DIFFICULTIES   Difficulties with adoption studies applied to psychiatric disorders include:

- few cases fulfil the criteria for adoption studies
- adoption studies take a long time to carry out
- information about the biological father may not be available
- adoption may cause indeterminate psychological sequelae for the adoptees
- the process of adoption is unlikely to be random
- in monozygotic twin studies it cannot be assumed that the environmental influences on each twin are more or less equivalent following adoption

TECHNIQUES IN MOLECULAR GENETICS

Restriction enzymes
Restriction enzymes, also known as restriction endonucleases, cleave DNA only at locations containing specific nucleotide sequences. Different restriction enzymes target different nucleotide sequences, but a given restriction enzyme targets the same sequence.

Gene library
This is a set of cloned DNA fragments representing all the genes of an organism or of a given chromosome.

Molecular cloning
This technique can be used to create a gene library. It can be carried out by splicing a given stretch of (human) DNA, cleaved using a restriction enzyme, into a bacterial plasmid having at least one antibiotic resistance gene. After the reintroduction of the resulting recombinant plasmid into bacteria, antibiotic selective pressure causes these bacteria to reproduce. Multiple recoverable copies of the original (human) DNA are contained in the resulting bacterial colonies.

Gene probes
These are lengths of DNA that are constructed so that they have a nucleotide sequence complementary, or almost complementary, to that of a given part of the genome, with which, therefore, they can hybridize under suitable conditions.

Oligonucleotide probes
These are small gene probes that can be used to detect single-base mutations.

Southern blotting
This is a technique that allows the transfer of DNA fragments from gel, where electrophoresis and DNA denaturation have taken place, to a nylon or nitrocellular filter. It involves overlaying the gel with the filter and in turn overlaying the filter with paper towels. A solution is then blotted through the gel to the paper towels. Autoradiography can then be used to identify the fragments of interest on the filter. The technique is named after its inventor, Edwin Southern.

Restriction fragment length polymorphisms
Restriction fragment length polymorphisms, or RFLPs, are polymorphisms at restriction enzyme cleavage sites that give rise to fragments of different lengths following restriction enzyme digestion. They can be used as DNA markers and are usually inherited in a simple Mendelian fashion.

Recombination
As mentioned above, recombination takes place during prophase I of meiosis. There is alignment and contact of homologous chromosome pairs during prophase I, allowing genetic information to cross-over between adjacent chromatids. This process of cross-over or recombination causes a change in the alleles carried by the chromatids at the end of the first meiotic division.

LINKAGE ANALYSIS

Genetic markers
A DNA polymorphism, such as a restriction fragment length polymorphism, if linked to a given disease locus, can be used as a genetic marker in linkage analysis

without its precise chromosomal location being known. Genetic markers can also be used in presymptomatic diagnosis and prenatal diagnosis.

Linkage

This is the phenomenon whereby two genes close to each other on the same chromosome are likely to be inherited together.

Linkage phases

For two alleles occuring at two linked loci in a double heterozygote, the following linkage phases can occur:

- coupling: the two alleles are on the same chromosome
- repulsion: the two alleles are on opposite chromosomes of a pair

Recombinant fraction

This is a measure of how often the alleles at two loci are separated during meiotic recombination. Its value can vary from zero to 0.5.

Lod scores

The lod score for a given recombinant fraction is the logarithm to base 10 of the odds $P_1:P_2$, where P_1 is the probability of there being linkage for a given recombinant fraction, and P_2 is the probability of there being no measurable linkage. Thus the lod score gives a measure of the probability of two loci being linked. The lod score method was devised by Morton.

Maximum likelihood score

This is the value of the recombinant fraction that gives the highest value for the lod score. It represents the best estimate that can be made for the recombinant fraction from the given available data.

CONDITIONS ASSOCIATED WITH CHROMOSOMAL ABNORMALITIES

AUTOSOMAL ABNORMALITIES

Down syndrome

The causes of Down syndrome are as follows:

- approximately 95 per cent of cases result from trisomy 21 (47, +21) following non-disjunction during meiosis
- approximately 4 per cent result from translocation involving chromosome 21; exchange of chromosomal substance may occur between chromosome 21 and

  - chromosome 13
  - chromosome 14
  - chromosome 15
  - chromosome 21
  - chromosome 22

- the remaining cases are mosaics

Edwards syndrome

This is caused by trisomy 18 (47, +18).

Patau syndrome

This is caused by trisomy 13 (47, +13).

Cri-du-chat syndrome

This partial aneusomy results from the partial deletion of the short arm of chromosome 5. Its characteristic kitten-like high-pitched cry has been localized to 5p15.3. Its other clinical features have been localized to 5p15.2, known as the cri-du-chat critical region of CDCCR.

SEX CHROMOSOME ABNORMALITIES

Klinefelter syndrome

In this syndrome phenotypic males possess more than one X chromosome per somatic cell nucleus. Genotypes include:

- 47,XXY (i.e. one extra X chromosome per somatic cell nucleus): the most common genotype in Klinefelter syndrome
- 48,XXXY
- 49,XXXXY
- 48,XXYY

XYY syndrome

In this syndrome phenotypic males have the genotype 47,XYY.

Triple X syndrome

In this syndrome phenotypic females have the genotype 47,XXX.

Tetra-X syndrome

In this syndrome (also referred to as super-female syndrome) phenotypic females have the genotype 48,XXXX.

Turner syndrome

In this syndrome phenotypic females have the genotype 45,X (= 45,XO).

PRINCIPAL INHERITED CONDITIONS ENCOUNTERED IN PSYCHIATRIC PRACTICE

Autosomal dominant disorders

Disorders that can be inherited in an autosomal dominant manner include:

- Huntington disease
- acrocephalosyndactyly type I
- phacomatoses
    - tuberous sclerosis
    - neurofibromatosis
    - von Hippel–Lindau syndrome
    - Sturge–Weber syndrome
- acrocallosal syndrome
- acrodysostosis
- De Barsey syndrome
- periodic paralyses

Autosomal recessive disorders

DISORDERS OF PROTEIN METABOLISM Disorders of protein metabolism that can be inherited in an autosomal recessive manner include:

- argininaemia
- cystathioninuria
- cystinuria
- Hartnup disease
- histidinaemia
- homocystinuria
- hydroxyprolinaemia
- hyperlysinaemia
- maple syrup urine disease
- non-ketotic hyperglycinaemia
- ornithinaemia
- phenylketonuria
- Stimmler syndrome
- type II tyrosinaemia
- urea cycle disorders

  - hyperammonaemia
  - citrullinaemia
  - arginosuccinic aciduria

- valinaemia

DISORDER OF CARBOHYDRATE METABOLISM   Disorders of carbohydrate metabolism that can be inherited in an autosomal recessive manner include:

- fucosidosis
- galactosaemia
- Gaucher disease
- generalized gangliosidosis
- hereditary fructose intolerance
- Hurler syndrome
- Krabbe disease
- mannosidosis
- metachromatic leucodystrophy
- mucolipidoses
- Niemann–Pick disease
- Pompe disease
- Tay–Sachs disease
- von Gierke disease

OTHERS   There are many other disorders inherited in an autosomal recessive manner. These include:

- Alexander disease
- cerebelloparenchymal disorders
- Coat disease
- Cohen syndrome
- Crome syndrome
- Friedrich's ataxia
- Laurence–Moon syndrome
- macrocephaly
- oculocerebral syndrome
- oculorenocerebellar syndrome
- Rubinstein syndrome

- Turcot syndrome
- Wilson disease (hepatolenticular degeneration)

X-linked dominant disorders

Disorders that can be inherited in an X-linked dominant manner include:

- Aicardi syndrome
- Coffin–Lowry syndrome
- Rett syndrome

X-linked recessive disorders

Disorders that can be inherited in an X-linked recessive manner include:

- cerebellar ataxia
- fragile X syndrome
- Hunter syndrome
- hyperuricaemia
- Lesch–Nyhan syndrome
- Lowe syndrome
- testicular feminization syndrome
- X-linked spastic paraplegia
- W syndrome

BIBLIOGRAPHY

McGuffin, P., Owen, M.J., O'Donovan, M.C., Thapar, A. and Gottesman, I.I. 1994: *Seminars in psychiatric genetics*. London: Gaskell.

Puri, B.K. and Tyrer, P.J. 1998: *Sciences basic to psychiatry*, 2nd edn. Edinburgh: Churchill Livingstone.

20
Epidemiology

DISEASE FREQUENCY

Incidence
The incidence of a disease is the rate of occurrence of new cases of the disease in a defined population over a given period of time. It is equal to the number of new cases over the given period of time divided by the total population at risk (see below) during the same period of time.

Prevalence
The prevalence of a disease is the proportion of a defined population that has the disease at a given time.

POINT PREVALENCE   This is the proportion of a defined population that has a given disease at a given point in time.

PERIOD PREVALENCE   This is the proportion of a defined population that has a given disease during a given interval of time.

LIFETIME PREVALENCE   This is the proportion of a defined population that has or has had a given disease (at any time during each individual's lifetime thus far) at a given point in time.

BIRTH DEFECT RATE   This is the proportion of live births that has a given disease.

Population at risk
This is the population of individuals free of a given disease, who have not already had the disease by the time of the commencement of a given period of time, who are at risk of becoming new cases of the disease.

CASE IDENTIFICATION, CASE REGISTERS, MORTALITY AND MORBIDITY STATISTICS

Case identification
CASENESS   An overall threshold is ideally defined in order to establish caseness: that is, to differentiate cases of a given psychiatric disorder from non-cases. Classification systems and screening can be used to help identify cases.

CLASSIFICATION   Classification systems that are useful in case identification are those that provide specific operational diagnostic criteria as guides for making each psychiatric diagnosis. A widely used example is that of DSM-IV.

SCREENING   Screening, by means of psychiatric assessment instruments, can be used to identify cases. The instruments used should have good sensitivity and specificity:

$$\text{Sensitivity} = (\text{true } +\text{ve})/((\text{true } +\text{ve}) + (\text{false } -\text{ve}))$$

$$\text{Specificity} = (\text{true } -\text{ve})/((\text{true } -\text{ve}) + (\text{false } +\text{ve}))$$

Case registers

Examples of case registers that have proved useful in epidemiological studies and psychiatric research generally include:

- Swedish and Danish twin registers
- psychiatric case registers: containing records of those who have been treated for psychiatric disorders in certain hospitals or catchment areas

Limitations of case registers include:

- the registered individuals may move out of the defined geographical area
- the registers may not be kept up-to-date for other reasons

Mortality rate

This is the number of deaths in a defined population during a given period of time divided by the population size during that time period.

STANDARDIZED MORTALITY RATE   This is the mortality rate adjusted to compensate for a confounder.

AGE-STANDARDIZED MORTALITY RATE   This is the mortality rate adjusted to compensate for the confounding effect of age.

STANDARDIZED MORTALITY RATIO   The standardized mortality ratio, or SMR, is the ratio of the observed standardized mortality rate, derived from the population being studied, to the expected standardized mortality rate, derived from a comparable standard population. It may be expressed as a percentage by multiplying the ratio by 100.

Life expectancy

This is a measure of the mean length of time that an individual can be expected to live based on the assumption that the mortality rates used remain constant. It is calculated from the ratio of the total time a hypothetical group of people is expected to live to the size of that group.

Morbidity rate

This is the rate of occurrence of new non-fatal cases of a given disease in a defined population at risk during a given period of time.

STANDARDIZED MORBIDITY RATE   This is the morbidity rate adjusted to compensate for a confounder.

AGE-STANDARDIZED MORBIDITY RATE   This is the morbidity rate adjusted to compensate for the confounding effect of age.

STANDARDIZED MORBIDITY RATIO   The standardized morbidity ratio is the ratio of the observed standardized morbidity rate, derived from the population being studied, to the expected standardized morbidity rate, derived from a comparable standard population. It may be expressed as a percentage by multiplying the ratio by 100.

BIBLIOGRAPHY

Puri, B.K. and Tyrer, P.J. 1998: *Sciences basic to psychiatry*, 2nd edn. Edinburgh: Churchill Livingstone.

21

Medical ethics and principles of law

Advocacy

An advocate enters into a relationship with the patient, to speak on their behalf and to represent their wishes or stand up for their rights. An advocate has no legal status and the patient should have an idea of their preferences in order that the advocate truly represents the patients wishes.

Appointeeship

An appointee is someone authorized by the Department of Social Security to receive and administer benefits on behalf of someone else, who is not able to manage their affairs. It can only be used to administer money derived from social security benefits, and cannot be used to administer any other income or assets. If benefits accumulate application may need to be made to the Public Trust Office or the Court of Protection to gain access to the accumulated capital.

Powers of attorney

A power of attorney is a means whereby one person (the donor) gives legal authority to another person (the attorney) to manage their affairs. The donor has sole responsibility in the decision as to whether power of attorney is given provided they fully understand the implications of what they are undertaking.

An ordinary power of attorney allows the attorney to deal with the donor's financial affairs generally, or it can be limited to specific matters. An ordinary power of attorney is automatically revoked by law when the donor loses their mental capacity to manage their own affairs.

An Enduring Power of Attorney allows people to decide who should manage their affairs if they become mentally incapable. This has been possible since 1985. An Enduring Power of Attorney continues in force after the donor has lost the mental capacity to manage their affairs, provided it is registered with the Public Trust Office. It is thus of use in patients with early dementia who can set their affairs in order early in the illness provided the illness has not already progressed to a point where they are unable to manage their own affairs. Once the donor is unable to manage their own affairs, the attorney must apply to the Public Trust Office for registration of the Enduring Power of Attorney to allow the attorney authority to continue to act.

Court of protection

This is an office of the Supreme Court. It exists to protect the property and affairs of persons who through mental disorder are incapable of managing their own financial affairs. The Court's powers are limited to dealing with the financial and legal affairs of the person concerned. Only one medical certificate is required, from a registered medical practitioner who has examined the patient. Guidance to medical practitioners accompanies the certificate of incapacity.

The Court appoints somebody to manage the patient's affairs on their behalf. This person is called the **receiver**. These may be relatives, friends, solicitors or others. The receiver must keep accounts and spend the patient's money on things that will benefit the patient. The Court must give permission before the disposal of capital assets such as the sale of property.

Testamentary capacity
To make a will a person must be of **sound disposing mind**. This entails that they must:

1   understand to whom they are giving their property;
2   understand and recollect the extent of their property;
3   understand the nature and extent of the claims upon them, both of those included and those excluded from the will.

A valid will is not invalidated by the subsequent impairment of testamentary capacity.

Driving
The responsibility for making the decision about whether or not a person should continue to drive is that of the Driver and Vehicle Licensing Authority (DVLA), with the doctor acting only as a source of information and advice. The driver has a duty to keep the DVLA informed of any condition that may impair the ability to drive. The doctor is responsible for advising the patient to inform the DVLA of a condition likely to make driving dangerous. If the patient fails to take this advice, the doctor may then contact the DVLA directly. Table 21.1 summarizes the advice of the DVLA to British doctors with respect to fitness to drive in patients with psychiatric disorders. In this Table, two types of licence are referred to:

GROUP 1 LICENCE   A driver with a Mobility Allowance may drive from the age 16. Licences are normally issued until aged 70, unless restricted to a shorter duration for medical reasons. There is no upper age limit but after the age of 70 licences are renewable every three years.

GROUP 2 LICENCE   Group 2 licences are issued at the age of 21 and valid until the age of 45. They are then issued every five years to the age of 65 unless restricted to a shorter duration for medical reasons. From the age of 65 the licence is issued annually.

Table 21.1 Advice of the DVLA to doctors with respect to fitness to drive in patients with psychiatric disorders

PSYCHIATRIC DISORDERS	GROUP 1 ENTITLEMENT	GROUP 2 ENTITLEMENT
NEUROSIS e.g. Anxiety state/Depression	DVLA need not be notified. Driving need not cease. Patients must be warned about the possible effects of medication which may affect fitness. However, serious psychoneurotic episodes affecting or likely to affect driving should be notified to DVLA and the person advised not to drive.	Driving should cease with serious *acute* mental illness from whatever cause. Driving may be permitted when the person is symptom free and stable for a period of 6 months. Medication must not cause side effects which would interfere with alertness or concentration. Driving may be permitted also if the mental illness is long standing but maintained symptom free on small doses of psychotropic medication with no side effects likely to impair driving performance. Psychiatric reports may be required.
PSYCHOSIS Schizo-Affective Acute Psychosis Schizophrenia	6 months off the road after an acute episode requiring hospital admission. Licence restored after freedom from symptoms during this period, and the person demonstrates that he/she complies safely with recommended medication and shows insight into the condition. 1, 2, or 3 year licence with medical review on renewal. Loss of insight or judgement will lead to recommendation to refuse/revoke.	Recommended refusal or revocation. At least 3 years off driving, during which must be stable and symptom free, and not on major psychotropic or neuroleptic medication, except Lithium. Consultant Psychiatric examination required before restoration of licence, to confirm that there is no residual impairment, the applicant has insight and would be able to recognise if he became unwell. There should be no significant likelihood of recurrence. Any psychotropic medication necessary must be of low dosage and not interfere with alertness or concentration or in any way impair driving performance.

PSYCHIATRIC DISORDERS	GROUP 1 ENTITLEMENT	GROUP 2 ENTITLEMENT
MANIC DEPRESSIVE PSYCHOSIS	6–12 months off the road after an acute episode of hypomania requiring hospital admission, depending upon the severity and frequency of relapses. Licence restored after freedom from symptoms during this period and safe compliance with medication. 1, 2 or 3 year licence with medical review on renewal. Loss of insight or judgement will lead to recommendation to refuse/revoke.	AS ABOVE
DEMENTIA - Organic Brain Disorders e.g. Alzheimer's disease NB: There is no single marker to determine fitness to drive but it is likely that driving may be permitted if there is retention of ability to cope with the general day to day needs of living, together with adequate levels of insight and judgement.	If early dementia, driving may be permitted if there is no significant disorientation in time and space, and there is adequate retention of insight and judgement. Annual medical review required. Likely to be recommended to be refused or revoked if disorientated in time and space, and especially if insight has been lost or judgement is impaired.	Recommended permanent refusal or revocation if the condition is likely to impair driving performance.
SEVERE MENTAL HANDICAP means a state of arrested or incomplete development of mind which includes severe impairment of intelligence and social functioning.	Severe mental handicap is a *prescribed disability*, licence must be refused or revoked. If stable, mild to moderate mental handicap it may be possible to hold a licence, but he/she will need to demonstrate adequate functional ability at the wheel, and be otherwise stable.	Recommended permanent refusal or revocation if severe. Minor degrees of mental handicap when the condition is stable with no medical or psychiatric complications may be able to have a licence. Will need to demonstrate functional ability at the wheel.

PSYCHIATRIC DISORDERS	GROUP 1 ENTITLEMENT	GROUP 2 ENTITLEMENT
PERSONALITY DISORDER (including post head injury syndrome and psychopathic disorders)	If seriously disturbed such as evidence of violent outbreaks or alcohol abuse and likely to be a source of danger at the wheel, licence would be refused or revoked. Licence restricted after medical reports that behaviour disturbances have been satisfactorily controlled.	Recommended refusal or revocation if associated with serious behaviour disturbance likely to be a source of danger at the wheel. If the person matures and psychiatric reports confirm stability supportive, licence may be permitted/restored. Consultant Psychiatrist report required.

N.B. A person holding entitlement to Group I (i.e. motor car/motor bike) or Group II (i.e. LGV/PCV), who has been relicensed following an acute psychotic episode, of whatever type, should be advised as part of follow up that if the condition recurs, driving should cease and DVLA be notified. General guidance with respect to psychotropic/neuroleptic medication is contained under the appropriate section in the text.

Alcohol and illicit drug misuse/dependency are dealt with under their specific sections.

Reference is made in the introductory page to the current GMC guidance to doctors concerning disclosure in the public interest without the consent of the patient.

ALCOHOL PROBLEMS	GROUP 1 ENTITLEMENT	GROUP 2 ENTITLEMENT ALCOHOL MISUSE
ALCOHOL MISUSE/ ALCOHOL DEPENDENCY There is no single definition which embraces all the variables in these conditions. But as a guideline the following is offered: - 'a state which because of consumption of alcohol, causes disturbance of behaviour, related disease or other consequences, likely to cause the patient his family or society harm now or in the future and which may or may not be associated with dependency. In addition assessment of the alcohol consumption with respect to current national advised guidelines is necessary.'	*ALOCHOL MISUSE* Alcohol misuse, confirmed by medical enquiry and by evidence of otherwise unexplained abnormal blood markers, requires licence revocation or refusal for a minimum six month period, during which time controlled drinking should be attained with normalisation of blood parameters. *ALCOHOL DEPENDENCY* Including detoxification and/or alcohol related fits. Alcohol dependency, confirmed by medical enquiry, requires a recommended one year period of licence revocation or refusal, to attain abstinence or controlled drinking and with normalisation of blood parameters if relevant. *LICENCE RESTORATION* Will require satisfactory independent medical examination, arranged by DVLA with satisfactory blood results and medical reports from own doctors. Patient recommended to seek advice from medical or other sources during the period off the road.	*ALCOHOL MISUSE* Alcohol misuse, confirmed by medical enquiry and by evidence of otherwise unexplained abnormal blood markers, will lead to revocation or refusal of a vocational licence for at least one year, during which time controlled drinking should be attained with normalisation of blood parameters. *ALCOHOL DEPENDENCY* Vocational licensing will not be granted where there is a history of alcohol dependency within the past three years. *LICENCE RESTORATION* On reapplication, independent medical examination arranged by DVLA, with satisfactory blood results and medical reports from own doctors. Consultant support/referral may be necessary. If an alcohol related seizure or seizures have occurred, the vocational Epilepsy Regulations apply.
*Alcohol Related Seizure(s)	A licence will be revoked or refused for a minimum one year period from the date of the event. Where more than one seizure occurs, consideration under the Epilepsy Regulations may be necessary. Before licence restoration, medical enquiry will be required to confirm appropriate period free from alcohol misuse and/or dependency.	Vocational Epilepsy Regulations apply (see DVLA Guidelines).

ALCOHOL PROBLEMS	GROUP 1 ENTITLEMENT	GROUP 2 ENTITLEMENT ALCOHOL MISUSE
ALCOHOL RELATED DISORDERS - e.g. severe hepatic cirrhosis, Wernicke's encephalopathy, Korsakoffs Psychosis, et alia.	Licence recommended to be refused/revoked.	Recommended to be refused/revoked.

NB: A person who has been relicensed following alcohol misuse or dependancy must be advised as part of their follow up that if their condition recurs they should cease driving and notify DVLA Medical Branch.

HIGH RISK OFFENDER SCHEME for drivers convicted of certain drink/driving offences

1. *One* disqualification for drink/driving when the level of alcohol is $2\frac{1}{2}$ or more times the legal limit.
2. *One* disqualification that he/she failed, without reasonable excuse to provide a specimen for analysis.
3. *Two* disqualifications within 10 years for being unfit through drink.
4. *Two* disqualifications within 10 years when the level of alcohol exceeds the legal limit.
   DVLA will be notified by courts. On application for licence, satisfactory *independent* medical examination with completion of structured questionnaire with satisfactory liver enzyme tests and MCV required. If favourable, Till 70 restored for Group I and can recommend issue Group II.
   If High Risk Offender associated with previous history of alcohol dependancy or misuse, after above satisfactory examination and blood tests, short period licence only for ordinary and vocational issued, depending on time interval between previous history and reapplication.
   High Risk Offender found to have current unfavourable alcohol misuse history and/or abnormal blood test analysis would have application refused.

DRUG MISUSE AND DEPENDENCY	GROUP 1 ENTITLEMENT	GROUP 2 ENTITLEMENT
Cannabis Ecstasy and other 'recreational' psychoactive substances, including LSD and Hallucinogens	The regular use of these substances, confirmed by medical enquiry, will lead to licence revocation or refusal for a six month period. Independent medical assessment and urine screen arranged by DVLA, may be required.	Regular use of these substances will lead to refusal or revocation of a vocational licence for at least a one year period. Independent medical assessment and urine screen arranged by DVLA, may be required.
Amphetamines Heroin Morphine Methadone* Cocaine Benzodiazepines	Regular use of, or dependency on, these substances, confirmed by medical enquiry, will lead to licence refusal or revocation for a minimum one year period. Independent medical assessment and urine screen arranged by DVLA, may be required. In addition favourable Consultant or Specialist report will be required on reapplication. * Applicants or drivers on Consultant supervised oral Methadone withdrawal programme may be licensed, subject to annual medical review and favourable assessment.	Regular use of, or dependency on, these substances, will require revocation or refusal of a vocational licence for a minimum three year period. Independent medical assessment and urine screen arranged by DVLA, may be required. In addition favourable Consultant or Specialist report will be required before relicensing.
Seizure(s) associated with illicit drug usage	A seizure or seizures associated with illicit drug usage may require a licence to be refused or revoked for a one year period. Thereafter, licence restoration will require independent medical assessment, with urine analysis, together with favourable report from own doctor, to confirm no ongoing drug misuse. In addition, patients may be assessed against the Epilepsy Regulations.	Vocational Epilepsy Regulations apply.

NB: A person who has been relicensed following illicit drug misuse or dependency must be advised as part of their follow up that if their condition recurs they should cease driving and notify DVLA Medical Branch.

22

Legal aspects of psychiatric care

The Mental Health Act 1983 for England and Wales is detailed in this chapter; the equivalent Scottish treatment orders are also given. The mental health legislation relevant to your country of practice should be obtained and you should be familiar with its contents and use. The Misuse of Drugs legislation for England and Wales is considered in Chapter 26.

ENGLAND AND WALES: MENTAL HEALTH ACT 1983

Section 1: Definitions
MENTAL DISORDER   Mental illness, arrested or incomplete development of mind, psychopathic disorder and any other disorder or disability of mind.

SEVERE MENTAL IMPAIRMENT   A state of arrested or incomplete development of mind which includes the severe impariment of intelligence and social functioning and is associated with abnormally aggressive or seriously irresponsible conduct on the part of the person concerned.

MENTAL IMPAIRMENT   A state of arrested or incomplete development of mind (not amounting to severe mental impairment) which includes significant impairment of intelligence and social functioning and is associated with abnormally aggressive or seriously irresponsible conduct on the part of the person concerned.

PSYCHOPATHIC DISORDER   A persistent disorder or disability of mind (whether or not including significant impairment of intelligence) which results in abnormally aggressive or seriously irresponsible conduct on the part of the person concerned.

PATIENT   A person suffering from or appearing to suffer from mental disorder.

MEDICAL TREATMENT   Includes nursing, and care and rehabilitation under medical supervision.

RESPONSIBLE MEDICAL OFFICER (RMO)   The registered medical practitioner in charge of the treatment of the patient: that is, the consultant psychiatrist; if they are not available the doctor who for the time being is in charge of the patient's treatment may deputize.

APPROVED DOCTOR   A registered medical practitioner approved under Section 12 of the Act by the Secretary of State (with authority being delegated to the Regional Health Authority) as having special experience in the diagnosis or treatment of mental disorder.

APPROVED SOCIAL WORKER (ASW)   An officer of a local social services authority with appropriate training who may make applications for compulsory admission; hospital senior social workers usually hold lists of approved social workers.

Table 22.1 Civil treatment orders under Mental Health Act 1983

Civil treatment order under Mental Health Act 1983	Grounds	Application by	Medical recommendations	Maximum duration	Eligibility for appeal to Mental Health Review Tribunal
Section 2 Admission for assessment	Mental disorder	Nearest relative or approved social worker	Two doctors (one approved under Section 12)	28 days	Within 14 days
Section 3 Admission for treatment	Mental illness, psycho-pathic disorder, mental impairment, severe mental impairment (If psycho-pathic disorder or mental impairment, treatment must be likely to alleviate or prevent deterioration)	Nearest relative or approved social worker	Two doctors (one approved under Section 12)	6 months	Within first 6 months. If renewed, within second 6 months, then every year. Mandatory every 3 years.
Section 4 Emergency admission for assessment	Mental disorder (urgent necessity)	Nearest relative or approved social worker	Any doctor	72 hours	
Section 5 (2) Urgent detention of voluntary in-patient	Danger to self or to others		Doctor in charge of patient's care	72 hours	
Section 5 (4) Nurses holding power of voluntary in-patient	Mental disorder (danger to self, health or others)	Registered mental nurse or registered nurse for mental handicap	None	6 hours	
Section 136 Admission by police	Mental disorder	Police officer	Allows patient in public place to be removed to 'place of safety'	72 hours	
Section 135	Mental disorder	Magistrates	Allows power of entry to home and removal of patient to place of safety	72 hours	

Reproduced with permission from Puri, B.K., Laking, P.J. and Treasaden, I.H. 1996: *Textbook of psychiatry.* Edinburgh: Churchill Livingstone.

NEAREST RELATIVE   The first surviving person in the following list, with full blood relative taking preference over half blood relatives, and the elder of two relatives of the same description or level of kinship taking preference also:

(a)   husband or wife
(b)   son or daughter
(c)   father or mother
(d)   brother or sister
(e)   grandparent
(f)   grandchild
(g)   uncle or aunt
(h)   nephew or niece

Preference is also given to a relative with whom the patient ordinarily lives or by whom they are cared for.

Note that the term **mental illness** is not formally defined; its operational definition is a matter of clinical judgement in each case. The Act states that a person may *not* be dealt with under the Mental Health Act as suffering from **mental disorder** 'by reason only of promiscuity or other immoral conduct, sexual deviancy or dependence on alcohol or drugs'.

Civil treatment orders
See Table 22.1

Supervision registers
The three categories of risk for inclusion on a supervision register are that a patient should be at:

- significant risk of suicide and/or
- significant risk of serious violence to others and/or
- significant risk of severe self-neglect

The decision to include a patient on a supervision register is made by the RMO in consultation with the multidisciplinary team.

Consent to treatment

Table 22.2 Consent to treatment under Mental Health Act 1983 Consent to treatment should be informed and voluntary (implies mental illness, e.g. dementia, does not affect judgement)

Type of treatment	Informal	Detained
Urgent treatment	No consent	No consent
Section 57	Consent and	Consent and
Irreversible, hazardous or non-established treatments, e.g. psychosurgery (e.g. leucotomy), hormone implants (for sex offenders), surgical operations (e.g. castration)	second opinion	second opinion
Section 58	Consent	Consent or
Psychiatric drugs, ECT		second opinion

1. For first 3 months of treatment a detained patient's consent is not required for Section 58 medicines, but is for ECT.
2. Patients can withdraw voluntary consent at any time.
Reproduced with permission from Puri, B.K., Laking, P.J. and Treasaden, I.H. 1996: *Textbook of psychiatry.* Edinburgh: Churchill Livingstone.

Table 22.3 Forensic treatment orders for mentally abnormal offenders

	Grounds	Made by	Medical recommendations	Maximum duration	Eligibility for appeal to Mental Health Review Tribunal
Section 35 Remand to hospital for report	Mental disorder	Magistrates or Crown Court	Any doctor	28 days. Renewable at 28-day intervals. Maximum 12 weeks	
Section 36 Remand to hospital for treatment	Mental illness, severe mental impairment (not if charged with murder)	Crown Court	Two doctors: one approved under Section 12	28 days. Renewable at 28-days intervals. Maximum 12 weeks	
Section 37 Hospital and guardianship orders	Mental disorder. (If psychopathic disorder or mental impairment must be likely to alleviate or prevent deterioration.) Accused of, or convicted for, an imprisonable offence	Magistrates or Crown Court	Two doctors, one approved under Section 12	6 months. Renewable for further 6 months and then annually	During second 6 months. Then every year. Mandatory every 3 years.
Section 41 Restriction order	Added to Section 37. To protect public from serious harm	Crown Court	Oral evidence from one doctor	Usually without limit of time. Effect: leave, transfer, or discharge only with consent of Home Secretary	As Section 37
Section 38 Interim hospital order	Mental disorder For trial of treatment	Magistrates or Crown Court	Two doctors: one approved under Section 12	12 weeks. Renewable at 28-day intervals Maximum 6 months	None

	Grounds	Made by	Medical recommendations	Maximum duration	Eligibility for appeal to Mental Health Review Tribunal
Section 47 Transfer of a sentenced prisoner to hospital	Mental disorder	Home Secretary	Two doctors: one approved under Section 12	Until earliest date of release from sentence	Once in the first 6 months. Then once in the next 6 months. Thereafter, once a year.
Section 48 Urgent transfer to hospital of remand prisoner	Mental disorder	Home Secretary	Two doctors: one approved under Section 12	Until date of trial	Once in the first 6 months. Then once in the next 6 months. Thereafter, once a year.
Section 49 Restriction direction	Added to Section 47 or Section 48	Home Secretary	–	Until end of Section 47 or 48. Effect: leave, transfer or discharge only with consent of Home Secretary	As for Section 47 and 48 to which applied

Reproduced with permission from Puri, B.K., Laking, P.J. and Treasaden, I.H. 1996: *Textbook of psychiatry*. Edinburgh: Churchill Livingstone.

Forensic treatment orders
See Table 22.3

MENTAL HEALTH (SCOTLAND) ACT 1984

Table 22.4 Equivalent Scottish and English Mental Health Act treatment orders

Treatment Order *Treatment Order*	*Mental Health (England & Wales) Act 1983*	*Mental Health (Scotland) 1984*
Emergency admission	Section 4	Section 24
Short-term detention	Section 2	Section 26
Admission for treatment	Section 3	Section 22
Nurses holding power of a voluntary inpatient	Section 5(4) (for 6 hours)	Section 25(2) for 2 hrs
Guardianship	Section 37	Section 37
Committal to hospital pending trial	Section 36	Sections 25 & 330 of the 1975 Act
Remand for enquiry into mental condition	Section 35	Sections 180 & 381 of the 1975 Act
Removal to hospital of persons in prison awaiting trial or sentence	Section 48	Section 70
Interim hospital order	Section 38	Sections 174a & 375a of the 1975 Act amended by the Mental Health (Amendment) (Scotland) Act 1983.
Hospital order	Section 37	Sections 175 & 376 of the 1975 Act
Restriction order	Section 41	Sections 178 & 379 by the 1975 Act
Transfer of prisoner under sentence to hospital	Section 47	Section 71

Reproduced with permission from Puri, B.K., Laking, P.J. and Treasaden, I.H. 1996: *Textbook of psychiatry*. Edinburgh: Churchill Livingstone.

23
Classification

ICD-10

Organic, including symptomatic, mental disorders

F00 Dementia in Alzheimer's disease
F01 Vascular dementia
F02 Dementia in other diseases classified elsewhere
F03 Unspecified dementia
F04 Organic amnesic syndrome, not induced by alcohol and other psychoactive substances
F05 Delirum, not induced by alcohol and other psychoactive substances
F06 Other mental disorders caused by brain damage and dysfunction and by physical disease
F07 Personality and behavioural disorders caused by brain disease, damage and dysfunction
F09 Unspecified organic or symptomatic mental disorder

Mental and behavioural disorders caused by psychoactive substance use

F10 Mental and behavioural disorders caused by the use of alcohol
F11 Mental and behavioural disorders caused by the use of opioids
F12 Mental and behavioural disorders caused by the use of cannabinoids
F13 Mental and behavioural disorders caused by the use of sedatives or hypnotics
F14 Mental and behavioural disorders caused by the use of cocaine
F15 Mental and behavioural disorders caused by the use of other stimulants, including caffeine
F16 Mental and behavioural disorders caused by the use of hallucinogens
F17 Mental and behavioural disorders caused by the use of tobacco
F18 Mental and behavioural disorders caused by the use of volatile solvents
F19 Mental and behavioural disorders caused by multiple drug use and the use of other psychoactive substances

Schizophrenia, schizotypal and delusional disorders

F20 Schizophrenia
F21 Schizotypal disorder
F22 Persistent delusional disorders
F23 Acute and transient psychotic disorders
F24 Induced delusional disorder
F25 Schizoaffective disorders
F28 Other nonorganic psychotic disorders
F29 Unspecified nonorganic psychosis

Mood [affective] disorders

F30   Manic episode
F31   Bipolar affective disorder
F32   Depressive episode
F33   Recurrent depressive disorder
F34   Persistent mood [affective] disorders
F35   Other mood [affective] disorders
F39   Unspecified mood [affective] disorder

Neurotic, stress-related and somatoform disorders

F40   Phobic anxiety disorders
F41   Other anxiety disorders
F42   Obsessive–compulsive disorder
F43   Reaction to severe stress, and adjustment disorders
F44   Dissociative (conversion) disorders
F45   Somatoform disorders
F48   Other neurotic disorders

Behavioural syndromes associated with physiological disturbances and physical factors

F50   Eating disorders
F51   Nonorganic sleep disorders
F52   Sexual dysfunction, not caused by organic disorder or disease
F53   Mental and behavioural disorders associated with the puerperium, not elsewhere classified
F54   Psychological and behavioural factors associated with disorders or diseases classified elsewhere
F55   Abuse of non-dependence-producing substances
F59   Unspecified behavioural syndromes associated with physiological disturbances and physical factors

Disorders of adult personality and behaviour

F60   Specific personality disorders
F61   Mixed and other personality disorders
F62   Enduring personality changes, not attributable to brain damage and disease
F63   Habit and impulse disorders
F64   Gender identity disorders
F65   Disorders of sexual preference
F66   Psychological and behavioural disorders associated with sexual development and orientation
F68   Other disorders of adult personality and behaviour
F69   Unspecified disorder of adult personality and behaviour

Mental retardation

F70   Mild mental retardation
F71   Moderate mental retardation
F72   Severe mental retardation
F73   Profound mental retardation
F78   Other mental retardation
F79   Unspecified mental retardation

Disorders of psychological development

F80   Specific developmental disorders of speech and language
F81   Specific developmental disorders of scholastic skills
F82   Specific developmental disorder of motor function
F83   Mixed specific developmental disorders
F84   Pervasive developmental disorders
F88   Other disorders of psychological development
F89   Unspecified disorder of psychological development

Behavioural and emotional disorders with onset usually occurring in childhood and adolescence

F90   Hyperkinetic disorders
F91   Conduct disorders
F92   Mixed disorders of conduct and emotions
F93   Emotional disorders with onset specific to childhood
F94   Disorders of social functioning with onset specific to childhood and adolescence
F95   Tic disorders
F98   Other behavioural and emotional disorders with onset usually occurring in childhood and adolescence

Unspecified mental disorder

F99   Mental disorder, not otherwise specified

DSM-IV

The fourth edition of the *Diagnostic and statistical manual of mental disorders* (DSM-IV), published by the American Psychiatric Association in 1994, is a multiaxial classification with the following five axes:

Axis I   Clinical disorders
           Other conditions that may be a focus of clinical attention
Axis II   Personality disorders
           Mental retardation
Axis III   General medical conditions
Axis IV   Psychosocial and environmental problems
Axis V   Global assessment of functioning

In the following summary, NOS stands for 'not otherwise specified'.

AXIS I: CLINICAL DISORDERS; OTHER CONDITIONS THAT MAY BE A FOCUS OF CLINICAL ATTENTION

Disorders usually first diagnosed in infancy, childhood, or adolescence (excluding mental ratardation, which is diagnosed on Axis II)

- Learning disorder
- Motor skills disorder
- Communication disorders
- Pervasive developmental disorders

- Autistic disorder
- Rett's disorder
- Childhood disintegrative disorder
- Asperger's disorder
- NOS

- Attention-deficit and disruptive behaviour disorders
- Feeding and eating disorders of infancy and early childhood
- Tic disorders
- Elimination disorders

  - Encopresis
  - Enuresis

- Other disorders of infancy, childhood, or adolescence

Delirium, dementia, and amnestic and other cognitive disorders

- Delirium
- Dementia
- Amnestic disorders
- Other cognitive disorders

Mental disorders caused by a general medical condition

Substance-related disorders

- Alcohol-related disorders
- Amphetamine (or amphetamine-like)-related disorders
- Caffeine-related disorders
- Cannabis-related disorders
- Cocaine-related disorders
- Hallucinogen-related disorders
- Inhalant-related disorders
- Nicotine-related disorders
- Opioid-related disorders
- Phencyclidine (or phencyclidine-like)-related disorders
- Sedative-, hypnotic-, or anxiolytic-related disorders
- Polysubstance-related disorders
- Other (or unknown) substance-related disorders

Schizophrenia and other psychotic disorders

- Schizophrenia
- Schizophreniform disorder
- Schizoaffective disorder
- Delusional disorder
- Brief psychotic disorder
- Shared psychotic disorder
- Psychotic disorder caused by a general medical condition
- Substance-induced psychotic disorder
- Psychotic disorder NOS

Mood disorders

- Depressive disorders
- Bipolar disorders

Anxiety disorders

- Panic disorder without agoraphobia
- Panic disorder with agoraphobia
- Agoraphobia without history of panic disorder
- Specific phobia
- Social phobia
- Obsessive–compulsive disorder
- Post-traumatic stress disorder
- Acute stress disorder
- Generalized anxiety disorder
- Anxiety disorder caused by a general medical condition
- Substance-induced anxiety disorder
- NOS

Somatoform disorders

- Somatization disorder
- Undifferentiated somatoform disorder
- Conversion disorder
- Pain disorder
- Hypochondriasis
- Body dysmorphic disorder
- NOS

Factitious disorders

Dissociative disorders

- Dissociative amnesia
- Dissociative fugue
- Dissociative identity disorder
- Depersonalization disorder
- NOS

Sexual and gender identity disorders

- Sexual dysfunctions
  - Sexual desire disorders
  - Sexual arousal disorders
  - Orgasmic disorders
  - Sexual pain disorders
  - Sexual dysfunction caused by a general medical condition
- Paraphilias
  - Exhibitionism
  - Fetishism
  - Frotteurism
  - Pedophilia

- Sexual masochism
- Sexual sadism
- Transvestic fetishism
- Voyeurism
- NOS

- Gender identity disorders

Eating disorders

- Anorexia nervosa
- Bulimia nervosa
- NOS

Sleep disorders

- Primary sleep disorders

  - Dyssomnias
  - Parasomnias

- Sleep disorders related to another medical disorder
- Other sleep disorders

Impulse-control disorders not elsewhere classified

Adjustment disorders

Other conditions that may be a focus of clinical attention

AXIS II: PERSONALITY DISORDERS; MENTAL RETARDATION

PERSONALITY DISORDERS

- Paranoid personality disorder
- Schizoid personality disorder
- Schizotypal personality disorder
- Antisocial personality disorder
- Borderline personality disorder
- Histrionic personality disorder
- Narcissistic personality disorder
- Avoidant personality disorder
- Dependent personality disorder
- Obsessive–compulsive personality disorder
- NOS

Mental retardation

- Mild mental retardation
- Moderate mental retardation
- Severe mental retardation
- Profound mental retardation
- Mental retardation, severity unspecified

AXIS III: GENERAL MEDICAL CONDITIONS

Infectious and parasitic diseases

Neoplasms

Endocrine, nutritional, and metabolic diseases and immunity disorders

Diseases of the blood and blood-forming organs

Diseases of the nervous system and sense organs

Diseases of the circulatory system

Diseases of the respiratory system

Diseases of the digestive system

Diseases of the genitourinary system

Complications of pregnancy, childbirth, and the puerperium

Diseases of the skin and subcutaneous tissue

Diseases of the musculoskeletal system and connective tissue

Congenital anomalies

Certain conditions originating in the perinatal period

Symptoms, signs, and ill-defined conditions

Injury and poisoning

AXIS IV: PSYCHOSOCIAL AND ENVIRONMENTAL PROBLEMS

Problems with primary support group

Problems related to the social environment

Educational problems

Occupational problems

Housing problems

Economic problems

Problems with access to healthcare services

Problems related to interaction with the legal system/crime

Other psychosocial and environmental problems

AXIS V: GLOBAL ASSESSMENT OF FUNCTIONING

BIBLIOGRAPHY

American Psychiatric Association 1994: *Diagnostic and statistical manual of mental disorders.* Washington DC: American Psychiatric Association.

World Health Organization 1992: *The ICD-10 classification of mental and behavioural disorders.* Geneva, Switzerland: World Health Organization.

24
Physical therapies

PHARMACOTHERAPY

This is considered in Chapters 15 to 18.

ECT

History
Key historical points in the development of electroconvulsive therapy (ECT) include:

- during the early twentieth century it was hypothesized that schizophrenia and epilepsy are more or less mutually exclusive disorders
- 1934: Meduna, on the basis of this hypothesis, attempted to treat schizophrenia by inducing seizures chemically
- 1938: Cerletti and Bini induced seizures electrically

Indications
The main indications for ECT are:

- severe depressive illness
- puerperal depressive illness
- mania
- catatonic schizophrenia
- schizoaffective disorder

Contraindications
Raised intracranial pressure is an absolute contraindications to ECT. Relative contraindications include:

- cerebral aneurysm
- recent myocardial infarction
- cardiac arrhythmia
- intracerebral haemorrhage
- acute/impending retinal detachment
- pheochromocytoma
- raised anaesthetic risk
- unstable vascular aneurysm or malformation

Administration

- a patient receiving ECT in the morning should remain 'nil by mouth' from the previous midnight
- a muscle relaxant is administered in order to prevent violent movements during the convulsion

- atropine is administered in order to reduce secretions and prevent the muscarinic actions of the muscle relaxant
- if there is any possibility that the patient may have low or atypical plasma pseudocholinesterase enzymes, the anaesthetist must be informed as this could lead to prolonged muscle paralysis with the muscle relaxant
- bilateral or unilateral (to the non-dominant cerebral hemisphere) ECT is administered under a short-acting general anaesthetic
- a bite is placed in the patient's mouth in order to prevent damage from biting during the convulsion

Side-effects
The main early side-effects include:

- headache
- temporary confusion
- some loss of short-term memory

ECT may cause depressed patients with bipolar mood disorder to become manic. In the long term, patients may complain of memory impairment.

PHOTOTHERAPY

This is treatment with high-intensity artificial light, and may be used to treat patients suffering from seasonal affective disorder (SAD).

SLEEP DEPRIVATION

Indications
The clinical indications for sleep deprivation in mood disorders include:

- as an antidepressant in treatment-resistant patients
- to augment the response to antidepressants
- to hasten the onset of action of antidepressant medication or of lithium
- as a prophylaxis in recurrent mood cycles
- as an aid to diagnosis
- to predict the response to antidepressants or ECT

Administration
In total sleep deprivation, the patient is kept awake for 36 hours. One variation is late partial sleep deprivation, in which the patient is kept awake from two in the morning until ten in the evening. Another variation entails depriving the patient only of rapid eye movement sleep.

PSYCHOSURGERY

History

- 3000–2000 BC: trepanation
- nineteenth century: Burckhardt removed postcentral, temporal, and frontal cortices from patients

- 1910: Pusepp resected fibres between the frontal and parietal lobes in patients with bipolar mood disorder
- 1936: Ody resected the right prefrontal lobe of a patient with so-called childhood-onset schizophrenia
- 1935 (published 1936): after learning of the work of Fulton and Jacobsen involving bilateral ablation of the prefrontal cortex in chimpanzees, Moniz carried out human frontal leucotomy

Indications

Psychosurgery is a last-resort treatment for:

- chronic severe intractable depression
- chronic severe intractable obsessive–compulsive disorder
- chronic severe intractable anxiety states

Administration

Current methods for making sterotaxic lesions include:

- electrocautery
- radioactive yttrium implantation
- thermocoagulation
- gamma knife

Types of operation

Some of the specific operations that may be used currently include:

- frontal-lobe lesioning
- cingulotomy
- capsulotomy
- subcaudate tractotomy
- limbic leucotomy

BIBLIOGRAPHY

Puri, B.K., Laking, P.J,. and Treasaden, I.H. 1996: *Textbook of psychiatry.* Edinburgh: Churchill Livingstone.
Trimble, M.R. 1996: *Neuropsychiatry* 2nd edn. Chichester: John Wiley.

25
Organic psychiatry

DEFINITION

In ICD-10 organic mental disorders are grouped on the basis of a common demonstrable aetiology being present in the form of cerebral disorder, injury to the brain, or other insult leading to cerebral dysfunction, which may be:

- primary: disorders, injuries and insults affecting the brain directly or with predilection, such as Alzheimer's disease
- secondary: systemic disorders affecting the brain only in so far as it is one of the multiple organs or body systems involved, for example hypothyroidism

By convention the following disorders are excluded from the category or organic mental disorders and considered separately:

- psychoactive substance use disorders (including brain disorder resulting from alcohol and other psychoactive drugs)
- certain sleep disorders
- the causes of learning disability (mental retardation)

The dementias and delirium are considered in Chapters 11 and 38, while Wernicke's encephalopathy and Korsakov's syndrome are considered in Chapter 26. The clinical features of focal cerebral disorders have been outlined in Chapter 10. The causes of dementia are conveniently summarized here:

- degenerative diseases of the central nervous system

    - Alzheimer's disease
    - Pick's disease
    - Huntington's disease
    - Creutzfeldt–Jakob disease
    - normal pressure hydrocephalus
    - multiple sclerosis
    - Lewy body disease

- intoxication

    - alcohol
    - heavy metals such as lead, arsenic, thallium and mercury
    - carbon monoxide
    - withdrawal from drugs
    - withdrawal from alcohol

- intracranial

    - space-occupying lesions such as tumours, chronic subdural haematomas, aneurysms and chronic abscesses
    - infections

  - head injury
  - punch-drunk syndrome
- endocrine disorders
  - Addison's disease
  - Cushing's syndrome
  - hyperinsulinism
  - hypothyroidism
  - hypopituitarism
  - hypoparathyroidism
  - hyperparathyroidism
- metabolic disorders
  - hepatic failure
  - renal failure
  - respiratory failure
  - hypoxia
  - renal dialysis
  - chronic uraemia
  - chronic electrolyte imbalance ($\uparrow Ca^{2+}$, $\downarrow Ca^{2+}$, $\downarrow K^{+}$, $\uparrow Na^{+}$, $\downarrow Na^{+}$)
  - porphyria
  - Paget's disease
  - remote effects of carcinoma or lymphoma
  - hepatolenticular degeneration (Wilson's disease)
  - vitamin deficiency (thiamine, nicotinic acid, folate, B_{12})
  - vitamin intoxication (A, D)
- vascular
  - multi-infarct (vascular) dementia
  - cerebral artery occlusion
  - cranial arteritis
  - arteriovenous malformation
  - Binswanger's disease

ORGANIC MENTAL DISORDERS

The treatment, course and prognosis for the following disorders are essentially those of the underlying pathology.

Organic hallucinosis
In ICD-10 organic hallucinosis is defined as being a disorder of persistent or recurrent hallucinations, in any modality but usually visual or auditory, that occur in clear consciousness without any significant intellectual decline and that may or may not be recognized by the subject as such; delusional elaboration of the hallucinations may occur, but often insight is preserved. The causes of organic hallucinosis are shown in Table 25.1.

Organic catatonic disorder
In ICD-10 organic catatonic disorder is defined as being a disorder of diminished (stupor) or increased (excitement) psychomotor activity associated with catatonic symptoms; the extremes of psychomotor disturbance may alternate. The

Table 25.1 Causes of organic hallucinosis

Psychoactive substance use	Alcohol abuse (alcoholic hallucinosis) Amphetamine and related sympathomimetics Cocaine Hallucinogens, e.g. LSD Flashback phenomena – following the use of hallucinogens
Intoxication	Drugs – amantadine, bromocriptine, ephedrine, levodopa, lysuride
Intracranial causes	Brain tumours Head injury Migraine Infections, e.g. neurosyphilis Epilepsy – particularly temporal lobe epilepsy
Sensory deprivation	Deafness Poor vision, e.g. cataracts Torture, e.g. in prisoners of war
Endocrine	Hypothyroidism – 'myxoedematous madness'
Huntington's disease	

Reproduced with permission from Puri, B.K., Laking, P.J. and Treasaden, I.H. 1996: *Textbook of psychiatry*. Edinburgh: Churchill Livingstone.

stuporose symptoms may include complete mutism, negativism and rigid posturing, while excitement manifests as gross hypermotility. Other catatonic symptoms include sterotypies and waxy flexibility. Important causes of organic catatonic disorder include:

- encephalitis
- carbon monoxide poisoning

Organic delusional or schizophrenia-like disorder
In ICD-10 organic delusional or schizophrenia-like disorder is defined as a disorder in which the clinical picture is dominated by persistent or recurrent delusions, with or without hallucinations. The delusions are most often persecutory, but grandiose delusions or delusions of bodily change, jealousy, disease, or death may occur. Memory and consciousness are unaffected. Causes include:

- psychoactive substance use
    - amphetamine and related substances
    - cocaine
    - hallucinogens
- intracranial causes affecting the temporal lobe, e.g. tumours and epilepsy
- Huntington's disease

Organic mood disorder
Organic mood disorder is a disorder characterized by a change in mood, usually accompanied by a change in the overall level of activity, caused by organic pathology. Table 25.2 gives the main causes of organic mood disorder.

Organic anxiety disorder
Organic anxiety disorder is characterized by the occurrence of the features of generalized anxiety disorder and/or panic disorder caused by organic pathology.

Table 25.2 Causes of organic mood disorder

Psychoactive substance use	Amphetamine and related sympathomimetics Hallucinogens, e.g. LSD
Medication	Corticosteroids Levodopa Centrally acting antihypertensives – clonidine, methyldopa, reserpine and rauwolfia alkaloids Cycloserine Oestrogens – hormone replacement therapy, oral contraceptives Clomiphene
Endocrine disorders	Hypothyroidism, hyperthyroidism Addison's disease Cushing's syndrome Hypoglycaemia, diabetes mellitus Hyperparathyroidism Hypopituitarism
Other systemic disorders	Pernicious anaemia Hepatic failure Renal failure Rheumatoid arthritis Systemic lupus erythematosus Neoplasia – particularly carcinoma of the pancreas, carcinoid syndrome Viral infections – e.g. influenza, pneumonia, infec- tions mononucleosis (glandular fever), hepatitis
Intracranial causes	Brain tumours Head injury Parkinson's disease Infections, e.g. neurosyphilis

Reproduced with permission from Puri, B.K., Laking, P.J. and Treasaden, I.H. 1996: *Textbook of psychiatry*. Edinburgh: Churchill Livingstone.

Some of the symptoms of anxiety, which include tremor, paraesthesia, choking, palpitations, chest pain, dry mouth, nausea, abdominal pain, loose motions and increased frequency of micturition, are secondary to hyperventilation. Secondary cognitive impairment may occur. Table 25.3 shows the main causes of organic anxiety disorder; of these, it is particularly important to exclude hyperthyroidism, phaeochromocytoma and hypoglycaemia in clinical practice.

Organic personality disorder
In ICD-10 organic personality disorder is defined as being characterized by a significant alteration of the habitual patterns of behaviour displayed by the subject premorbidly. Such alteration always involves more profoundly the expression of emotions, needs and impulses. Cognition may be defective mostly or exclusively in the areas of planning one's own actions and anticipating their likely personal and social consequences. The causes of organic personality disorder include:

- intracranial (particularly affecting the frontal or temporal lobes)

    - head injury
    - tumours
    - abscesses
    - subarachnoid haemorrhage

Table 25.3 Causes of organic anxiety disorder

Psychoactive substance use	Alcohol and drug withdrawal Amphetamine and related sympathomimetics Cannabis
Intoxication	Drugs – penicillin, sulphonamides Caffeine and caffeine withdrawal Poisons – aresenic, mercury, organophosphates, phosphorus, benzene Aspirin intolerance
Intracranial causes	Brain tumours Head injury Migraine Cerebrovascular disease Subarachnoid haemorrhage Infections – encephalitis, neurosyphilis Multiple sclerosis Hepatolenticular degeneration (Wilson's disease) Huntington's disease Epilepsy
Endocrine	Pituitary dysfunction Thyroid dysfunction Parathyroid dysfunction Adrenal dysfunction Phaeochromocytoma dysfunction Hypoglycaemia Virilization disorders of females
Inflammatory disorders	Systemic lupus erythematosus Rheumatoid arthritis Polyarteritis nodosa Temporal arteritis
Vitamin deficiency	Vitamin B_{12} deficiency Pellagra (nicotinic acid deficiency)
Other systemic disorders	Hypoxia Cardiovascular disease Cardiac arrhythmias Pulmonary insufficiency Anaemia Carcinoid syndrome Systemic neoplasia Febrile illnesses and chronic infections Porphyria Infectious mononucleosis (glandular fever) Posthepatic syndrome Uraemia Premenstrual syndrome

Based on Cummings, J. 1985: *Clinical neuropsychiatry.* Orlando. Grune & Stratton.
Reproduced with permission from Puri, B.K., Laking, P.J. and Treasaden, I.H. 1996: *Textbook of psychiatry.* Edinburgh: Churchill Livingstone.

- neurosyphilis
- epilepsy

- Huntington's disease
- hepatolenticular degeneration (Wilson's disease)

- medication e.g. corticosteroids
- psychoactive substance use
- endocrinopathies

BIBLIOGRAPHY

Cummings, J. 1985: *Clinical neuropsychiatry*. Orlando, Florida:. Grune & Stratton.

Lishman, W.A. 1997. *Organic psychiatry: the psychological consequences of cerebral disorder*, 3rd edn. Oxford: Blackwell Scientific.

Marsden, C.D. and Fowler, T.J. 1989: *Clinical neurology*. London: Edward Arnold.

Yudofsky, S.C. and Hales, R.E. (eds) 1992: *The American Psychiatric Press textbook of neuropsychiatry*, 2nd edn. Washington, DC: American Psychiatric Press.

26
Psychoactive substance use disorders

DRUG AND ALCOHOL ABUSE

ICD-10
MENTAL AND BEHAVIOURAL DISORDERS CAUSED BY PSYCHOACTIVE SUBSTANCE USE (F10–19)

F10   Mental and behavioural disorders caused by the use of alcohol;
F11   caused by the use of opioids;
F12   caused by the use of cannabinoids;
F13   caused by the use of sedatives or hypnotics;
F14   caused by the use of cocaine;
F15   caused by the use of other stimulants, including caffeine;
F16   caused by the use of hallucinogens;
F17   caused by the use of tobacco;
F18   caused by the use of volatile solvents;
F19   caused by the use of multiple drug use and use of other psychoactive substances.

Specific clinical conditions are additionally coded as follows:

0.   Acute intoxication
1.   Harmful use
2.   Dependence syndrome
3.   Withdrawal state
4.   Withdrawal state with delirium
5.   Psychotic disorder
6.   Amnesic syndrome
7.   Residual and late-onset psychotic disorder
8.   Other mental and behavioural disorders
9.   Unspecified mental and behavioural disorder

ACUTE INTOXICATION   This is transient condition following the use of psychoactive substance, resulting in disturbed conscious level, cognition, perception, affect or behaviour. Its intensity is closely related to dose, lessening with time, and the effects disappear when stopped. Recovery is usually complete.

PATHOLOGICAL INTOXICATION   This applies only to alcohol, and refers to sudden aggressive behaviour, out of character, after drinking small amounts which would not produce intoxication in most people.

HARMFUL USE   This is use that is causing damage to physical or mental health. It does not refer to adverse social consequences.

DEPENDENCE SYNDROME   This is diagnosed if three or more of the following have been present together at some time in the previous year:

■ compulsion to take the substance
■ difficulties in controlling substance-taking behaviour: onset, termination or levels of use
■ characteristic physiological withdrawal state when substance reduced or withdrawn; use of substance to avoid or relieve withdrawal symptoms
■ tolerance: increased doses required to achieve effect originally produced by lower doses
■ progressive neglect of other activities with increasing time spent in acquiring, taking or recovering from the effects of the substance
■ persisting with substance use despite evidence of harmful consequences

WITHDRAWAL STATE   Symptoms occur upon withdrawal or reduction of a substance after repeated, usually high dose and prolonged use. Onset and course are time-limited, dose-related and differ according to the substance involved. Convulsions may complicate withdrawal.

WITHDRAWAL STATE WITH DELIRIUM   Withdrawal state is complicated by delirium.

Alcohol induced **delirium tremens** is a short-lived sometimes life-threatening toxic confusional state precipitated by relative or absolute alcohol withdrawal in severely dependent users. Classic symptoms include:

■ clouding of consciousness
■ hallucinations and illusions
■ marked tremor

It involves prodromal symptoms of insomnia, tremulousness and fearful affect. Delusions, agitation, insomnia and autonomic overactivity usually accompany it; convulsions may occur.

PSYCHOTIC DISORDER   Psychotic symptoms occur during or immediately after psychoactive substance use, in relatively clear sensorium (some clouding of consciousness but not severe confusion). It is not a manifestation of drug withdrawal or a functional psychosis. The characteristics of the psychosis vary according to the substance used, but vivid hallucinations in more than one modality, delusions, psychomotor disturbances and abnormal affect are common. Stimulant-induced psychotic disorders are generally related to prolonged high-dose use. Typically it resolves at least partially within one month and fully within six months.

In ICD-10 further subdivisions may be specified:

■ schizophrenia-like
■ predominantly delusional
■ predominantly hallucinatory (includes alcoholic hallucinosis)
■ predominantly polymorphic
■ predominantly depressive symptoms
■ predominantly manic symptoms
■ mixed

AMNESIC SYNDROME   This is induced by alcohol or other psychoactive substances. Requirements for diagnosis include:

- chronic prominent impairment of **recent** memory; remote memory may be impaired. Difficulty learning new material; disturbance of time sense
- immediate recall preserved; other cognitive functions are usually relatively preserved and consciousness is clear
- history of chronic and usually high-dose use of alcohol or drugs

Confabulation may be present, but not invariably so. **Korsakov's psychosis** is included here.

RESIDUAL AND LATE-ONSET PSYCHOTIC DISORDER   Alcohol- or psychoactive substance-induced changes of cognition, affect, personality, or behaviour persist beyond the period during which the substance might reasonably be assumed to be operating. Onset is directly related to substance use.

Further subdivided by ICD-10 into:

- flashbacks: episodic psychotic experiences which duplicate previous drug-related experiences and are usually very short-lived (seconds or minutes)
- personality or behaviour disorder
- organic mood disorder
- dementia: may be reversible after an extended period of abstinence
- other persisting cognitive impairment

ALCOHOL

The concentration of alcohol in beverages is stated in terms of 'proof' scales. In the United States one degree ($1°$) proof is equal to a concentration of 0.5 per cent by volume (v/v). In Britain $1°$ proof is equal to 0.5715 per cent by volume.

EXCESSIVE CONSUMPTION

Units of alcohol
One unit of alcohol is approximately 10 g, and is the amount contained in a standard measure of spirits, a standard glass of sherry or fortified wine, a standard glass of table wine, and in one half-pint of beer or lager of standard strength (3 to 3.5 per cent by volume).

Levels of consumption
Up to 21 units of alcohol per week for men, and up to 14 units of alcohol per week for women, not consumed in one go and not consumed every day, are considered to be **low risk levels** of intake. Women are more susceptible to the harmful effects of alcohol because their lower lean body mass results in higher blood alcohol levels per unit taken.

Consumption in greater amounts constitutes **excessive consumption**, carrying much greater risks of developing alcohol-related disability and alcohol dependence.

Abstinence or minimal alcohol intake is recommended in pregnancy, because of the risk of the development of fetal alcohol syndrome.

ALCOHOL-RELATED DISABILITIES

Excessive alcohol intake can lead to physical, psychiatric and social morbidity.

Physical morbidity
Alcohol accounts for one-fifth to one-third of medical admissions to hospital.

GASTROINTESTINAL DISORDERS

- Nausea and vomiting, particularly in the morning, prevented by drinking more alcohol
- Gastritis, peptic ulcers, diarrhoea
- Mallory–Weiss tears, oesophageal varices

MALNUTRITION   This results from poor intake, malabsorption, and impaired metabolism.

- Thiamine deficiency presenting with Wernicke's encephalopathy acutely, leading in a high proportion of cases to Korsakov's psychosis. May also present with high output heart failure of beri-beri
- Niacin deficiency (vitamin B3) presenting with pellagra, causing confusion, diarrhoea and light sensitive rash
- Vitamin C deficiency presenting with skin haemorrhages and gingivitis

HEPATIC DAMAGE   Fatty infiltration leading to an acute increase in the size of the liver occurs within a few days of excessive intake; it may cause pain in right hypochondrium, nausea and vomiting but is usually not detected. It is reversible with abstinence. Alcoholic hepatitis secondary to long-term heavy daily drinking. Liver cell necrosis and inflammation occurs, presenting with right hypochondrial pain and jaundice, sometimes accompanied by ascites and encephalopathy.

Cirrhosis with permanent fibrotic changes occurs. This may present with signs of liver failure: ascites, encephalopathy and bleeding oesophageal varices, but it may be symptomless initially.

ACUTE AND CHRONIC PANCREATITIS   This leads to food malabsorption and diabetes in some.

CARDIOVASCULAR SYSTEM

- Hypertension, poorly responsive to conventional treatment but responsive to abstinence
- Cardiac arrhythmias particularly after binge-drinking (**holiday heart syndrome**)
- Cardiomyopathy, presenting with gradual onset of heart failure. Prognosis poor with continued drinking
- Haemorrhagic and thrombotic CVA, even in the young

HAEMATOLOGICAL   Alcohol is a bone marrow toxin, resulting in the following:

- Macrocytosis
- Folate deficiency
- Impaired clotting caused by vitamin K deficiency and/or reduced platelet functioning
- Iron deficiency anaemia, often as a result of gastrointestinal haemorrhage

ENDOCRINE AND SEXUAL DISORDERS

There is gonadal atrophy which affects both sexes. Direct toxic effects upon the gonads result in reduced sex hormone synthesis. Liver disease results in oestrogenization in men resulting in gynacomastia. Fertility may recover with abstinence. Autonomic nervous system dysfunction may result in erectile impotence and central effects cause anorgasmia. This is an increased risk of miscarriage and recurrent abortion in women.

Alcoholic pseudo-Cushing's syndrome, causing obesity, hirsuitism and hypertension.

CANCER   Increased incidence of:

- oropharygeal
- oesophageal
- colorectal
- pancreatic
- hepatic
- lung

FETAL ALCOHOL SYNDROME   Excessive alcohol consumption in **pregnancy** can lead to permanent fetal damage. It comprises low IQ (mean 70), cardiac abnormalities and characteristic facies with low-set ears, absent philtrum and a depressed bridge of the nose.

ACCIDENTS AND TRAUMA   These include road accidents, assaults, falls, drowning, burns and death by fire. The most common traumatic injuries include rib fractures, head injuries, subdural/extradural haematomata, and long bone fractures.

There is an increased risk of **infections** such as tuberculosis and pneumonia, particularly in the homeless.

METABOLIC

- Alcohol-induced lactic acidosis
- Alcoholic ketoacidosis
- Hyperlipidemia in one-third of alcohol-dependent subjects. Low levels of intake appear protective, however
- Hypoglycaemia
- Hyperuricaemia
- Haemochromatosis
- Porphyria cutanea tarda

SKIN

- Acne
- Rhinophyma

MUSCULOSKELETAL DISORDERS

- Myopathy, presenting acutely with pain and tenderness of swollen muscles. Usually symmetrical. If severe may cause renal failure due to myoglobinuria
- Proximal muscle weakness and wasting is common in alcoholics
- Osteoporosis
- Avascular necrosis

NEUROLOGICAL DISORDERS

- Peripheral neuropathy resulting in numbness and parasthesias in glove and stocking distribution
- Cerebellar degeneration, affecting mainly the vermis, resulting in ataxia of gait
- Convulsions occurring mainly secondary to alcohol withdrawal, within the first 48 hours. Also secondary to brain damage or hypoglycemia
- Optic atrophy
- Central pontine myelinolysis
- Marchiafava–Bignami disease, a rare fatal demyelinating disease characterized neuropathologically by widespread demyelination affecting the central corpus callosum, and often also the middle cerebellar peduncles, the white matter of the cerebral hemispheres, and the optic tracts. Present clinically with emo-

tional disturbance and cognitive impairment followed by epilepsy, delirium, paralysis and coma.

Psychiatric morbidity

MOOD DISORDERS   Chronic heavy drinking can itself produce severe, usually transient depressive symptoms, which generally improve with abstinence. If symptoms persist with abstinence, antidepressants should be considered. Suicide rate is at least 50 times greater in alcoholics than in the general population. Between one-quarter and one-third of completed suicides occur in alcoholics and up to four-fifths of those who kill themselves have been drinking.

PERSONALITY DISORDER   Those with sociopathic personality disorder engage in excessive drinking and those who drink heavily often engage in antisocial acts. If antisocial behaviour predates alcoholism by several years then the primary diagnosis is of personality disorder.

Cloninger (1987) described two types of alcoholic:

Type 1 (milieu limited)   Less severe, occuring in men and women, in dependent, anxious, rigid, less aggressive types, whose biological father or mother may have a mild adult onset alcohol problem. It is thought that genetic predisposition and postnatal provocation are required to provoke this type of alcoholism.

Type 2   Severe, early onset, occurring in men who are socially detached and confident, whose biological fathers (but not mothers) often have teenage onset alcoholism and criminality. This type is thought by some to be alcoholism secondary to sociopathic personality disorder. Genetic predisposition has a powerful aetiological effect, with little contribution from the environment.

PSYCHOSIS   There is no relationship between schizophrenia and alcoholism other than that occurring by chance. Genetic studies find that people suffering from alcoholism and schizophrenia have a predisposition to each condition separately.

A rarer disorder caused by chronic alcohol intake is **alcoholic hallucinosis**, characterized by auditory hallucinations in clear consciousness. It is distinguished from schizophrenia by the association with alcohol abuse, lack of family history, onset at an older age (40 or 50), more acute presentation with resolution commonly within a month (if abstinent), absence of thought disorder and more appropriate affect. It may follow abstinence but can present or recur in those who are still drinking. If it persists for longer than six months the likely diagnosis is schizophrenia.

PATHOLOGICAL JEALOUSY   This is a well-recognized association with alcoholism, but may occur with other conditions such as schizophrenia and depression.

NEUROTIC DISORDERS   These may predispose to alcoholism in an attempt by the patient to self-medicate. Generalized anxiety, panic attacks and phobic disorders, particularly agarophobia, may precede alcoholism. The patient should be reassessed once abstinent and any underlying condition should be appropriately managed.

PSYCHOSEXUAL DISORDERS   In men intoxication leads to erectile impotence and delayed ejaculation. Chronic heavy drinking in men can cause the loss of libido, reduction in the size of the testes and penis, loss of body hair and gynaecomastia; in women it can lead to menstrual cycle abnormalities, the loss of breast tissue and vaginal dryness.

Heavy drinking is often associated with gambling and the use of other psychoactive substances.

ORGANIC BRAIN SYNDROMES

Acute / subacute syndromes

ALCOHOLIC BLACKOUTS   Intoxication frequently leads to episodes of short-term amnesia or blackouts. These may occur after just one bout of heavy drinking, and is estimated to have been experienced by 15 to 20 per cent of those who drink.

Three types of blackout are recognized, of increasing severity:

1. **State dependent** memory loss, in which memory for events occurring while intoxicated are lost when sober, but return when next intoxicated.
2. **Fragmentary** blackouts in which there is no clear demarcation of memory loss, and islets of memory exist within the gap. Some recovery occurs with time.
3. **En bloc** blackouts in which there is a clearly demarcated total memory loss, with no recovery of this lost memory over time. If this memory loss extends for days the subject experiences a fugue-like state in which they may travel some distance before coming around, with no memory of the events occurring during this time.

DELIRIUM TREMENS   In chronic heavy drinkers a fall in the blood alcohol concentration leads to withdrawal symptoms including **delirium tremens**. Peak onset is within two days of abstinence and it usually lasts for about five days. There is a prodromal period with anxiety, insomnia, tachycardia, tremor and sweating. The onset of delirium is marked by disorientation, fluctuating conscious level, intensely fearful affect, hallucinations, misperceptions, tremor, restlessness and autonomic overactivity. Hallucinations are often visual and are commonly Lilliputian in nature. Auditory and tactile hallucinations, and secondary delusions may also be present.

Mortality of 5 per cent is associated with cardiovascular collapse or infection. Treatment is supportive with sedation, fluid and electrolyte replacement, high potency vitamins (especially thiamine to prevent an unrecognized Wernicke's encephalopathy progressing to Korsakov's psychosis).

Another important withdrawal symptom is **withdrawal fits** which may take place within 48 hours of stopping drinking.

WERNICKE'S ENCEPHALOPATHY   Wernicke's encephalopathy is caused by severe deficiency of thiamine (vitamin B_1), which is usually caused by alcohol abuse in Western countries. Other causes include: lesions of the stomach (e.g. carcinoma), duodenum, or jejunum causing malabsorption; hyperemesis; and starvation. The most important clinical features of Wernicke's encephalopathy are:

- ophthalmoplegia
- nystagmus
- ataxia
- clouding of consciousness
- peripheral neuropathy may also be present

Wernicke's encephalopathy and Korsakov's psychosis have overlapping pathology and the former may culminate in the latter if untreated. Wernicke's encephalopathy is a medical emergency and should be treated with intravenous thiamine plus other B vitamins.

Post-mortem examination of the brains of those dying of Wernicke'e encephalopathy reveal petechial haemorrhages in the mammillary bodies and less commonly in the walls of the third ventricle, periaqueductal grey matter, floor of the fourth ventricle and inferior colliculi.

Nicotinic acid depletion can sometimes give rise to pellagra encephalopathy, a confusional state resembling Wernicke's encephalopathy.

b) Chronic syndromes

KORSAKOV'S SYNDROME   This alcohol-induced amnesic syndrome is frequently preceded by **Wernicke's encephalopathy,** 'An abnormal state in which memory and learning are affected out of all proportion to other cognitive functions in an otherwise alert and responsive patient' (Victor *et al.* 1971).

It is retrograde and anterograde amnesia (sparing of immediate memory) with disorientation in time and an inability to recall the temporal sequence of events. Patients may confabulate and may have peripheral neuropathy.

Neuropathologically there is scarring and atrophy of the mammillary bodies and anterior thalamus, with substantial frontal lobe dysfunction on neuroimaging.

Improvement may occur with abstinence and high dose thiamine and vitamin B replacement which should be continued for six months.

ALCOHOLIC DEMENTIA   Those who have abused alcohol for some years commonly suffer mild to moderate cognitive impairment, which may improve over a number of years of abstinence. Women, who are known to suffer physical complications of alcohol abuse earlier than men, also develop cognitive impairment earlier in their drinking histories. A CT scan of the brain in alcoholics commonly shows ventricular enlargement and sulcal widening, which does not correlate with the degree of cognitive impairment and largely reverses with abstinence.

Chronic alcoholics show a coarsening of personality which appears to be related to frontal lobe atrophy.

SOCIAL MORBIDITY   The social costs of excessive alcohol consumption are high. They include:

BREAKDOWN OF FAMILIES   One-third of problem drinkers cite marital discord as one of their problems; one-third of divorce petitions cite alcohol as a contributory factor; three-quarters of battered wives describe their husbands as frequently drunk or subject to heavy drinking. Children of alcoholics often suffer neglect, poverty or physical violence.

CRIME   Alcohol misuse is strongly associated with crime particularly against the person and against property.

Half of those committing homicide have been drinking at the time of the offence, and half of victims are intoxicated. Half of rapists were drinking at the time of the offence. One- to two-thirds of burglaries are committed under the influence of alcohol.

ACCIDENTS AND TRAUMA   In 1978 31 per cent of drivers and 29 per cent of motorcyclists killed in accidents had blood alcohol levels above the legal limit of 80 mg per 100 ml, as did 30 per cent of passengers and 21 per cent of pedestrians. It is estimated that 1200 deaths each year, representing one-fifth of all deaths on the road, result from drink-driving.

Alcohol is implicated in one-third of accidents at home and deaths by drowning, and 40 per cent of deaths by fire and falling.

ECONOMIC HARM   Major costs to the country are incurred through lost productivity, damage, medical, legal and social costs associated with the use of alcohol.

Alcohol dependence

Edwards and Gross (1976) described the alcohol-dependence syndrome which was later also applied to other psychoactive substances:

1. Increased tolerance.
   Repeated doses of drug produce less effect, resulting in escalating doses of the drug to achieve the original effect. Rate at which tolerance develops varies with substance used: it is generally rapid with heroin, but much slower with alcohol.

2. Repeated withdrawal symptoms.
    A fall in blood-alcohol concentration leads to unpleasant withdrawal symptoms within 12 hours of the last intake, relieved by drinking more alcohol.
3. Subjective awareness of compulsion to drink.
    Attempted abstinence leads to tension and an increased craving for alcohol.
4. Salience of drink-seeking behaviour.
    Acquiring and drinking alcohol take primacy over other activities such as family, career and social position.
5. Relief or avoidance of withdrawal symptoms, by further drinking.
6. Narrowing of the drinking repertoire.
    The pattern of drinking becomes increasingly stereotyped with increasing dependence. A daily routine develops and a certain drink will be favoured over others.
7. Rapid reinstatement following abstinence.
    After a period of abstinence the drinker may attempt to drink in moderation. The intake is likely to escalate rapidly as tolerance and dependence reappear within a few days.

Epidemiology

There is a close association between liver-cirrhosis mortality and the national consumption of alcohol. Mortality figures are a useful index of national alcohol consumption. Other indices include the number of arrests for drunkenness, drunken driving, cases of assault and battery, and deaths from alcohol poisoning.

Ten per cent of the drinking population drinks half of all the alcohol drunk.

Price greatly affects levels of drinking. Countries with cheap alcohol consume more than countries with more expensive alcohol. As the prices of alcohol rise, the quantity drunk by even chronic dependent drinkers falls, and the amount of alcohol-related morbidity falls.

It is estimated that of the 55 million UK population, 36 million are regular drinkers; 2 million are heavy drinkers (> 80 g alcohol daily for men, and > 40 g for women); 700 000 are problem drinkers and 200 000 are dependent drinkers.

Men outnumber women, but the sex ratio of alcohol-related problems is falling. Ten years ago alcoholic cirrhosis was five times as common in men as in women, but the sex ratio has fallen to 2:1.

The age of first drinking has fallen to between 12 and 14 in both sexes. The highest rates of heavy drinking are seen between adolescence and the early twenties.

Certain occupational groups are at greater risk of drinking problems. Those with jobs in the drink industry are at highest risk, including publicans, bartenders and brewers. Those whose jobs take them away from home, such as fishermen, armed servicemen and executives, and those with professional autonomy, such as doctors, are also at higher risk.

Aetiology

GENETIC   There is good evidence that heavy drinking runs in families.

The relatives of alcoholics have higher rates of alcoholism than the relatives of controls.

Twin studies indicate that monozygotic twins have a higher concordance rate than dizygotic twins. In normal twins approximately one-third of the variance in drinking habits has been estimated to be genetic in origin.

Adoption studies support the hypothesis of the genetic transmission of alcoholism. The sons of alcoholic parents are three to four times more likely to become alcoholic than the sons of non-alcoholics, irrespective of the home environment.

Strains of rats have been bred which voluntarily consume large quantities of alcohol. These rats appear to have abnormalities in brain levels of serotonin, noradrenaline and dopamine.

PERSONALITY   It has been suggested that some problem drinkers are predisposed to harmful drinking by their personality; however, studies in this area give contradictory results. It is known that those with sociopathic personality disorder have a high prevalence of heavy drinking and alcoholism. However, there is no typical pre-alcoholic personality.

BIOLOGICAL   The EEG of sober, awake alcoholics shows an excess of fast activity and a deficiency of alpha, theta and delta activity. The sons of alcoholics also show an excess of fast activity when compared to controls, leading to speculation that this may be a specific marker for alcoholism.

Electrically evoked responses show reduced P3 voltage in both abstinent chronic alcoholics and in the young sons of alcoholics when compared to controls.

The metabolism of alcohol is genetically determined and varies between individuals. Over half of Orientals develop an unpleasant flushing response when alcohol is ingested, related to the accumulation of acetaldehyde, caused by the absence of the isoenzyme ALDH2: aldehyde dehydrogenase. It is thought that this intolerance of alcohol protects them from developing alcoholism, since it is much less prevalent in those of oriental heritage.

Ethanol at low concentrations (5–10 mmol L^{-1}), inhibits the action of the NMDA-glutamate controlled ion channels, and potentiates the actions of GABA type A controlled ion channels. These are the main excitatory and inhibitory systems of the brain; the overall effect of ethanol is therefore as a central nervous depressant.

At slightly higher ethanol concentrations the actions of voltage-sensitive calcium channels and channels controlled by serotonin are affected.

Ethanol given *in vivo* promotes the CNS release of dopamine particularly from the nucleus accumbens.

Chronic administration of ethanol produces alterations in the GABA, NMDA and voltage-sensitive calcium channel systems. Reduction in the production of subunits of the GABA receptors are seen particularly in mice prone to withdrawal convulsions. Chronic ethanol administration also causes an up-regulation of NMDA receptors in mouse hippocampus, more evident in mice prone to withdrawal convulsions. Both of these receptor changes promote CNS excitability and increase the likelihood of convulsions.

Excessive glutamate stimulation is toxic to the nerve cell and results in damage or cell death. Although ethanol exposure is the cause of increased numbers of NMDA receptors, its presence protects against the neurotoxicity of glutamate over-stimulation. The acute withdrawal of ethanol in the dependent subject results in convulsions and neurotoxicity.

PSYCHOLOGICAL   There are three main components to psychological theories of dependence:

Withdrawal avoidance   Prolonged drug use results in tolerance, with CNS adaptation to allow normal functioning despite the chronic presence of the psychoactive drug. If the drug is suddenly withdrawn, this adaptation results in drug-withdrawal symptoms, which are usually opposite to the effects of the drug. Thus in terms of this theory the dependent person continues drug use in order to avoid the adverse effects of drug withdrawal.

Positive effects of the drug   According to this theory, the pleasant effects of the drug reinforce drug-taking behaviour, despite adverse social and physical consequences.

Motivational distortion   According to this theory the repetition of drug-taking behaviour, or the effects of the drugs themselves, change the motivational system supporting that behaviour. Habit strength is a term describing the strength of the link between a stimulus that cues a behaviour. It is possible that it involves habituation at the neuronal level.

Each of these theories accounts for some but not all aspects of addiction.

CULTURAL FACTORS   There are high rates of alcoholism in countries where alcohol is drunk routinely with family meals, and in places where it is cheap.

PSYCHIATRIC ILLNESS   This can predispose patients to harmful drinking, particularly anxiety disorders, phobic disorders, depression and bereavement and mania.

MANAGEMENT

HISTORY

For screening purposes the CAGE questionnaire is widely used. Positive answers to two or more of the four questions is indicative of problem drinking.

CAGE questionnaire:

- Have you ever felt you should **c**ut down on your drinking?
- Have people ever **a**nnoyed you by criticizing your drinking?
- Have you ever felt **g**uilty about your drinking?
- Have you ever had a drink first thing in the morning to steady your nerves or get over a hangover? (**e**ye-opener)

The alcohol history should include the average number of units of alcohol consumed weekly and the drinking pattern.

An alcohol history should include: information about the evolution of the problem (drinking career, drink-related problems, dependence); typical recent drinking day (initial, then hourly quantification of alcohol intake, waking nausea, tremor, nightmares and night sweats), and an interview with the spouse.

When alcohol dependence is suspected or diagnosed it is essential to carry out a full physical examination bearing in mind the multiple organ systems damaged by this substance.

INVESTIGATIONS   Blood investigations include alcohol levels in the intoxicated (breathalyzers can be useful to give an indication of levels of recent drinking). Alcoholism is the most common cause of raised mean corpuscular volume (MCV), and it is raised in 60 per cent of alcohol abusers. Since the life of a red blood cell is 120 days, the MCV should return to normal four months after continued abstinence. Raised gamma glutamyl transferase may occur; this is good for screening as an indication of recent alcohol use, but it can be raised after only one heavy drinking session. Liver function tests (e.g. aspartate transaminase) may be abnormal, particularly during acute alcoholic hepatitis, less so in fatty liver, and may be normal in cirrhosis.

TREATMENT   Detoxification can usually be conducted as an outpatient unless severe withdrawal effects such as delirium tremens or convulsions are likely to occur; the patient's mental state causes concern; or there are severe social problems, in which case inpatient care should be organized. The aim should be for abstinence; education, support and counselling will be required.

After the assessment of the severity of withdrawal symptoms, a substitute sedative is started. Benzodiazepines such as diazepam or chlordiazepoxide are commonly used in a reducing regimen. Attention should be paid to the state of hydration and nutrition of the patient. Thiamine should always be given. If malabsorption is likely, intravenous thiamine and other B vitamins should be given in the first instance. A glucose load should be avoided as this can precipitate or exacerbate thiamine deficiency; ascorbic acid may also be required. The suicide risk should be assessed.

Alcoholics Anonymous is a self-help group which some alcoholics find helpful. Al-Anon supports the families of alcoholics, and Al-Ateen the teenage children of alcoholics.

Supportive therapy is helpful. Other forms of psychotherapy are also useful. Cognitive-behavioural models appear to be particularly effective in relapse prevention. Such therapies include cue exposure, relapse prevention strategies, contingency management, social skills and assertiveness training.

Medication can be used in the detoxified alcoholic to help maintain abstinence.

Aversive agents disulfiram (Antabuse) and citrated calcium carbimide both inhibit aldehyde dehydrogenase leading to the accumulation of aldehyde if alcohol is ingested. The patient experiences very unpleasant symptoms of flushing, headache, palpitations, tachycardia, nausea and vomiting with ingestion of small amounts of alcohol, and air hunger, arrhythmias and severe hypotension with large amounts of alcohol. These agents are contraindicated in ischaemic heart disease, in pregnancy or if there is a history of convulsions. Patients must be well motivated and aware of the risks of taking alcohol with these agents. Efficacy requires compliance with taking the aversive agent; involving the spouse in administration can improve the success rate.

Prognosis

Good prognostic factors include good insight, strong motivation, and good social and family support. Relapse can be precipitated by emotional stress, interpersonal conflict and social pressures.

Follow-up of alcoholics over a period of ten years finds that 25 per cent continue troubled drinking, 12 per cent are abstinent, and the remainder follow a pattern of intermittent troubled drinking and abstinence.

OTHER PSYCHOACTIVE SUBSTANCES

Colloquial names for some abused drugs are given in Table 26.1.

Table 26.1 Colloquial names for some abused drugs

Drug	Colloquial name
Heroin	Smack
Cannabinoids	Grass, hash, ganja, pot
Temazepam capsules	Jellies
Barbiturates	Downers
Cocaine	Snow, coke, girl, lady
Amphetamines	Speed, whizz
LSD	Acid
PCP	Angel dust, Peace Pill
MDMA	Ecstacy, XTC, Adam, E

Opioids

Drugs derived from opium poppies are known as opiates. Synthetically derived opiates are known as opioids.

Heroin (gear, smack, scag)

Heroin (3,6-diacetylmorphine) is produced from morphine which is derived from the sap of the opium poppy.

It is smoked or chased by heating on tin foil and inhaling the sublimate. It is injected intravenously, and much less commonly subcutaneously (skin-popping). Street heroin is usually between 30 and 60 per cent pure, and between 1/4 g–3/4 g is a common daily consumption for addicts.

Misuse of Drugs Act 1971

This specifies the classes of controlled drugs according to perceived dangerousness:

Class A   This includes most opiates (heroin; morphine; opium; pethidine; methadone), cocaine, and hallucinogens and psychotomimetics (LSD; mescaline, PCP).
Class B   This includes cannabis, codeine, amphetamines and barbiturates. Injectable preparations of Class B drugs are designated as Class A.
Class C   This includes dextropropoxyphene, benzodiazepines, meprobamate, pemoline and others.

The penalties for drug use and supply are related to these classes.

Home Office Notification

The Misuse of Drugs (Notification of and supply to addicts) Regulations 1973 required any doctor to notify the Chief Medical Officer at the Home Office in writing within seven days of attending to a patient who is considered or suspected (on reasonable grounds) to be addicted to any of the following controlled drugs:

- cocaine
- dextromoramide (Palfium)
- diamorphine (heroin)
- dipipanone (Diconal)
- hydrocodone
- hydromorphone
- levorphanol
- methadone
- morphine
- opium
- oxycodone
- pethidine
- phenazocine and piritramide

Notifications are compiled in the Addicts Index which provides epidemiological information for use in the planning of services. Doctors can also contact the Index by telephone to check whether a patient presenting to them is currently known to another service. It thus acts as a safeguard against multiple scripting. About one-fifth of addicts are notified to the Home Office at any one time.

From 1st May 1997 the Addicts Index was closed and the statutory duty for doctors to notify details of addicts to the Addicts Index was removed.

In addition to the compulsory national reporting of addicts, there are local voluntary schemes in which information of a similar nature is held on Regional Drug Misuse Databases. These include in addition to the above controlled drugs information about other drug use.

Prescribing controlled drugs

The Misuse of Drugs Regulations 1985 require that prescriptions for controlled drugs in schedules 1, 2 and 3 (except phenobarbitone) must be:

- In indelible ink
- In the doctor's own handwriting and signed by the doctor
- Inclusive of the patient's name, address, dose, form and strength of preparation; and the total quantity to be dispensed

If dispensed in instalments e.g. daily, the number of instalments, total dose per instalment, and intervals must be specified in the doctor's own handwriting. Doctors prescribing for ten or more addicts can apply to get a handwriting dispensation from the Home Office.

A special licence is required from the Home Secretary for doctors who wish to prescribe cocaine, diamorphine or dipipanone to an addict. This does not apply to the other notifiable drugs, and does not apply to the prescription of cocaine, diamorphine or dipipanone for the purposes of treating organic disease or injury.

Epidemiology

The numbers of addicts notified to the Home Office has increased dramatically over the last 30 years. This is thought to be related to the wider availability of cheap opiates imported from the Middle East. Youth culture has become much more accepting of drug use, and poly-drug use is much more common than it used to be.

	Number of notifications (approximate)
1960	500
1980	5000
1990	15000

Most heroin users are aged between 20 and 30 years. The steepest increase has occurred in those aged 16 to 24 years. The male: female ratio is 2:1.

Drug action

The stimulation of opiate receptors produces analgesia, euphoria, miosis, hypotension, bradycardia and respiratory depression.

Opioid receptors fall into different types, each of which has subtypes. The main types are mu, kappa and delta receptors. The effects of a particular opiate drug depend upon the combination of receptors stimulated. Most of the effects of morphine are mediated through mu receptors.

Euphoria is initially intense and is related in part to the method of administration. Thus methods delivering a large bolus quickly to the CNS are associated with a greater initial rush. Intravenous and inhalational techniques fulfil these conditions, oral and subcutaneous methods do not.

Dependence may arise within weeks of regular use.

Effects of drug withdrawal

This begins within 4–12 hours of last heroin use. Peak intensity is at about 48 hours, and the main symptoms disappear within a week of abstinence. Physical symptoms include intense dysphoria; aching limbs; nausea; diarrhoea; dilated pupils; shivering; sweating; yawning; sneezing; rhinorrhoea; lacrimation; fatigue; insomnia and craving for the drug which may continue for weeks. Although it is unpleasant, opiate withdrawal is not generally dangerous (exceptions include pregnancy, when abortion may result from precipitous withdrawal).

Harmful effects

Those using opiates are at risk from:

The effects of the drug itself   Overdose caused by the uncertain concentration of street drugs, or to reduced tolerance following a period of abstinence e.g. upon release from prison.

The clinical features of opiate overdose include stupor or coma; pinpoint pupils; pallor; severe respiratory depression; pulmonary oedema. Supportive treatment and administration of an opioid antagonist such as nalaxone is indicated. The half-life of opioid antagonists is less than that of most opiate drugs, therefore the patient must be observed for several hours to ensure that the underlying opiate overdose has passed.

The effects of intoxication, such as accidents

The effects of administration   The inhalation of heroin commonly exacerbates or causes lung conditions such as asthma. There are increased rates of pneumonia and tuberculosis in those who are HIV positive.

The hazards of intravenous use are many, and include the transmission of infection through the use of shared needles. HIV and hepatitis B, C and D are commonly transmitted through this route. Those who are HIV positive have a poorer outcome if they continue to inject.

Bacterial infection results from the lack of aseptic technique; the risk is not eliminated by using clean needles since the drug itself is not of pharmaceutical quality, has often been adulterated with other substances, and is often not suitable for intravenous administration because of the presence of non-soluble components.

Skin infection at injection sites leads to abscess formation, and thrombophlebitis. *Staphylococcus aureus* and *Streptococcus pyogenes* are often responsible.

Most injecting results in transient bacteremia. This can result in septicemia and/or bacterial endocarditis, even in those with previously normal heart valves. Septic emboli may be carried to distant sites.

Systemic fungal infections have been reported which are difficult to treat and result in death or blindness because of ophthalmic involvement.

Vascular complications include the obliteration of the lung vascular bed with continued prolonged injection of particulate matter. The same effect is seen in the lymphatic system, resulting in puffy hands. DVT may develop at the site of femoral administration. Arterial administration can result in occlusion caused by spasm or embolism. The loss of a limb may result.

Long-term users may develop membranous glomerulonephritis or amyloid disease.

Septic embolism can result in osteomyelitis.

Social effects   Because of the effects of tolerance and dependence, heroin users usually escalate the dose of drug taken in an attempt to continue to achieve the euphoriant effects and to keep the unpleasant withdrawal effects of the drug at bay. The result is often that the addict turns to acquisitive crime in order to fund their growing drug habit.

It is estimated that the stabilization of heroin addicts on to methadone costs the NHS approximately £1000 per year, but that this saves society approximately £30 000 in drug-related crime.

Relationships and family commitments usually come second to drug-related activities, and family breakdown often results. It is difficult to continue in employment when seriously addicted to heroin.

Methadone (physeptone)

This is a synthetic opiate which can be taken orally or intravenously. Its half-life is longer than that of heroin (16–24 hours) allowing once daily oral prescribing. It has little euphoric effect when administered orally, but has some street value, particularly in injectable form. It is frequently prescribed in the management of opiate dependence. In this case the elixir is the preferred preparation as it is less likely to be abused. Tablet form and sugar-free elixir should not be used routinely as both are more likely to be injected.

Dipipanone (Diconal)

Diconal consists of a combination of the opiate analgesic dipipanone and cyclizine. Intravenous use produces intense euphoria, but there is a danger of CVA, arterial spasm and gangrene if injected into an artery.

Codeine

Misuse of codeine preparations is common. Includes DF118 (dihydrocodeine 30 mg), and codeine linctus (codeine phosphate 15 mg/5 ml).

The management of opiate dependence

AIMS OF MANAGEMENT

- help patient to deal with drug-related problems
- reduce damage occurring during drug use
- reduce duration of episodes of drug use
- reduce the chance of relapse
- help patient to remain healthy until they manage to attain a drug-free state

Before any treatment is initiated it is essential to establish that the patient is in fact drug dependent. A history of drug use, past and current, an account of withdrawal symptoms experienced upon cessation of the drug, a social history including sources of support, accommodation and employment, the funding of the drug habit, and a medical and psychiatric history are all considered necessary.

Physical examination should seek signs of current drug use and of complications related to the route of administration. It is essential to test urine for a drug screen, to establish that on two separate occasions the patient was taking the drugs claimed. Most drugs will show up on urine screens for at least 24 hours after ingestion.

Once it is established that the patient is opiate dependent, it is necessary to assess their motivation for treatment, and to reach an agreement with them about the aims of treatment.

The Home Office should be notified; the patient should be informed that there is a legal obligation upon the doctor to do this, but that the information will not be made available to the police.

Patients should receive information about harm minimization, and HIV and hepatitis testing should be arranged after counselling and with the patient's consent.

The ultimate aim of treatment is to achieve opiate abstinence. However, this is unacceptable to some patients, in which case the aim is to minimize the harm associated with opiate abuse (harm minimization)

Harm minimization

The aims are to stop or reduce the use of contaminated injecting equipment, to prevent the sharing of injecting equipment, to stop or reduce drug use, to stop or reduce unsafe sexual practices, to encourage health consciousness and a more stable lifestyle, and to establish and retain contact with the drug services.

To achieve these aims, education about the potential hazards is important. Sterile injecting equipment and condoms should be provided, non-immune individuals should be offered hepatitis B vaccination, and substitute oral opiates such as methadone should be prescribed.

Substitute prescribing

If dependence is not severe, reassurance, support and symptomatic treatment with non-opiate drugs may suffice.

The following may be used:

- clonidine: an alpha adrenergic antagonist can give some symptomatic relief in opiate withdrawal. Hypotension can be a problem
- lofexidine; like clonidine it acts centrally to reduce sympathetic tone, but reduction in blood pressure is less marked than that produced by clonidine. It is used to alleviate the symptoms of opiate withdrawal
- propranolol: for somatic anxiety
- thioridazine: relieves anxiety in low doses
- promethazine: sedative antihistamine effective for mild withdrawal
- benzodiazepines: for anxiety; do not give for longer than a fortnight

Substitute opioids

Oral methadone mixture 1 mg/ml is the usual choice. Any doctor can prescribe methadone to a drug misuser. Daily dispensing reduces the risk of overdose and abuse.

MAINTENANCE Substitute opiate is prescribed indefinitely in an effort to stabilize the addict's life, and reduce risks of intravenous use.

LONG-TERM WITHDRAWAL Substitute prescribing takes place over a period of months to years with the long-term aim of opiate abstinence.

RAPID WITHDRAWAL This is withdrawal over a period of weeks by the use of a substitute drug in decreasing doses.

GRADUAL WITHDRAWAL As above but takes place over a period of months.

Treatment should be undertaken initially by the general practitioner, possibly with help from the local community drugs team. If these approaches fail, referral to the more specialized drug dependency unit may be required.

Patients who are dependent on more than one drug, those with a history of several failed attempts, those with coexisting mental or physical disease, those who are violent or highly manipulative and those requiring injectable or high doses of substitute drugs should be considered for specialist referral.

Psychological methods

Therapeutic outcome is improved if substitute prescribing is combined with various forms of behaviour therapy.

MOTIVATIONAL INTERVIEWING Confrontational approaches have traditionally been used to deal with issues of denial. However, it seems that confrontational techniques increase rather than reduce resistance in treatment. Motivational interviewing is a cognitive–behavioural approach that takes into account the patient's stage of preparedness for change, and prompts the patient to consider the favourable reasons to change.

RELAPSE PREVENTION Described by Marlatt, this is a short-term intervention with extensive follow-up and preparation of the patient to anticipate urges to return to the drug-taking behaviour for a considerable period after abstinence has been achieved.

Those patients undergoing relapse prevention therapy are more likely to internally attribute change, and are more likely to remain opiate free during follow-up, or to contain a temporary relapse. The internal attribution of control over drug use maximizes treatment effects.

Naltrexone is a long-acting opioid antagonist which precipitates a withdrawal syndrome in the opiate-dependent person. It is used in the detoxified addict who requires additional help to remain drug free. The euphoriant effects of opiates are abolished, thus aiding abstinence. It is particularly helpful if a partner administers it, and if used in conjunction with cognitive–behavioural therapy.

Prognosis

The mortality rate for intravenous drug abusers is twenty times that of their non-drug-using peers. Since the 1980s the prevalence of HIV infection among intravenous drug users has increased to approximately 50–60 per cent in some groups (e.g. New York, Edinburgh), and mortality among this group has increased further.

Stimulants

COCAINE (COKE, SNOW, CRACK)   Cocaine is derived from the leaves of the coca shrub. Coca leaves are chewed, and the paste derived from the leaves is smoked.

Cocaine hydrochloride, a white powder usually snorted, may be injected. Crack cocaine (rock) and freebase, alkaloid forms may also be smoked. This provides a powerful hit which produces strong psychological dependence.

It is a Class A drug, requiring notification.

EPIDEMIOLOGY   There has been an epidemic of cocaine use in the USA. It remains relatively expensive in the UK, although its use increasing. Amphetamines tend to be the preferred stimulant of abuse in the UK.

Fewer than 10 per cent of cocaine addicts are notified to the Home Office.

DRUG ACTION   Cocaine blocks dopamine uptake at the dopamine reuptake site. Extracellular levels of dopamine are markedly increased. Dopaminergic activity, particularly at the nucleus accumbens, has been found to have a major role in the pleasurable and reinforcing effects of cocaine, amphetamine, phencyclidine, nicotine and alcohol. Genetic polymorphisms at the dopamine reuptake site may contribute to an individual's liability to become dependent.

Acute effects last about twenty minutes and include euphoria, reduced hunger tirelessness, agitation, tachycardia, raised blood pressure, sweating, nausea, vomiting, dilated pupils, impairment of judgement and social functioning. High doses may lead to an acute toxic psychosis with marked agitation, paranoia and auditory, visual and tactile hallucinations (cocaine bug).

Chronic use leads to tolerance, withdrawal symptoms and a chronically anxious state, possibly caused by dopamine depletion.

DRUG WITHDRAWAL   Following the initial rush of wellbeing and confidence, when the effects of the drug wear off there follows a rebound crash. This consists of dysphoria, anxiety, irritability, depression,fatigue and intense craving for the drug. The crash phase lasts nine hours to four days. The withdrawal phase of one to ten weeks is the period of the greatest risk of relapse. The final phase is of unlimited duration, when stimuli can trigger craving.

HARMFUL EFFECTS   At higher doses convulsions, hyperthermia, coma and death may occur. Excessive use can also lead to hypertension with cardiac failure, myocardial infarction, subarachnoid haemorrhage and CVA.

Perforation of the nasal septum can follow long-term administration by the nasal route because of the vasoconstriction caused by cocaine. Intravenous use carries with it the risks described above.

Cocaine abusers often take sedatives, including heroin, alcohol and benzodiazepines. As well as taking the edge off the high produced by cocaine, some of the metabolites of the cocaine-alcohol interaction have been found to have a much longer half-life than cocaine alone. It is possible that this prolongation of the effects of cocaine contributes to its use with alcohol.

Long-term stimulant abuse results in a stereotyped compulsive repetitive pattern of behaviour and paranoid psychosis resembling schizophrenia.

Amphetamines (speed, whizz, sulphate)

These are cheap and widely available in UK. They are used clinically in the treatment of narcolepsy, as appetite suppressants and selectively in the hyperkinesis of childhood. They are administered orally and intravenously. Methamphetamine may be inhaled.

Drug action, clinical effects, and withdrawal effects are similar to those of cocaine.

The toxic psychosis produced by amphetamine abuse can be indistinguishable from schizophrenia. It usually resolves with abstinence, but may continue for some months. Marked tolerance can develop. Following chronic use profound depression and fatigue occur. Long-term use leads to CNS 5HT neurone destruction.

Caffeine

This is widely available in coffee, tea and chocolate, and is added to soft drinks and proprietary cold preparations.

Coffee contains about 80–150 mg of caffeine per cup depending upon the brewing method. Peak blood levels occur 15–45 minutes following oral administration; half-life is six hours. Metabolism is increased by smoking, and reduced by oral contraceptives and pregnancy. Neonates cannot metabolize caffeine, therefore there is a very long half-life.

DRUG EFFECTS   A dose of 80–200 mg produces mood elevation, increased alertness and clarity of thought, increased gastric secretion, tachycardia, raised blood pressure, diuresis, and increased productivity.

In overdose (greater than 250 mg per day) caffeinism occurs. This results in anxiety, restlessness and nausea, and facial flushing.

At levels of intake in excess of 600 mg per day dysphoria replaces euphoria, anxiety and mood disturbances become prominent, insomnia, muscle-twitching, tachycardia and sometimes cardiac arrhythmias occur.

DRUG WITHDRAWAL   At high daily doses a withdrawal syndrome occurs with abstinence. This comprises restlessness, irritability, dizziness, severe headache, rhinorrhoea, depression and poor work performance.

MANAGEMENT OF STIMULANT DEPENDENCE   There is no case for substitute prescribing since these drugs do not produce a major withdrawal syndrome. Drugs should be withdrawn abruptly. Following stimulant withdrawal insomnia, depression and intense craving for the drug may occur. Antidepressants may be helpful. Desipramine has been found to reduce the intensity of cocaine craving irrespective of other psychopathology. Most patients can be managed as outpatients, but some become acutely suicidal and need observation.

Psychological support is helpful and relapse prevention techniques incorporated into treatment packages increase the chances of success.

Sedatives

Central nervous system sedatives depress CNS activity with little analgesic effect. They include alcohol (see above), barbiturates, benzodiazepines and carbamates. All the CNS depressants have abuse potential and cause both psychological and physical dependence. Cross-tolerance between groups occurs, and the withdrawal syndromes are similar. When taken repeatedly in high doses all these drugs produce sadness/depression, a worsening of confusional states, and withdrawal syndromes in which anxiety is prominent.

Benzodiazepines

Widely prescribed, these have widespread physical dependence among licit users, and are very popular with illicit substance abusers.

The most common route of administration is oral, but some abusers attempt to inject the contents of capsules or ground tablets intravenously.

EPIDEMIOLOGY   Over one million of the UK population use benzodiazepines continuously for more than one year.

DRUG ACTION   Potentiates the inhibitory actions of the GABA-A receptor in the limbic areas of the brain.

They have anxiolytic, hypnotic and anticonvulsant properties at normal doses.

The clinical signs of intoxication include slurred speech, uncoordination, unsteady gait, impaired attention or memory, psychological effects such as paradoxical aggression and disinhibition, lability of mood, impaired judgement and impaired social or occupational functioning.

DRUG WITHDRAWAL   Tolerance occurs rapidly. There is rebound anxiety after four weeks of use; dependence is seen in 45 per cent of users after three months.

The onset and intensity of withdrawal symptoms are related in part to the half-life of the drug used (shorter half-lives lead to a more abrupt and intense withdrawal syndrome). The withdrawal syndrome is also related to the dose used. Onset is usually within 1–14 days after drug reduction/cessation, and may last for months.

Withdrawal symptoms include somatic effects such as autonomic hyperactivity (tachycardia, sweating, anorexia, weight loss, pyrexia, tremor of hands, tongue and eyelids, GI disturbance, sleep disturbance with vivid dreams due to REM rebound), malaise and weakness, tinnitus and grand mal convulsions .

There are cognitive effects with impaired memory and concentration.

There are also perceptual effects with hypersensitivity to sound, light and touch, depersonalization and derealization. Delirium may develop within a week of cessation, associated with visual, auditory and tactile hallucinations, and delusions.

Affective effects such as irritability, anxiety and phobic symptoms may also occur.

HARMFUL EFFECTS   In high-dose abusers severe withdrawal symptoms occur if they are unable to acquire their usual dose of drug. As in these doses the drugs have usually been acquired illicitly, supply cannot be guaranteed. Withdrawal from sedative drugs is potentially lethal and should usually be managed on a medical ward.

Benzodiazepines are relatively safe in overdose, but are liable to produce respiratory depression, and in combination with other drugs they can be lethal.

The injection of street benzodiazepines incurs all the dangers of injecting described above, but is particularly liable to cause limb ischaemia and gangrene, with resulting amputation.

Barbiturates

Although the prescribing of barbiturates has largely been superceded by the safer benzodiazepines, they still appear in the form of phenobarbitone, amylobarbitone and quinalbarbitone (Tuinal) and are widely available.

DRUG ACTION   Potentiate action at the GABA-A receptor thus increasing CNS depression. This is particularly marked in the reticular activating system and cerebral cortex.

Clinical effects include impaired concentration, reduced anxiety and dysphoria. In increasing doses dysarthria, ataxia, drowsiness, coma, respiratory depression and death occur.

Chronic use results in tolerance caused by hepatic enzyme induction, cross-tolerance with alcohol, personality change, persistent intoxication, labile affect, poor concentration, impaired judgement and incoordination.

DRUG WITHDRAWAL   This causes anxiety, tremor, sweating, insomnia with marked REM rebound, irritability, agitation, twitching, vomiting, nausea, tachycardia, orthostatic hypotension, delirium and convulsions.

HARMFUL EFFECTS   Barbiturates are dangerous in overdose. Their therapeutic index is low. Tolerance to psychotropic effects exceeds tolerance to respiratory depression.

Parenteral administration of oral preparations is attempted by some addicts, incurring all the risks described.

MANAGEMENT   A gradual tapering of the dose is considered to be the most appropriate way to manage barbiturate dependence. Short-acting compounds should first be substituted by long-acting compounds, diazepam being the most commonly used form for the purposes of withdrawal. After stabilizing on diazepam, dose reduction is commenced. At high doses this can occur quite rapidly e.g. 5mg per week, until the patient starts to complain of unpleasant effects, when the rate of reduction can be reduced. If symptoms of depression are present an antidepressant is indicated. Propranolol may help with some of the somatic symptoms of anxiety.

Psychological support is very important, with weekly contact initially. The family should be involved in the process.

The withdrawal of barbiturates similarly needs phased withdrawal; inpatient admission is often necessary.

Hallucinogens

These are substances which give rise to marked perceptual disturbances when taken in relatively small quantities.

LYSERGIC ACID DIETHYLAMINE (LSD, ACID, MICRODOTS, SUPERMANS)   This is chemically related to 5HT, is available in tablets or absorbed onto paper; minute amounts (<100 micrograms) produce marked psychoactive effects. These peak at 2–4 hours and subside after about 12 hours. It is taken orally; intravenous use not common because the onset of the trip is very rapid with oral ingestion (15 minutes) therefore having no advantage. Tolerance develops rapidly; sensitivity to its effects returns rapidly with abstinence.

DRUG ACTION   This acts at multiple sites in CNS; the effects are thought to be related to 5HT antagonism.

The effects are dose related. Psychic effects include the heightening of perceptions, with perceptual distortion of shape, intensification of colour and sound, movement of stationary objects, and changes in sense of time and place. Hallucinations may occur, but are relatively rare. The user usually retains insight into the nature of their experiences. Delusions (e.g. belief in the ability to fly) may occur. Emotional lability, heightened self-awareness and ecstatic experiences can occur. Synaesthesias in which a stimulus in one sensory modality is experienced in another modality (e.g. hearing colours) are common.

The physical effects are sympathomimetic, with tachycardia, hypertension and dilated pupils.

Unpleasant experiences may occur (bad trips), and these are more likely in the inexperienced, or if the ambient mood is disturbed. Users generally avoid being alone, in case of bad trips or dangerous behaviour while under the influence. The features of adverse experiences include anxiety, depression, dizziness, and disorientation, and a short-lived psychotic episode characterized by hallucinations and paranoid delusions.

With heavy use an acute schizophreniform psychosis may persist.

Flashback phenomena (posthallucinogen perception disorder) occur, in which aspects of the LSD experience occur spontaneously some time after LSD use. These are usually fleeting.

DRUG WITHDRAWAL   Physical withdrawal symptoms do not occur following the abrupt discontinuation of LSD or other hallucinogens.

HARMFUL EFFECTS   Accidents may occur while under the influence of hallucinogens, such as jumping from a height because of the delusional belief that the user can fly.

Flashback phenomena occur many months after drug elimination giving rise to the possibility that these substances may cause permanent neurological changes.

Hallucinogenic mushrooms (magic mushrooms)
A number of different fungi grow in the UK which contain psychoactive substances e.g. psilocybin and psilocin. Liberty cap and fly agaric mushrooms are the ones most commonly used for their psychoactive effects. Ingestion of these in the raw state is legal, but any attempt to process them such as cooking, drying or freezing them is illegal.

DRUG ACTION   Ingestion causes mild LSD-like effects, with marked euphoria. At high doses hallucinations, bad trips and acute psychoses can occur.

Mescaline
This is the active component of the Mexican peyote cactus. Mescaline is similar to noradrenaline. It is hallucinogenic, and is orally administered.

LSD is 200 times as potent as psilocybin, which is 30 times as potent as mescaline.

Phencyclidine (PCP, Angel dust)
This is an arylcyclohexylamine related to ketamine. It is taken by smoking, snorting and injecting.

DRUG ACTION   It produces stimulant, anaesthetic, analgesic and hallucinogenic effects. At low doses it induces euphoria, and a feeling of weightlessness. At high doses visual hallucinations and synaesthesias occur.

Psychosis, violence, paranoia and depression can occur following a single dose.

Physical effects include uncoordination, slurred speech, blurred vision, convulsions, coma and respiratory arrest.

DRUG WITHDRAWAL   Prolonged use can result in a withdrawal syndrome upon cessation.

3,4-Methylenedioxymethamphetamine (MDMA, Ecstasy, XTC, E, Adam)
This is an hallucinogenic amphetamine. It possesses both stimulant and mild hallucinogenic properties. It is widely used at parties or raves by young people, particularly in the last decade. Taken orally in tablet or capsule form, it is often impure. Its effects last 4–6 hours; multiple dosing is tried, but tolerance develops rapidly, and subsequent doses have less potency. Physical dependence does not occur.

DRUG ACTION   It produces a positive mood, with feelings of euphoria, intimacy and closeness to others. The stimulant effects resemble those of amphetamine, and hallucinogenic effects resemble those of LSD. The physical effects include anorexia, tachycardia, jaw-tightening and bruxism, and sweating.

HARMFUL EFFECTS   Deaths have occurred in those with pre-existing cardiac disease caused by cardiac arrhythmias. In the fit user at normal doses deaths have occurred as a result of hyperpyrexia, resulting in disseminated intravascular coagulation, rhabdomyolysis, and renal failure.

Convulsions can also occur. Most deaths of this nature occur when the user has been dancing vigorously for a considerable period, in high ambient temperatures, with inadequate fluid replacement. MDMA has a direct effect upon the thermo-regulatory mechanisms which compound these conditions.

Hypertensive crises may occur leading to CVA in some.

Toxic hepatitis has been reported in MDMA users possibly related to impurities in the preparation.

Psychiatric conditions (psychosis, depression, anxiety) in previously vulnerable individuals can occur following MDMA use.

Neurotoxicity is an established fact. Serotonergic nerve terminals are damaged by this drug, and although rat studies indicate that this is reversible, primate studies indicate the opposite. The long-term consequences of MDMA-induced serotonergic neurotoxicity in man are not known.

MANAGEMENT   Abrupt discontinuation is recommended, there being no advantage to gradual withdrawal. Psychiatric disturbance should be treated accordingly.

CANNABINIODS

Cannabis (grass, hash, ganja, pot)

The major active constituent in cannabis is 9-tetrahydrocannabinol. It is derived from cannabis salva, the Indian hemp plant; the dried leaves contain 1–10 per cent (marijuana); the resin contains 8–15 per cent (hashish). It is usually smoked, but it can be eaten, and it is widely used. It is highly lipophilic, therefore it can be detected in the blood 20 hours following a single dose.

DRUG ACTION   Tetrahydrocannabinol has anticholinergic effects, and its action is particularly marked in the hippocampus. It thus has adverse effects on memory, cognition and other higher mental functions. The psychological effects include euphoria, relaxation, suspiciousness, a feeling that time has slowed down, impaired judgement, heightened sensory awareness and social withdrawal. Hunger and anxiety may occur. Physical effects include tachycardia, raised blood pressure, dry mouth, thirst, constipation, reduced intraocular pressure, ataxia and, rarely, photophobia and nystagmus. In high-dosage perceptual distortions, confusion, drowsiness, bradycardia, hypotension, hypothermia, bronchodilatation and peripheral vasoconstriction can occur. An acute toxic psychosis which resolves with abstinence may occur.

DRUG WITHDRAWAL   In chronic users, cessation of cannabis is often followed by a withdrawal syndrome consisting of irritability, restlessness, anorexia, nausea, and insomnia. Craving and psychological dependence do not occur.

HARMFUL EFFECTS   Chronic cannabis use can lead to a deterioration in personality. An increase in aggressiveness may also occur.

Flashbacks, and prolonged depersonalization and derealization may occur.

Cognitive and psychomotor impairment resulting from even small amounts of cannabis make the performance of skilled tasks (such as driving) hazardous.

Volatile solvents (glue-sniffing)

Volatile substances are inhaled in order to experience their psychoactive effects. Solvents from glue (e.g. toluene), correction fluids (e.g. trichloroethane), butane gas and other aerosol propellants are popular.

Solvents have been tried by 3–5 per cent of 15-year-olds. Often fumes are rebreathed from a plastic bag, but sometimes an aerosol is sprayed directly into the oropharynx (this is particularly dangerous). Rapidly absorbed, its effects last about 30 minutes.

DRUG ACTION   The clinical effects include euphoria, disinhibition, dizziness, perceptual distortions and frank hallucinations, tinnitus, ataxia, confusion, slurred speech, nystagmus, decreased reflexes, tremor and muscle weakness. High doses cause stupor and death. Aspiration of vomit can occur at any time.

DRUG WITHDRAWAL   There is no physical withdrawal syndrome.

HARMFUL EFFECTS   Acute intoxication can lead to fatal accidents, particularly through falling or drowning.

The greatest risk of death is during an episode of sniffing. Butane squirted directly into the mouth can cause cardiac arrest. Propellants squirted directly into the mouth are cooled to $-20°C$, which can cause burns to the throat and lungs, and may freeze the larynx, causing cardiac arrest through vagal nerve stimulation.

Rebreathing from plastic bags can result in asphyxiation.

There are approximately 100 deaths per annum in the UK, with 20 per cent of these occurring in first-time users, and the majority in those aged under 20 years.

There are reports of long-term damage to the CNS, heart, liver and kidneys. Chronic use may cause a persistent cerebellar syndrome, and peripheral neuropathy.

MANAGEMENT   Abrupt discontinuation is recommended. Advice from social services and/or a child psychiatrist may be needed.

PREGNANCY

Drug use often results in poor antenatal care and the risk of infection.

Women at this time may have an increased motivation to change their behaviour, and it is important to take this opportunity to engage them in services. Education and harm minimization should be attempted.

ANTENATAL CARE   Drug misusers are at a high risk of obstetric complications. There is a high incidence of intrauterine growth retardation and premature labour. HIV-positive women need counselling about risks to themselves and their fetus.

Drug withdrawal is best attempted gradually during the second trimester of pregnancy. If this is not possible then attempts should be made to ensure that the practice is as safe as possible, e.g. changing to non-injecting modes of administration. Sudden withdrawal should be avoided because of the risk of intrauterine death. Abstinence 4–6 weeks before birth minimizes the risks of neonatal withdrawal symptoms.

If the mother is HIV-positive or receiving high doses of opioids, breast-feeding should be avoided.

Following the birth, an assessment of the amount social support the mother is likely to need should be made. Continuing support after delivery is essential.

BIBLIOGRAPHY

Cloninger, C.R. 1987: Neurogenetic adaptive mechanisms in alcoholism. *Science* 23, 410–15.

Department of Health, Scottish Office Home and Health Department, Welsh Office 1991: *Drug misuse and dependence: guidelines on clinical management.* London: HMSO.

Edwards, G. and Gross, M. 1976: Alcohol dependence: provisional description of a clinical syndrome. *British Medical Journal* i: 1058.

Glass, I.B. 1991: *The international handbook of addiction behaviour.* London: Routledge.

Jarman, C.M.B. and Kellett, J.M. 1979: Alcoholism in the general hospital. *British Medical Journal* i, 469–71.

Jaswrilla, A.G., Adams, P.H. and Hore, B.D. 1979: Alcohol and acute general medical admissions. *Health Trends* 11, 95–7.

Kendler, K.S. 1985: A twin study of individuals with both schizophrenia and alcoholism. *British Journal of Psychiatry* 147, 48–53.

Mattick, R.P. and Heather, N. 1993: Developments in cognitive and behavioural approaches to substance misuse. *Current Opinion in Psychiatry* 6, 424–9.

Paton, A. 1988: *ABC of alcohol*, 2nd edn. London: British Medical Journal.

Raistrick, D.S. and Davidson, R. 1986: *Alcoholism and drug addiction*, Current Reviews in Psychiatry. Edinburgh: Churchill Livingstone.

Solowij, N. 1993: Ecstasy (3,4-methylenedioxymethamphetamine). *Current Opinion in Psychiatry* 6, 411–15.

Tabakoff, B. and Hoffman, P.L. 1993: The neurochemist. *Psychiatry* 6, 388–94.

Taylor, C., Brown, D., Duckitt, A. *et al.* 1985: Patterns of outcome: drinking histories over ten years among a group of alcoholics. *British Journal of Addiction* 80, 45–50.

The Royal College of Psychiatrists 1986: *Alcohol: our favourite drug*. London: Tavistock Publications.

Victor, M., Adams, R.D. and Collins, G.H. 1971: *The Wernicke–Korsakoff syndrome*. Oxford: Blackwell.

27
Schizophrenia and delusional (paranoid) disorders

SCHIZOPHRENIA

HISTORY

1860 Morel used the term *démence précoce* for a disorder of deteriorating adolescent psychosis.

1863 Kahlbaum described katatonie.

1871 Hecker described hebephrenie.

1894 Sommer included deteriorating paranoid syndromes in the concept of primary dementia.

1868 Griesinger believed that insanity could develop in the absence of mood disturbance, primary insanity (*primäre Verrücktheit*), and that all functional psychoses were expressions of single disease entity (*Einheitspsychoses*).

1896 Emil Kraepelin grouped together catatonia, hebephrenia and the deteriorating paranoid psychoses under the name dementia praecox. He differentiated dementia praecox with its poor prognosis from the manic depressive psychoses with their relatively better prognoses. He considered dementia praecox to be a disease of the brain.

1911 Bleuler introduced the term schizophrenia, applied it to Kraepelin's cases of dementia praecox, and expanded the concept to include what today may be considered schizophrenic spectrum disorders. He considered symptoms of **ambivalence, autism, affective incongruity and disturbance of association of thought** to be fundamental, (the 'four As'); delusions and hallucinations assumed secondary status. He was influenced by the writings of Sigmund Freud. He added schizophrenia simplex to Kraepelin's list.

1931 Hughlings-Jackson considered positive symptoms as 'release phenomena' occurring in healthy tissue; negative symptoms were attributed to neuronal loss.

1959 Kurt Schneider emphasized the importance of delusions and hallucinations in defining his **first rank symptoms**.

1960 Langfeldt sought to distinguish between schizophrenia and the better prognosis schizophreniform psychoses; process versus non-process schizophrenia.

1972 Cooper compared patients admitted to psychiatric hospitals in New York and London. He found identical symptomatology, but schizophrenia was diagnosed nearly twice as often in New York compared to London.

1973 WHO conducted their *International Pilot Study of Schizophrenia*. Using narrow criteria, they found one-year incidence of schizophrenia of 0.7–1.4 per 10 000 population aged 15–54, across all countries. They confirmed that psychiatrists in the USA and the USSR diagnosed schizophrenia twice as often as those in seven other countries (Columbia, Czechoslovakia, Denmark, Nigeria, India, Taiwan and the UK). This led to the realization that psychiatric diagnoses had to be **operationally defined**.

CLASSIFICATION

Schneiderian first rank symptoms
In defining his first rank symptoms Schneider stated that in the absence of organic brain disease the following are highly suggestive of schizophrenia:

- auditory hallucinations

  - repeat the thoughts out loud (e.g. *Gedankenlautwerden, écho de la pensée*)
  - in the third person
  - in the form of a running commentary

- delusions of passivity

  - thought insertion, withdrawal and broadcasting
  - made feelings, impulses and actions

- somatic passivity
- delusional perception

Second rank symptoms include perplexity, emotional blunting, other hallucinations and other delusions.

First rank symptoms can occur in other psychoses. Although they are highly suggestive of schizophrenia, they are not pathognomonic.

St. Louis criteria (Feighner *et al.* 1972)
The patient must be continuously ill for at least six months, with no prominent affective symptoms, presence of delusions, hallucinations or thought disorder. Personal and family history should be taken into account, e.g. marital status, age under 40, premorbid social adjustment.

CATEGO (Wing *et al.* 1974)
This uses Present State Examination to generate diagnoses from a computer programme. It is based on the Schneiderian concept of schizophrenia. No account is taken of symptom duration.

Research Diagnostic Criteria (Spitzer *et al.* 1975)
This applies to a two-week duration period, lack of affective symptoms, the presence of thought disorder, and hallucinations or delusions similar to Schneider's first rank symptoms.

International Classification of Diseases: Tenth revision: ICD-10 (WHO 1992)
These have fundamental, characteristic distortions of thinking and perception, and inappropriate or blunted affect; clear consciousness. Intellectual capacity is usually maintained; some cognitive deficits can evolve over time.

Symptoms can be divided into groups:

Table 27.1   ICD-10 classification of schizophrenia and delusional disorders

F20 Schizophrenia
        F20.0 Paranoid schizophrenia
        F20.1 Hebephrenic schizophrenia
        F20.2 Catatonic schizophrenia
        F20.3 Undifferentiated schizophrenia
        F20.4 Post-schizophrenic depression
        F20.5 Residual schizophrenia
        F20.6 Simple schizophrenia
        F20.8 Other schizophrenia
        F20.9 Schizophrenia, unspecified

F22 Persistent delusional disorders
        F22.0 Delusional disorder
        F22.8 Other persistent delusional disorders
        F22.9 Persistent delusional disorder, unspecified

F23 Acute and transient psychotic disorders
        F23.0 Acute polymorphic psychotic disorder without symptoms of
        schizophrenia
        F23.1 Acute polymorphic psychotic disorder with symptoms of
        schizophrenia
        F23.2 Acute schizophrenia-like psychotic disorder
        F23.3 Other acute predominantly delusional psychotic disorder
        F23.8 Other acute and transient psychotic disorders
        F23.9 Acute and transient psychotic disorder, unspecified

F24 Induced delusional disorder

F25 Schizoaffective disorders
        F25.0 Schizoaffective disorder, manic type
        F25.1 Schizoaffective disorder, depressive type
        F25.2 Schizoaffective disorder, mixed type
        F25.8 Other schizoaffective disorders
        F25.9 Schizoaffective disorder, unspecified

F28 Other nonorganic psychotic disorders

F29 Unspecified nonorganic psychosis

- thought echo and thought alienation
- delusions of passivity; delusional perception
- auditory hallucinations in the form of a running commentary, or discussing the patient, or hallucinatory voices coming from some part of the body
- persistent delusions, culturally inappropriate and impossible
- persistent hallucinations in any modality, accompanied by fleeting delusions without affective content, or by persistent over-valued ideas, or occurring every day for weeks
- formal thought disorder comprising interruptions in the train of thought, incoherence, irrelevant speech, or neologisms
- catatonic behaviour e.g. excitement, stupor, posturing, waxy flexibility, negativism and mutism
- negative symptoms e.g. apathy, paucity of speech, blunted or incongruous affect
- A significant and consistent change in the overall quality of some aspects of personal behaviour e.g. loss of interest, aimlessness, idleness, self-absorbed attitude, social withdrawal

Diagnostic guidelines require a minimum of one clear symptom (two if less clear-cut) belonging to groups (1) to (4), or symptoms from at least two of the groups (5) to (8) should have been present for most of the time during a period of one month or more.

The last symptom applies only to a diagnosis of simple schizophrenia; duration of at least one year is required.

Schizophrenia is not diagnosed if extensive affective symptoms are present, unless they postdate the schizophrenic syndrome. If both schizophrenic and affective symptoms develop together and are evenly balanced, the diagnosis of schizoaffective disorder is made.

Schizophrenia is not diagnosed in the presence of an overt brain disease or during drug intoxication or withdrawal.

The pattern of the course is classified as continuous; episodic, progressive deficit; episodic, stable deficit; episodic, remittent; incomplete remission; complete remission.

In ICD-10 the following subtypes of schizophrenia are distinguished:

PARANOID SCHIZOPHRENIA   This is the most common subtype. Hallucinations and/or delusions are prominent. Disturbances of affect, volition, speech and catatonic symptoms are relatively inconspicuous. There are auditory, olfactory, gustatory and somatic hallucinations; visual hallucinations may occur. There are commonly delusions of control, influence, passivity and persecution.

HEBEPHRENIC SCHIZOPHRENIA   The age of onset is usually between 15 and 25. The prognosis is poor. Affective changes are prominent, and fleeting and fragmentary delusions and hallucinations, irresponsible behaviour, fatuous, disorganized thought, rambling speech, and mannerisms are common. Negative symptoms, particularly flattening of affect and loss of volition, are prominent. Drive and determination are lost, goals are abandoned, and behaviour becomes aimless and empty. The premorbid personality is characteristically shy and solitary.

CATATONIC SCHIZOPHRENIA   Here, one or more of the following behaviours dominate: stupor, excitement, posturing, negativism, rigidity, waxy flexibility, command automatism and the perseveration of words or phrases. Catatonic symptoms alone are not diagnostic of schizophrenia; they may be provoked by brain disease, metabolic disturbance, alcohol and drugs and mood disorders. Psychomotor disturbances may alternate between extremes; violent excitement may occur. This may be combined with a dream-like state with vivid scenic hallucinations.

SIMPLE SCHIZOPHRENIA   This has an insidious onset of decline in functioning. Negative symptoms develop without preceding positive symptoms. Diagnosis requires changes in behaviour over at least a year, with a marked loss of interest, idleness and social withdrawal.

RESIDUAL OR CHRONIC SCHIZOPHRENIA   This is characterized by negative symptoms. There should be past evidence of at least one schizophrenic episode, a period of at least one year in which the frequency of positive symptoms has been minimal *and* negative schizophrenic syndrome has been present. There is an absence of depression, institutionalization, dementia or other brain disorder.

UNDIFFERENTIATED SCHIZOPHRENIA   Here the general criteria for schizophrenia are satisfied, but do not conform to above syndromes.

POST-SCHIZOPHRENIC DEPRESSION   This is a depressive episode arising after a schizophrenic illness. Schizophrenic illness must have occurred within the last 12 months, some symptoms still being present. Depressive symptoms fulfil at least those criteria for depressive episode, and are present for at least two weeks. There is an increased risk of suicide.

Type 1 and type 2 schizophrenia (Crow 1980)
This is a two syndrome hypothesis of schizophrenia: a categorical approach.

TYPE 1 SCHIZOPHRENIA   This is characterized by prominent positive symptoms, acute onset, good premorbid adjustment, good treatment response, intact cognition, intact brain structure and a reversible neurochemical disturbance.

TYPE 2 SCHIZOPHRENIA   This is characterized by prominent negative symptoms, insidious onset, poor premorbid adjustment, poor treatment response, impaired cognition, structural brain abnormalities (ventricular enlargement) and an underlying pathology based on neuronal loss. It is therefore irreversible.

SAPS and SANS
In 1983–1984 Andreasen developed structured scales for the assessment of positive and negative symptoms: the Scale for the Assessment of Positive Symptoms (SAPS) and the Scale for the Assessment of Negative Symptoms (SANS).

Liddle's syndromes (Liddle 1987)
Liddle found that the pattern of symptoms in schizophrenia segregated into three distinguishable syndromes: a dimensional approach:

PSYCHOMOTOR POVERTY SYNDROME   Poverty of speech, flatness of affect and decreased spontaneous movement.

DISORGANIZATION SYNDROME   Disorders of the form of thought and inappropriate affect.

REALITY DISTORTION SYNDROME   Delusions and hallucinations.

A subsequent PET study of regional cerebral blood flow (Liddle *et al.* 1992) showed that each of these three syndromes is associated with a specific pattern of perfusion:

PSYCHOMOTOR POVERTY SYNDROME   Hypoperfusion of the left dorsal prefrontal cortex, extends to medial prefrontal cortex and anterior cingulate cortex. Hyperperfusion in head of caudate nucleus which receives substantial projections from the dorsolateral prefrontal cortex. Some changes are also found on the right (laterality only a matter of degree). Hypofrontality in schizophrenia is more often seen in chronic patients and is associated with inactivity and catatonic symptoms. In normal subjects prefrontal activity increases when involved in the internal generation of action.

DISORGANIZATION SYNDROME   Hypoperfusion of the right ventral prefrontal cortex, and increased activity in the anterior cingulate and dorsomedial thalamic nuclei which project to the prefrontal cortex. Relative hypoperfusion of Broca's area and bilateral hypoperfusion of parietal association cortex. Evidence that in primates ventral prefrontal cortex plays a role in the suppression of interference from irrelevant mental activity. Anterior cingulate plays a role in attentional mechanisms. It suggests that these patients are engaged in an ineffective struggle to suppress inappropriate mental activity.

REALITY DISTORTION SYNDROME   Increased activity in left parahippocampal region and left striatum. Consistent with the proposal that delusions and hallucinations arise from a disorder of internal monitoring resulting in failure to recognize internally generated mental acts. Abnormalities of function underlying schizophrenic symptoms are not confined to single loci, but involve distributed neuronal networks.

Neurodevelopmental classification (Murray *et al.* 1992)
On the basis of genetic, epidemiological, neuropathological, neuroimaging and

gender difference studies, schizophrenia can be subdivided into the following three groups:

CONGENITAL SCHIZOPHRENIA   Abnormality is present at birth. It may be caused by genetic predisposition and/or environmental insult e.g. maternal influenza, obstetric complication, early brain injury or infection. It is more likely to involve minor physical abnormalities, abnormal personality or social impairment in childhood, present early, exhibit negative symptoms, show morphological brain changes and cognitive impairment. More likely to be male and to have a poor outcome.

ADULT-ONSET SCHIZOPHRENIA   More likely to exhibit positive and affective symptoms. May have genetic predisposition to manifest symptomatology anywhere along a continuum from bipolar mood disorder, schizoaffective disorder, to schizophrenia.

LATE-ONSET SCHIZOPHRENIA   Presents after the age of 60, good premorbid functioning. More common in females, often associated with auditory and visual sensory deprivation. Sometimes related to paranoid personality or to mood disorder. Organic brain dysfunction is often present.

EPIDEMIOLOGY

Incidence is between 15 and 30 new cases per 100 000 of the population per year.

Point prevalence is approximately 1 per cent.

Lifetime risk is approximately 1 per cent.

Age of onset is usually between 15 and 45 years, earlier in men than in women. It is equally common in males and females. There is a higher incidence in those who have not married. It is most common in social classes IV and V.

Prevalence varies geographically. Rates from urban areas are generally higher than in rural areas; marked exceptions e.g. highest prevalence measured (17.4 per 1000 population) was from a sparsely populated rural area in the west of Ireland.

Theories accounting for geographical variance in prevalence of schizophrenia:

Social drift: Goldberg and Morrison (1963) studied fathers' birth certificates, and found that schizophrenic males had lower social class distribution than their fathers. They attributed their findings to social drift i.e. migration of those affected to areas where social demands may be less. Men were more likely to drift into inner-city areas.

Social residue: the healthy migrate away from undesirable areas, leaving schizophrenics behind.

'Breeder', or social causation hypothesis: this assumes that environmental factors are either causative or have to be present for the predisposed individual to develop schizophrenia. Castle et al. (1993) found that schizophrenic patients in Camberwell were more likely to have been born in a socially deprived area and to have fathers with manual jobs. Those developing schizophrenia were more likely than controls to have been born into socially deprived households. Castle suggested that some environmental factor of aetiological importance in schizophrenia is more likely to affect those born into households of lower socioeconomic status and in the inner city.

Theories emphasizing environmental influences need not exclude the importance of biological factors e.g. exposure to toxins, the increased incidence of obstetric complications and a higher rate of infectious disease in cities. Social factors which are more common in cities include stressful life events, social isolation and social overstimulation.

AETIOLOGY

Genetics

Twin, family and adoption studies have consistently demonstrated the familial aggregation of schizophrenia, largely attributable to genetic factors.

FAMILY STUDIES

Table 27.2 Approximate lifetime risks for the development of schizophrenia in the relatives of patients with schizophrenia

Relationship	Lifetime expectancy rate to the nearest percentage point
Parents	6
All siblings	10
Siblings (when one parent has schizophrenia)	17
Children	13
Children (when both parents have schizophrenia)	46
Grandchildren	4
Uncles, aunts, nephews and nieces	3

TWIN STUDIES Higher concordance rate for monozygotic twins (MZ) of approximately 45 per cent, than for dizygotic twins (DZ) approximately 10 per cent (Gottesman and Shields 1972). Studying adult offspring of 21 MZ and 41 DZ twin pairs discordant for schizophrenia, Gottesman and Bertelsen found the risk of developing schizophrenia was 17 per cent among the adult children of the MZ and DZ probands, 17 per cent among the offspring of phenotypically normal MZ cotwins, and only 2 per cent among the offspring of phenotypically normal DZ cotwins. This suggests that the normal MZ cotwins carried and transmitted the relevant genotype without expressing it themselves.

ADOPTION STUDIES   When children of schizophrenic mothers have been adopted soon after birth by non-schizophrenic families, they have a similar likelihood of developing schizophrenia (approximately 13 per cent) as the rates suggested by family studies. No such increased risk of developing schizophrenia was seen in the children of non-schizophrenic parents who are similarly adopted (Kety et al. 1971).

Possible modes of inheritance:

1   **Single major locus**. Some forms possibly exist but they would account for a very small proportion of observed cases. To date no single genetic focus responsible for the development of schizophrenia has been reliably demonstrated.
2   **Polygenic**. A threshold of gene numbers is required for the expression of schizophrenia.
3   **Multifactorial**. Aetiological heterogeneity with various genetic and environmental subtypes. Probably a spectrum of causes ranging from the wholly genetic, through those with mixed aetiology, to the totally environmental.

LINKAGE STUDIES   Bassett et al. (1985) reported a man who presented with schizophrenia plus minor physical abnormalities, both shared by his maternal uncle. Cytogenetic analysis revealed translocation of part of chromosome 5; it led them to postulate this segment of chromosome 5 may be the site of a putative schizophrenia gene. Sherrington *et al.* (1988) collected seven extended schizo-phrenic families from Iceland and England, probed chromosome 5 and found evidence which was highly suggestive of a linkage between markers on chromo-some 5 and schizophrenia. However, this finding has never been replicated and the study has subsequently been criticized on methodological grounds.

Problems in applying linkage methodology to schizophrenia:

- schizophrenia probably genetically heterogeneous
- linkage analysis usually applied to conditions transmitted by simpler Mende-lian inheritance
- diagnostic and penetrance problems probably require a much higher LOD score than the usual +3 before linkage for psychiatric diagnoses can be regarded as proved

Prenatal factors

Persons developing schizophrenia as adults are born disproportionately more often during late winter and early spring. Similar, less marked season-of-birth effect is reported for bipolar affective disorders, but not for neurotic or person-ality disorders. Seasonally varying environmental causes have been sought. Pre-natal infection is currently the most favoured explanation.

An excess of minor physical abnormalities is reported in schizophrenics e.g. low-set ears, greater distance between the eyes, single transverse palmar crease. There are thought to originate early in the second trimester of pregnancy.

Dermatoglyphics are determined by genes; deleterious events in the second trimester of pregnancy can alter their form. Schizophrenics have deviations from normal in their ridge patterns of fingers, palms and soles. Schizophrenic probands of monozygotic twin pairs discordant for schizophrenia have significantly more finger and palm epidermal ridge anomalies than their healthy cotwins (Bracha *et al.* 1991).

Structural abnormalities in the brains of many schizophrenics suggest a neu-rodevelopmental process rather than a degenerative one. Most studies investigat-ing brain morphology in schizophrenia report non-progressive ventricular and cortical sulcal enlargement, and structural abnormalities in the limbic areas. Structural changes reflect an early acquired hypoplasia, not degeneration. Cytoarchitectural changes in limbic and prefrontal areas are strong indicators of early disordered brain development. Altered distribution of cortical layers of NADPH-d neurones is consistent with a disturbance of development, in which the normal pattern of programmed cell death is compromised resulting in the defective migration of neurones.

Murray suggests neural dysplasia results in premorbid cognitive deficits, abnor-mal personality, negative symptoms and abnormal CT scans in schizophrenia. Maturational brain changes in adolescence, possibly myelination or synaptic pruning, reveal immature neuronal circuitry with the consequent onset of hallu-cinations and delusions.

The neurodevelopmental model of schizophrenia accounts for the following findings:

- Individuals who were in their second trimester of fetal life during the influenza epidemic in Finland in 1957 have an increased risk of later schizo-phrenia (Mednick *et al.* 1988)
- winter excess of births in schizophrenics caused by the seasonal prevalence of viral infection or other perinatal hazard
- males have an earlier onset of schizophrenia than females, possibly because of

increased vulnerability to neurodevelopmental damage (generally more common in males). Postulates that a smaller proportion of male schizophrenia is genetically determined; evidence that concordance rates for schizophrenia are lower in male than in female identical twins

Obstetric complications are more frequent in schizophrenics than in normal controls. This is noted particularly in schizophrenics without a positive family history for psychosis, implying that they may augment or substitute for a genetic cause.

Personality
Only **schizotypal personality disorder** is aetiologically related to schizophrenia. Among the schizotypal criteria, eccentricity, affect constriction, and excessive social anxiety are linked to schizophrenia. This may be a milder phenotype along the schizophrenia spectrum.

Social factors
In 1968 Brown and Birley found that schizophrenics had experienced significantly more independent life events in the three weeks before the onset of relapse than controls.

In 1976 Vaughn and Leff found increased relapse rate of schizophrenia in those who live with families in which the relatives display **high expressed emotion** (critical comments, over-involvement). Changes in physiological arousal may account for this effect.

Table 27.3   Relapse rates of 128 schizophrenics over a nine-month period (Vaughn and Leff 1976)

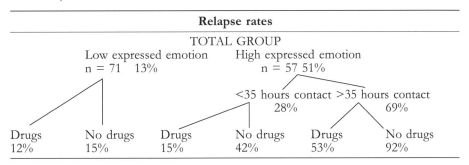

There was a **poverty of the social milieu** of patients with chronic schizophrenia associated with increased negative symptoms, particularly social withdrawal, affective blunting and poverty of speech. (Wing and Brown 1961 'Three hospitals study').

Neurotransmitters
DOPAMINE   The **mesolimbic–mesocortical system** is a **dopaminergic** system originating in the ventral tegmental area of the brain. The mesolimbic system projects to the limbic system, while the mesocortical system innervates the cingulate, entorhinal and medial prefrontal cortices. **Dopamine hypothesis of schizophrenia**: the clinical features are the result of central dopaminergic hyperactivity in the mesolimbic–mesocortical system. Evidence in favour of the dopamine hypothesis includes:

All clinically effective antipsychotic drugs occupy a substantial proportion of

D2 receptors in the brain (70–80 per cent D2 receptor occupancy in the striatum at normal doses).

- Amphetamine, a dopamine agonist, can cause a state similar to that of acute schizophrenia.
- Dopamine agonists exacerbate psychotic symptoms.
- Comparing actions of α and β isomers of flupenthixol in patients with acute schizophrenia, only those receiving the dopamine antagonist improved (Johnstone *et al*. 1978).
- Post-mortem studies have found increased D2 receptors in the basal ganglia and limbic regions of schizophrenics' brains.
- In animals, administration of dopamine agonists produces a behavioural picture said to be similar to human psychosis. This is reversed by giving dopamine antagonists.
- In drug naive schizophrenics, the number of D2 receptors in the striatum was 2–3 times that of controls as measured by PET (Wong *et al*. 1986).

Evidence against the dopamine hypothesis includes:

- The concentration of dopamine metabolite HVA (homovanillic acid) in the cerebrospinal fluid in schizophrenics has generally not been found to be higher than in control subjects.
- D2 receptor blockade caused by antipsychotics is an acute effect, but the therapeutic effect is observed three to four weeks later.
- 15–30 per cent of schizophrenics fail to respond to dopamine antagonists.
- Antipsychotics have a better effect on positive than on negative symptoms.
- Clozapine, an effective antipsychotic, has less D2 blocking activity than conventional antipsychotics.
- Some studies have failed to replicate Wong's findings of increased D2 receptors in the striatum of brains of living schizophrenics.

Explanations which may account for contradictory results:

- Schizophrenia is clinically complex, and the aetiology is heterogeneous.
- Schizophrenia may involve reduced dopaminergic activity in the prefrontal cortical area, and compensatory overactivity in subcortical or limbic areas.
- Problems in patient selection and study methodology.

Identification of D1, D3, D4 and D5 receptors has suggested that they alone or in addition to D2 receptor may be the appropriate target for antipsychotic drug therapy.

Clozapine acts in part by antagonism of D1, D2, and particularly D4 receptors; it is effective during long-term use in up to 60 per cent of neuroleptic resistant patients.

D1 antagonist alone failed to show antipsychotic efficacy. Specific D3 and D4 antagonists have not yet been studied.

During treatment with haloperidol the ratio of dopamine metabolite (HVA) to serotonin and noradrenaline metabolites in CSF of schizophrenics increased significantly and correlated with the reduction of symptoms. This supports the hypothesis that interactions between different monoamine neurotransmitters are involved in the expression of schizophrenic symptoms.

SEROTONIN (5HT)   There is evidence that serotonergic dysfunction may be associated with schizophrenia:

- Hallucinogen LSD acts at serotonin receptors.

- Antipsychotic risperidone is a potent 5HT2 receptor antagonist (also blocks D2 receptors, however).
- Ritanserin, a selective 5HT2 antagonist, reduced negative symptoms when given as adjunctive in neuroleptic treated schizophrenics.

GLUTAMATE This stimulates the NMDA receptor. Phencyclidine ('angel dust') causes schizophrenic-like effects by blocking NMDA receptors. A balance exists between excitatory glutamatergic and inhibitory dopaminergic terminals in corpus striatum, regulating GABAergic neurones. These function in the 'thalamic filter' which seems to be hypoactive in schizophrenia. According to this theory, the hypoactivity of GABA neurones is corrected by either reducing dopaminergic activity, or increasing glutamatergic activity.

Structural cerebral abnormalities

Johnstone *et al.* 1976 conducted a CT scan study, finding that chronically hospitalized schizophrenic patients had larger lateral ventricles than controls. This was confirmed by numerous subsequent neuroimaging studies.

Andreasen *et al.* 1990 conducted a large study, matched for age, sex, height, weight and level of education. Ventricle:brain ratio greater in schizophrenics than controls. The differences are small, overlap with the normal population, and are more marked in males.

Not caused by treatment, present at the onset of schizophrenic illness, usually nonprogressive. May be associated with poor premorbid adjustment.

Diffuse reduction in the volume of cortical grey matter has been found in schizophrenic patients using MRI, and is also associated with poor premorbid function. These findings are consistent with neurodevelopmental changes having taken place in such patients.

Other structural changes in schizophrenia found in some studies:

- reduced size of frontal lobes, or some division thereof
- reduced size of temporal lobe, particularly on the left
- reduced size of hippocampus and amygdala, particularly on the left
- reduced size of parahippocampal gyrus

Neuropathological abnormalities

POST-MORTEM STUDIES Compared with control subjects, the brains of schizophrenic patients have shown in some studies (see Chapter 11):

- lower fixed brain weight
- reduced brain length
- reduced size of parahippocampal gyrus

HISTOLOGICAL STUDIES Compared to controls, the brains of schizophrenics have shown in some studies:

- hippocampal pyramidal cell disarray
- reduced hippocampal cell numbers
- reduced cell numbers in the entorhinal cortex
- reduced hippocampal cell size
- disturbed cytoarchitecture in the entorhinal cortex

Functional brain abnormalities

Studies have found:

- hypofrontality: associated with the presence of negative symptoms and autism

Combining functional imaging with task activation:

- Weinberger *et al.* 1986 measured regional cerebral blood flow at rest and during Wisconsin Card Sorting Test (activates frontal lobes normally).
- Impaired performance by schizophrenics was mirrored by smaller increase in blood flow to prefrontal cortex.

MANAGEMENT

HOSPITALIZATION   Those with acute schizophrenia usually require admission to hospital, if necessarily compulsorily, for assessment, investigations and treatment. Before discharge Section 117 of the Mental Health Act 1983 for detained patients, and the care-programme approach for all patients requires that an 'assessment of needs' is made. A keyworker should be assigned to monitor the patient's progress and administer depot medication.

Attendance at a day hospital or centre may be considered, and communication with the GP should take place.

DRUG TREATMENT   Efficacy of neuroleptics on acute symptoms of schizophrenia has been demonstrated beyond doubt. 'Positive' symptoms respond better than 'negative' symptoms.

- 5–25 per cent of schizophrenics are unresponsive to conventional neuroleptics
- 5–10 per cent are intolerant because of adverse neurological effects (Parkinsonism, akathisia, dyskinesias)
- 40–60 per cent of schizophrenics are non-compliant with oral medication. Possible reasons are:
  - limited insight into disease
  - limited beneficial effect
  - side-effects
  - pressure from family, friends
  - poor communication from medical team

Depot neuroleptics increase compliance, and reduce relapse rates.

Continuous therapy is superior to intermittent treatment, and results in fewer relapses and lower overall dose of neuroleptics.

Of patients who stop medication, 60–70 per cent relapse within one year, and 85 per cent within two years, compared to 10–30 per cent of those who continue on active medication.

If a patient has failed to respond to a trial of three neuroleptics of different classes, using an adequate dose for an adequate duration, an atypical agent such as clozapine could be tried.

Clozapine can cause agranulocytosis, so regular blood counts are necessary. The incidence of agranulocytosis is 0.8 per cent at 12 months and 0.9 per cent at 18 months, with a peak risk in the third month. This is higher in women and older patients.

Atypical neuroleptics is distinguished from conventional neuroleptics by:

- not producing catalepsy in animals
- not elevating prolactin levels in man
- considerably lower potential for extrapyramidal side-effects and tardive dyskinesia

Kane *et al.* 1988 showed that clozapine was significantly better than chlorpromazine in the treatment of schizophrenics previously resistant to haloperidol. Improvement was observed in positive and negative symptoms.

Extrapyramidal side-effects occur in up to 90 per cent of patients taking neuroleptic medication; much less with clozapine.

Electroconvulsive therapy is used in the treatment of catatonic stupor.

Psychosocial treatments

SOCIAL MILIEU   Wing and Brown (1970) found that negative symptoms varied in intensity with social stimulation within psychiatric institutions.

The TAPS study (1993) of long-stay patients discharged into the community found that, providing reprovision is well resourced with staffed homes for the more disabled, at one and five-year follow-up, compared to matched controls, there was no increase in death rates, suicides, crime or vagrancy. Between discharge and five years negative symptoms reduced significantly in response to a more stimulating environment. Positive symptomatology remained stable.

EXPRESSED EMOTION   Psychoeducational family programmes to increase medi- cation compliance and coping with stressors are successful in reducing the risk of relapse. High expressed emotion (EE) families identified using the Camberwell Family Interview. Education and family sessions in the home were run in parallel with a relatives group. These aimed at teaching problem-solving skills, lowering criticism and over-involvement, reducing contact between patients and relatives and expanding social networks.

PROGNOSIS

Heterogeneous disorder, no reliable predictors of outcome.

Approximately one-quarter of cases of schizophrenia show good clinical and social recovery while most studies show that fewer than one-half of patients have a poor long-term outcome.

Factors associated with good prognosis include:

- female
- abrupt onset of illness
- married
- affective component to illness
- paranoid, compared with non-paranoid
- good premorbid social adjustment
- family history of affective disorder
- short duration of illness prior to treatment
- good initial response to treatment
- later onset
- lack of negative symptoms
- lack of cognitive impairment
- no ventricular enlargement

Ten per cent commit suicide.

Roy (1982) found it more likely if:

- early in illness
- males
- younger
- chronic illness, relapses and remissions
- unemployed
- high educational attainment prior to onset
- akathisia
- abrupt stoppage of drugs

- recent discharge from in-patient care
- paranoid three times more likely than non-paranoid

DELUSIONAL (PARANOID) DISORDERS

According to ICD-10:

- Ill-defined disorder, single delusion or a set of related delusions, persistent, sometimes lifelong and does not have an identifiable organic basis. Occasional or transitory auditory hallucinations, particularly in the elderly.
- Delusions are the most conspicuous or only symptom. They must be present for at least three months. There must be no evidence of schizophrenic symptoms or brain disease.

ICD-10 includes the previously used term of late paraphrenia.

There is evidence that there are differences between persistent delusional disorder and late paraphrenia. Howard *et al.* (1994) showed, using MRI scans in a group of late onset schizophrenics and late onset delusional disorders, that lateral ventricle volumes in the delusional disorder patients were much greater than those of schizophrenics, and almost twice those of controls.

Monodelusional disorders feature a stable, encapsulated delusional system, which takes over much of a person's life. The personality is preserved.

EPIDEMIOLOGY

Point prevalence 0.03 per cent, **lifetime risk** 0.05 to 0.1 per cent.

Munro (1991) reported from his series of patients with monodelusional disorder:

- Mean age of onset 35 years for males and 45 years for females
- Sex ratio equal
- Often unmarried, high marital breakdown, low fecundity
- Introverted, long-standing interpersonal difficulties
- Increased family history of psychiatric disorder, but not of delusional disorder or schizophrenia
- Onset gradual in 62 per cent
- Course unremitting, severity may fluctuate
- 16 per cent had evidence of minimal brain disorder

SPECIFIC DELUSIONAL (PARANOID) DISORDERS

Pathological (delusional) jealousy
The patient holds the delusional belief that their sexual partner is being unfaithful, and will go to great lengths to find evidence of infidelity. Underclothing may be examined for semen stains, belongings may be searched and the partner may be interrogated and followed.

This is also called the Othello syndrome, morbid jealousy, erotic jealousy, sexual jealousy, psychotic jealousy and conjugal paranoia; it is more common in men.

Pathological jealousy may be associated with the following conditions:

- **organic disorders** and **psychoactive substance use disorders** e.g. alcohol dependence, cerebral tumours, endocrinopathies, dementia, cerebral infection, and use of amphetamines and cocaine
- **paranoid schizophrenia**

- **depression**
- **neurosis and personality disorder**

Treatment should be directed at the underlying disorder. If no primary cause is identified, pharmacotherapy with a neuroleptic and/or psychotherapy may be helpful. There may be a risk of violence to the partner and it may be best to recommend that the couple separate.

Erotomania (de Clérambault's syndrome)

The patient holds the delusional belief that someone, usually of a higher social or professional status or a famous personality or in some other way 'unattainable', is in love with them. The patient may make repeated attempts to contact that person. Eventually, rejections may lead to animosity and bitterness on the part of the patient towards the object of their attention.

In hospital and outpatient clinical psychiatry, patients are more likely to be female than male, whereas in forensic psychiatry male patients are more common. Overall, females outnumber males.

Cotard's syndrome

Cotard's syndrome, also called *délire de négation*, is a nihilistic delusional disorder in which the patient believes that, for example, all their wealth has gone or that their relatives or friends do not exist. It may take a somatic form with the patient believing that parts of their body do not exist. It can be secondary to very severe depression or to an organic disorder.

Capgras syndrome

Although Capgras syndrome is also called *illusion des sosies* or illusion of doubles, it is not an illusion but a delusional disorder. The essential feature of this rare symptom is that a person who is familiar to the patient is believed to have been replaced by a double. It is more common in females. Common primary causes are schizophrenia, mood disorder and organic disorder. Derealization often occurs.

Fregoli syndrome

In this very rare delusional disorder the patient believes that a familiar person, who is often believed to be the patient's persecutor, has taken on different appearances. Primary causes include schizophrenia and organic disorder.

Induced psychosis (folie à deux)

This rare delusional disorder is shared by two, or, rarely, more than two people who are closely related emotionally. One of the people has a genuine psychotic disorder; their delusional system is induced in the other person, who may be dependent or less intelligent than the first. Geographical separation leads to the recovery of the well person.

SCHIZOAFFECTIVE DISORDERS

In 1933 Kasanin introduced the term 'schizoaffective psychosis'. It includes sudden acute onset, good premorbid functioning, both affective and schizophrenic symptoms and usually a complete recovery.

ICD-10: disorders in which both affective and schizophrenic symptoms are prominent within the same episode of illness, either simultaneously or within a few days of each other.

Schizoaffective disorder, manic type: patient usually makes a full recovery.

Schizoaffective disorder, depressive type: prognosis not as good as that of manic subtype; greater chance of developing 'negative' symptoms.

Schizoaffective disorder, mixed type: no consensus concerning nosological status of schizoaffective disorder. Opposing views: Kraepelinian binary system versus continuum theorists.

Binary theorists e.g. Winokur, Kendler: traditional notion that there are two separate illnesses, schizophrenia and manic depressive psychosis, with different treatments and different aetiologies.

Continuum theorists e.g. Crow, Kendall: doubt that there are distinct illnesses, rather that features of psychosis vary quantitatively along a continuum, with schizophrenia and manic depression at opposing poles and schizoaffective disorder somewhere in between.

Tsuang 1991 studied a subgroup of patients with strictly defined schizoaffective disorder. He found that the morbid risk of schizophrenia in relatives of schizoaffectives was similar to that of the schizophrenic group, and fell between schizophrenia and affective disorder for the risk of affective disorder in relatives. He concluded that this group was different from schizophrenia or manic depression.

Goldstein *et al.* 1993 found that, among probands with schizoaffective disorder, relatives had higher rates of schizophrenia and unipolar depression than the relatives of males. Among relatives, males were at higher risk for schizophrenia spectrum disorders than females. This suggests a stronger relationship for schizoaffective disorder to schizophrenia.

Relationship between schizophrenia and affective disorder:

1   At least one-third of schizophrenics have depressive symptoms.
2   Affective disorder is more frequent in schizophrenics families than in controls.
3   Unipolar depression is more common in families of schizoaffectives than schizophrenia only probands. Bipolar disorder is as frequent in families of both.
4   Affective disorder is frequently inherited from the same parental line as schizophrenia.
5   Bipolar disorder is more frequent in male relatives and unipolar disorder is more frequent in female relatives.

Concludes therefore that the same genes contribute to schizophrenia and affective disorder, and sex and phenotypic expression are related.

PROGNOSIS

The prognosis of schizoaffective disorders lies between that of mood disorders and schizophrenia.

BIBLIOGRAPHY

Andreasen, N.C. 1983: *The Scale for the Assessment of Negative Symptoms* (SANS). Iowa City Iowa: The University of Iowa.

Andreasen, N.C. 1984: *The Scale for the Assessment of Positive Symptoms* (SAPS). Iowa City Iowa: The University of Iowa.

Andreasen, N.C., Swayze, V.W., Flaum, M. *et al.* 1990: Ventricular enlargement in schizophrenia evaluated with computed tomographic scanning. *Archives of General Psychiatry* 47, 1008–15.

Bassett, A., McGillivray, B., Jones, B. and Pantzar, J. 1985: Partial trisomy chromosome 5 cosegregating with schizophrenia. *Lancet* i: 1023–6.

Bracha, H.S., Torrey, E.F., Bigelow, L.B. *et al.* 1991: Subtle signs of prenatal maldevelopment of the hand ectoderm in schizophrenia: a preliminary monozygotic twin study. *Biological Psychiatry* 30, 719–25.

Brown, G.W. and Birley, J.L.T. 1968: Crises and life changes and the onset of schizophrenia. *Journal of Health and Social Behaviour* 9, 203.

Castle, D.J., Scott, J., Wessely, S. and Murray, R.M. 1993: Does social deprivation during gestation and early life predispose to later schizophrenia? *Social Psychiatry and Psychiatric Epidemiology* 28, 1–4.

Chua, S.E. and McKenna, P.J. 1995: Schizophrenia – a brain disease? A critical review of structural and functional cerebral abnormality in the disorder. *British Journal of Psychiatry* 166, 563–82.

Crow, T.J. 1980: Molecular pathology of schizophrenia: more than one disease process? *British Medical Journal* 280, 66–8.

DeLisi, L.E., Henn, S., Bass, N. *et al.* 1994: *Depression in schizophrenia. Is the Kraepelinian binary system dead? Proceedings of the 9th World Congress of Psychiatry*, 1993. Macclesfield: Gardiner-Caldwell Communications.

Duinkerke, S.J., Botter, P.A., Jansen, AII. *et al.* 1993: Ritanserin, a selective 5–HT2/1c antagonist, and negative symptoms in schizophrenia: a placebo controlled double blind trial. *British Journal of Psychiatry* 163, 451–5.

Goldstein, J.M., Faraone, S.V., Chen, W.J. *et al.* 1993: The role of gender in understanding the familial transmission of schizoaffective disorder. *British Journal of Psychiatry* 163, 763–8.

Gottesman, I.I. and Shields, J. 1972: *Schizophrenia and genetics: a twin study vantage point.* New York: Academic Press.

Howard, R.J., Almeida, O., Levy, R. *et al.* 1994: Quantitative magnetic resonance imaging volumetry distinguishes delusional disorder from late onset schizophrenia. *British Journal of Psychiatry* 165, 474–80.

Johnstone, E.C., Crow, T.J., Frith, C.D., Husband, J. and Kreel, L. 1976: Cerebral ventricular size and cognitive impairment in chronic schizophrenia. *Lancet* ii, 924–6.

Johnstone, E.C., Crow, T.J., Frith, C.D. *et al.* 1978: Mechanism of the antipsychotic effect in the treatment of acute schizophrenia. *Lancet* ii, 848–51.

Jones, D. 1993: The TAPS Project II: The selection of patients for reprovision. *British Journal of Psychiatry* (suppl.) 19, 36–9.

Kahn, R.S., Davidson, M., Knott, P. *et al.* 1993: Effect of neuroleptic medication on cerebrospinal fluid monoamine metabolite concentrations in schizophrenia. *Archives of General Psychiatry* 50, 599–605.

Kane, J.M. and Freeman, H.L. 1994: Towards more effective antipsychotic treatment. *British Journal of Psychiatry* 165 (suppl. 25), 22–31.

Kane, J.M., Honigfield, G., Singer, J. *et al.* 1988: Clozapine for the treatment-resistant schizophrenic. A double blind comparison with chlorpromazine. *Archives of General Psychiatry* 45, 789–96.

Kety, S.S., Rosenthal, D., Wender, P.H. *et al.* 1971: Mental illness in the biological and adoptive families of adopted schizophrenics. *American Journal of Psychiatry* 128, 302.

Leff, J., Thornicroft, G., Coxhead, N. *et al* 1994: The TAPS project. 22: A five-year follow-up of long-stay psychiatric patients discharged to the community. *British Journal of Psychiatry* 165 (suppl. 25), 13–17.

Lewis, S.W. and Murray, R.M. 1988: Obstetric complications, neurodevelopmental deviance and risk of schizophrenia. *Journal of Psychiatric Research* 21, 473.

Liddle, P.F. 1987: The symptoms of chronic schizophrenia. A re-examination of the positive–negative dichotomy. *British Journal of Psychiatry* 151, 145–51.

Liddle, P.F., Friston, K.J., Frith, C.D., Hirsch, S.R., Jones, T. and Frackowiak, R.S.J. 1992: Patterns of cerebral blood flow in schizophrenia. *British Journal of Psychiatry* 160, 179–86.

Lieberman, J.A. and Sobel, S.N. 1993: Predictors of treatment response and course of schizophrenia. *Current Opinion in Psychiatry* 6, 63–9.

Mednick, S.A., Machon, R.A., Huttunen, M.O. and Bonnet, D. 1988: Adult schizophrenia following prenatal exposure to an influenza epidemic. *Archives of General Psychiatry* 189–192.

Meltzer, H.Y., Myung, A.L. and Ranjan, R. 1994: Recent advances in the pharmacotherapy of schizophrenia. *Acta Psychiatrica Scandinavica* 90 (suppl. 384), 95–101.

Munro, A. 1991: Phenomenological aspects of monodelusional disorders. *British Journal of Psychiatry* (suppl.) 14, 62–4.

Murray, R,M., Lewis, S,W., Owen, M.J. and Foester, A. 1988: Neurodevelopmental origins of dementia praecox. In Bebbington, P. and McGuffin, P. (eds) *Schizophrenia: the major issue*. London: Heinemann.

Murray, R.M., O'Callaghan, E., Castle, D.J. and Lewis, S.W. 1992: A neurodevelopmental approach to the classification of schizophrenia. *Schizophrenia Bulletin* 18, 319–32.

Roy, A. 1982: Suicide in chronic schizophrenia. *British Journal of Psychiatry* 141, 171–7.

Sherrington, R., Brynjjolfsson, J., Petursson, H. *et al.* 1988: Localisation of a susceptibility locus for schizophrenia on chromosome 5. *Nature* 336, 164–7.

Syvälahti, E.K.G. 1994: Biological factors in schizophrenia: Structural and functional aspects. *British Journal of Psychiatry* 164 (suppl. 23), 9–14.

Torgersen, S. 1994: Personality deviations within the schizophrenia spectrum. *Acta Psychiatrica Scandinavica* (suppl. 384), 40–44.

Tsuang, M.T. 1991: Morbidity risks of schizophrenia and affective disorders among first-degree relatives of patients with schizoaffective disorders. *British Journal of Psychiatry* 158, 165–70.

Vaughn, C.E. and Leff, J.P. 1976: Influence of family and social factors on the course of psychiatric illness. *British Journal of Psychiatry* 129, 125–37.

Weinberger, D.R., Berman, K.F. and Zec, R.F. 1986: Physiological dysfunction of dorsolateral prefrontal cortex in schizophrenia: I. Regional cerebral blood flow evidence. *Archives of General Psychiatry* 43, 114–24.

Wing, J.K., Brown, G.W. 1961: Social treatment of chronic schizophrenia: a comparative survey of three mental hospitals. *Journal of Mental Science* 107, 847.

Wing, J.K. and Brown, G.W. 1970: *Institutionalism and schizophrenia*. Cambridge: Cambridge University Press.

Wong, D.F., Wagner, H.N., Tune, L.E. *et al.* 1986: Positron emision tomography reveals elevated D2 dopamine receptors in drug naive schizophrenics. *Science* 234, 1558–63.

World Health Organization 1973: *Report of the International Pilot Study of Schizophrenia*. Geneva: WHO.

28
Mood disorders, suicide and parasuicide

HISTORY

1921   Kraepelin divided the functional psychoses into two broad categories, **dementia praecox** and **manic–depressive insanity**. He thought of the latter as a disorder in which discrete episodes of illness alternated with clearly defined well periods during which patients returned to their previous state of health.

1949   Cade first initiated the use of lithium, but it was not widely used until the 1960s.

1950s   Tricyclic and MAOI antidepressants were first introduced.

1970s   Anticonvulsants were first used for bipolar disorders. Specific psychological treatments e.g. cognitive therapy were introduced.

CLASSIFICATION

ICD-10

Bipolar affective disorder
Repeated episodes of mood disturbance, sometimes elevated, sometimes depressed. Repeated episodes of mania classified as bipolar (resemble those who also have depressive episodes in their family history, premorbid personality, age of onset and prognosis).

It includes:

- Bipolar affective disorder

  - current episode hypomanic
  - current episode manic without psychotic symptoms
  - current episode manic with psychotic symptoms

- Bipolar affective disorder

  - current episode mild or moderate depression
  - current episode severe depression without psychotic symptoms
  - current episode severe depression with psychotic symptoms

■   Bipolar affective disorder

■   current episode mixed

Manic episode

Fundamental disturbance is an elevation of mood to elation, with concomitant increase in activity level. Three degrees of manic episode specified by ICD-10, all used for a single manic episode only:

HYPOMANIA   Persistent elevated mood, increased energy and activity, feelings of wellbeing, reduced need for sleep. Irritability may replace elation; considerably disrupted work. No hallucinations or delusions.

MANIA WITHOUT PSYCHOTIC SYMPTOMS   Mood elevated, almost uncontrollable excitement. Overactivity, pressured speech, reduced sleep, distractible, inflated self-esteem, grandiose. Perceptual heightening may occur. Patient may spend excessively, become aggressive, amorous, or facetious.

MANIA WITH PSYCHOTIC SYMPTOMS   As above but with delusions and hallucinations, usually grandiose. Sustained physical activity, aggression, self-neglect may occur.

Depressive episode

Depression of mood, reduced energy and fatiguability. Mood is pervasively depressed. Reduced attention and concentration, lowered self-esteem, ideas of guilt and worthlessness, pessimistic thoughts, thoughts of self-harm or suicide, disturbed sleep.

Somatic changes include reduced appetite leading to weight loss (at least 5 per cent of body weight in a month), constipation, early morning wakening (>2 hours before usual), diurnal variation of mood, anhedonia, loss of normal reactivity of mood, reduced libido, amenorrhoea, psychomotor retardation or agitation.

Duration of two weeks is required for diagnosis.

Applies to first episode only. Graded severity, includes:

■   mild depressive episode
■   moderate depressive episode
■   severe depressive episode without psychotic symptoms
■   severe depressive episode with psychotic symptoms

Recurrent depressive disorder

Repeated episodes of depression, without episodes of mania. Recovery between episodes is usually complete, but a minority become chronic, especially the elderly.

It includes:

■   Recurrent depressive disorder

■   current episode mild
■   current episode moderate
■   current episode severe without psychotic symptoms
■   current episode severe with psychotic symptoms

■   Recurrent depressive disorder

■   currently in remission

Depression is variously classified; the usefulness of differing categories is still under debate.

Endogenous versus reactive depression (Roth and Newcastle school 1950s)

Endogenous form is thought to be of biological origin, with psychomotor retardation or agitation, loss of appetite and weight, anhedonia, early morning wakening and diurnal mood variation.

Reactive form is thought to be of psychological origin, depression moderate, anxiety, irritability, initial insomnia and mood remains reactive.

However, triggering events are present in both types.

Kendall (1965) failed to find a point of rarity in symptomatology between neurotic/psychotic depression, therefore concluded no essential differences between them.

Unipolar versus bipolar (Leonhard; Angst and Perris 1950s)

Unipolar depression is more common in females; episode is longer with somatic symptoms, anxiety, agitation, suicidal ideas, weight loss and initial insomnia.

In bipolar depression a seasonal pattern and hypersomnia tend to be more commonly present. More males, more family history of mania, earlier more acute onset (15 years earlier than unipolars on average), more episodes.

No difference is observed in sleep EEGs of these two groups.

Schneider's first rank symptoms have been reported in 8 to 23 per cent of cases of mania.

Bipolar I and Bipolar II

Bipolar I refers to major depression alternating with mania.
Bipolar II refers to major depression alternating with hypomania.

Rapid cycling bipolar disorder

This refers to those patients who experience four or more affective episodes in 12 months. It is more common in women, predicts poorer prognosis with more lifetime affective episodes and a poorer response to lithium and other treatments. Twenty per cent are antidepressant induced.

Dysthymia

A chronic, less severe depression, usually with an insidious onset. Symptoms include excessive guilt, difficulty concentrating, loss of interest, pessimism, low self-esteem, low energy, irritability and reduced productivity. Must be present for at least two years. ICD-10 and DSM IV criteria are similar.

Double depression

Major depression superimposed upon dysthymia.

Depressive stupor

Unresponsive, akinetic, mute and fully conscious. Following an episode, the patient can recall the events that took place at the time. Episodes of excitement may occur between episodes of stupor.

Recurrent brief depression

Angst 1990 proposed diagnostic criteria. Dysphoric mood or loss of interest for a duration of less than two weeks. At least four of the following: poor appetite, sleep problems, agitation, loss of interest, fatigue, feelings of worthlessness, difficulty concentrating and suicidality. One or two episodes per month for at least one year are characteristic.

Masked depression

Depressed mood is not always complained of, rather somatic or other complaints. It is more common in the undeveloped world and in those unable to articulate their emotions e.g. with learning disability, dementia. The presence of biological symptoms is helpful in making the diagnosis. Diurnal variation in abnormal behaviour may mirror diurnal variation in mood.

Seasonal affective disorder (SAD)

Regular temporal relationship between the onset of depressive episodes and a particular time of year. Depressive episodes commence in autumn or winter months and end in the spring or summer months as the hours of daylight increase. Onset of bipolar disorders may also be seasonal. Hyperphagia, hypersomnia and weight gain is more frequent than in matched non-seasonal patients.

Atypical depression

Depression characterized by reversed neurovegetative symptoms such as psychomotor retardation, hypersomnia and hyperphagia with weight gain.

Manic stupor

Unresponsive, akinetic, mute and fully conscious, elated. On recovery the patient remembers experiencing the flight of ideas typical of mania.

Mixed affective states

Kraepelin maintained that mood, cognition and behaviour may vary independently, producing mixed affective states which are usually transitional, but are sometimes persistent.

Bereavement reactions

Normal grief has three phases. **Stunned phase** lasts from a few hours to two weeks. This gives way to the **mourning phase**, with intense yearning and autonomic symptoms. After several weeks the **phase of acceptance and adjustment** takes over. Grief typically lasts about six months.

Atypical grief is divided by Parkes (1985) into:

- unexpected grief syndrome
- ambivalent grief syndrome
- chronic grief

EPIDEMIOLOGY

Depressive episodes

Problems are encountered in epidemiological studies in mood disorders because of the differing use of diagnostic categories, screening instruments and definitions of caseness.

Broadly: more common in females. **Incidence** between 80 and 200 new cases per 100 000 of the population per year in men, and between 250 and 7800 new cases per 100 000 of the population per year in women. **Point prevalence** in Western countries is between 1.8 and 3.2 per cent for men and between 2.0 and 9.3 per cent for women.

Point prevalence of depressive **symptoms** is 10–30 per cent. (women 18–34 per cent, men 10–19 per cent). **Lifetime risk** in the general population of Western countries of suffering from depressive episodes is 5–12 per cent in men and 9–26 per cent in women.

Average **age of onset** of depressive episodes is around the late thirties; however, they can start at any age.

There is a higher incidence in those who are not married.

Brown and Harris (1978) found that 15 per cent of urban women had severe depressive symptoms, and there was a higher prevalence in working-class than in middle-class women.

Bipolar mood disorder
Sex ratio equal. **Point prevalence** in Western countries between 0.4 per cent and 1.2 per cent in the adult population. **Lifetime risk** in the general population of Western countries of suffering from bipolar disorder is 0.6 per cent to 1.1 per cent.

Average **age of onset** is around the mid-twenties.

It is more common in the upper social classes.

AETIOLOGY

Genetics
FAMILY STUDIES   In unipolar probands there is an increased risk of unipolar depression in first degree relatives, but the amount of bipolar illness is virtually the same as the general population (combined risk 7–8 per cent). In bipolar probands there is an increased risk of both bipolar and unipolar disorder in first degree relatives (combined risk 18–20 per cent).

TWIN STUDIES   In a large Danish twin study of affective disorder (Bertelson *et al.* 1977), the concordance rate for monozygotic (MZ) twins was 67 per cent, compared with 20 per cent for dizygotic (DZ) twins. MZ:DZ concordance ratio for bipolar disorder of 79:19 compared with 54:24 for unipolar disorder.

ADOPTION STUDIES   In adoptees with bipolar disorder, 28 per cent of biological parents suffer from a mood disorder compared with 12 per cent of adoptive parents. By comparison, 26 per cent of the biological parents of bipolar non-adoptees were found to suffer from a mood disorder.

MOLECULAR GENETICS   In certain families manic depressive illness has been X-linked to colour blindness and glucose-6–phosphate deficiency.

Egeland *et al.* (1987) found linkage to chromosome 11 in an old order Amish pedigree. This finding is now thought to have been a statistical artefact and has not been replicated. In linkage studies of complex diseases such as manic depressive disorder, spurious linkage may be produced because of phenotypic misclassification and misspecification of the disease model.

Personality
CYCLOTHYMIC PERSONALITY DISORDER   This is characterized by persistent instability of mood with numerous periods of mild depression and mild elation. It may predispose to bipolar disorder.

DEPRESSIVE PERSONALITY DISORDER   This is related to the mood disorders, overlapping substantially with them, but not congruent with them. It often coexists with mood disorders. Core phenomena are excessive negative, pessimistic beliefs about oneself and others. Symptoms include unhappy, gloomy mood, low self-esteem, being self-critical, brooding, negativistic and judgemental towards others, pessimism and prone to feelings of guilt.

Psychosocial stressors
Vaughn and Leff (1976) showed that high expressed emotion (EE) increased the risks of relapse in depressed patients. Compared to schizophrenics, depressives were more sensitive to critical remarks. However, hostility and over-involvement did not add to the significant association. The effect of critical comments (criticism index) was not mitigated by reducing the number of hours depressed people spent in contact with their relatives (unlike schizophrenia, in which it was).

Excess life events occur in the six months before a depressive episode starts. Brown and Harris 1978 in a community survey in Camberwell, south London, identified **vulnerability factors** which increase the risk of depression if a **provoking agent** is present. Four vulnerability factors are:

- having three or more children at home under the age of 14
- not working outside the home
- lack of confiding relationship
- loss of mother before the age of 11

Vulnerability factors may operate by reducing self-esteem.

Kendler *et al.* (1995) compared stressful life events in twins with and without depression. He found that in those with the lowest risk (MZ cotwin unaffected) the probability of onset of major depression was 0.5 per cent and 6.2 per cent respectively for those unexposed and exposed to the life event. In those at highest genetic risk (MZ cotwin affected) these probabilities were 1.1 per cent and 14.6 per cent respectively. He concluded that genetic factors influence the risk of the onset of major depression in part by altering the sensitivity of individuals to the depression-inducing effect of stressful life events.

Physical illness

Viral infection, particularly influenza, hepatitis A and brucellosis, are sometimes accompanied or followed by depressed mood.

Endocrine disorders commonly predispose to depression. Eighty-three per cent of patients with Cushing's syndrome develop affective disorder during the course of their disorder. It is also seen in hypothyroidism and hypo- and hyperparathyroidism.

Psychological factors

Seligman gave naïve dogs unavoidable electric shocks and found that, after learning that there was nothing that could be done to influence the outcome of events, the dogs finally developed a condition which he thought resembled depression in humans, with reduced appetite, reduced sex drive and disturbed sleep. He called this condition **learned helplessness.**

It has been suggested that in humans depression is more likely to occur if the helplessness is perceived to be attributable to a personal source, thus leading to lowered self-esteem. Global stable attributions are likely to be the longest lasting.

Beck *et al.* (1979) has proposed a cognitive model of depression from which cognitive therapy has developed. Three concepts seek to explain the psychological substrate of depression:

1. Cognitive triad
   The depressed patient has:

   - a negative view of themselves
   - a tendency to interpret their ongoing experiences in a negative way
   - a negative view of the future

2. Schemas
   These are stable cognitive patterns forming the basis for the interpretation of situations.
3. Cognitive errors
   These are systematic errors in thinking that maintain depressed peoples' beliefs in negative concepts.

Cognitive distortions include:

- arbitrary inference
- selective abstraction
- overgeneralization
- personalization
- magnification and minimization
- dichotomous thinking

Neurotransmitters

Schildkraut in 1965 found that the monoamine hypothesis of mood disorders stated that depression was associated with a depletion, and mania with an excess of central monoamine. Evidence favouring this hypothesis:

- Tricyclic antidepressants inhibit the reuptake of noradrenaline and serotonin by presynaptic neurones, leading to an increase in the availability of these monoamines in the synaptic cleft.
- Monoamine oxidase inhibitors increase the availability of monoamines, by inhibiting their metabolic degradation by monoamine oxidase.
- Selective serotonin re-uptake inhibitors (SSRIs) increase the availability of serotonin by inhibiting the reuptake of serotonin.
- Use of antidepressants in bipolar disorder can precipitate mania.
- Amphetamine releases catecholamines from the neurones; it is a central nervous system stimulant that lifts mood.
- Reserpine, an antihypertensive drug derived from the Indian plant *Rauwolfia*, depletes central monoaminergic neuronal stores of catecholamines and serotonin. Its use can lead to severe depression and suicide.
- The cerebrospinal fluid level of the serotonin metabolite 5-hydroxyindole-acetic acid (5-HIAA) is often reported as being reduced in depressed patients.

Evidence against the monoamine hypothesis includes:

- Antidepressant pharmacotherapy takes at least a fortnight to effect a clinical improvement. This time interval is much greater than the relatively rapid onset of biochemical action.
- Not all drugs that act as monoamine reuptake inhibitors have a therapeutic antidepressant action e.g. cocaine.

SEROTONIN

Evidence for abnormal serotonergic function in mood disorders includes:

- Low CSF 5-HIAA in subgroups of depressed patients.
- Low density of brain and platelet serotonin transporter sites in depressed patients.
- High density of brain and platelet serotonin binding sites in depressed patients.
- Induction by dietary tryptophan depletion of a prompt relapse in depressed patients who have responded to SSRIs.
- Low plasma tryptophan in depressed patients.
- All SSRIs are clinically effective antidepressants.
- Serotonin function is reduced in depression and may be normalized with active treatment.

ADAPTIVE CHANGES IN RECEPTORS During antidepressant treatment, changes take place in cerebral alpha- and beta-adrenergic and serotonin receptors, showing only after two weeks of treatment, at the same time as the therapeutic effect. A decrease in the sensitivity (down regulation) of adrenergic beta receptors is particularly evident.

Neuroendocrine factors

BRAIN–STEROID AXIS   Disturbances of the hypothalamic–pituitary–adrenal axis are reported in depression. In normal humans cortisol secretion is episodic and follows a circadian rhythm. Peak cortisol secretion is in the morning; between noon and 4 a.m. secretion remains low, being lowest just after the onset of sleep.

In biological depression, there is disruption in the normal circadian rhythm of cortisol secretion, the morning peak being increased and longer lasting. A phase shift with the morning peak occurring earlier has been reported.

In depressed patients increased secretion has been reported in corticotrophin (ACTH), cortisol, β-endorphin and prolactin.

In the **dexamethasone suppression test** (DST) plasma cortisol levels are measured following the administration of the long-acting potent synthetic steroid dexamethasone the previous evening. In normal subjects dexamethasone leads to a suppression in the level of cortisol over the next 24 hours through negative feedback. In depressed patients with biological symptoms, non-suppression of cortisol has been reported in over 60 per cent. The DST has not proved to be a useful laboratory test for depression because a relatively high level of cortisol non-suppression has been found in other psychiatric disorders. The DST can be affected by factors such as age, body weight, drugs, ECT and endocrinopathies. The DST is usually state-dependent and in most subjects normalizes as the patient recovers.

Corticotropin-releasing factor (CRH or CRF) is an important hypothalamic peptide in the regulation of appetite and eating. In the **CRH stimulation test** the administration of CRH to normal humans leads to the release of corticotropin. In depression there is a consistent reduction of corticotropin response.

The noradrenergic neurones of the locus coeruleus express glucocorticoid receptors, through which corticosteroids can regulate its functioning. It is hypothesized that steroids may be important in causing and perpetuating depression.

BRAIN–THYROID AXIS   Thyroid-releasing hormone (TRH) causes the release of thyroid-stimulating hormone (TSH) from the adenohypophysis. In normal subjects there is a circadian pattern of TSH secretion, with a nocturnal rise which is blunted in depression and returns with sleep deprivation. In the **TRH stimulation test** the TSH response to intravenous TRH is measured. About 25 per cent of depressed patients show a blunted TSH response to TRH stimulation. This does not often normalize as the subject recovers from depression. Blunting is also found in panic disorder. TRH stimulation studies in depression have also shown that approximately 15 per cent of patients have a raised TSH response; many of these patients have been found to have antimicrosomal thyroid and antithyroglobulin antibodies, indicating that depression can be associated with symptomless autoimmune thyroiditis.

MELATONIN   Patients with depression have disordered biological rhythms i.e. short REM latency (time from falling asleep to onset of REM sleep), early morning wakening, and diurnal mood variation. The suprachiasmatic nucleus (SCN) of the hypothalamus plays a major role in regulating diurnal rhythms. Information about light conditions from the retina, via the retinohypothalamic pathway, controls the SCN. This influences the pineal which excretes melatonin. The biosynthesis of melatonin from its precursor, serotonin, occurs via *N*-acetylation followed by *O*-methylation. The step involving serotonin *N*-acetyl-transferase is probably rate limiting and is stimulated at night. Melatonin receptors are numerous in the SCN and parts of the hypothalamus where releasing and inhibiting hormones end. Darkness stimulates melatonin release and light blocks its synthesis. When compared with normal subjects, patients with SAD have been found to have an increased sensitivity of melatonin biosynthesis to inhibition by phototherapy.

Water and electrolyte changes

There are increases in the body's **residual sodium** (which is an index of intracellular sodium ion concentration) in both depression and mania. Erythrocyte sodium ion concentrations decrease following recovery from depression or mania as a result of increased sodium-potassium ATPase activity.

MANAGEMENT

Physical treatments

PHARMACOTHERAPY

UNIPOLAR DEPRESSION   Frank *et al.* (1991) have categorized outcomes of treatment according to the '5 Rs':

- Response.
- Remission: a return to the patients premorbid self.
- Relapse: a return of depressive symptoms in the time between initial response and recovery. Risk is particularly high following the withdrawal of antidepressants within the first four months of achieving a response (40–60 per cent). The risk of relapse is reduced to 10–30 per cent by continuation pharmacotherapy.
- Recovery: a patient who has achieved a stable remission for at least 4–6 months is assumed to have recovered from the index episode.
- Recurrence: a return of depression after recovery from index episode. Risk factors for recurrent depression include frequent and/or multiple prior episodes, seasonal pattern, and a family history of mood disorder.

ACUTE TREATMENT   This is initial treatment which aims to achieve a response.

CONTINUATION TREATMENT   This begins when a patient has achieved a significant response to treatment. The aim is to prevent relapse and consolidate response into remission.

MAINTENANCE TREATMENT   This follows continuation treatment for those patients with a history of recurrent depression. A recurrence rate of 85 per cent is seen in those patients with recurrent depression within three years following the discontinuation of pharmacotherapy. After six months continuation becomes maintenance treatment by arbitrary definition.

First line treatment of depression is with antidepressants. It is important that patients receive an adequate dose for an adequate duration, conventionally six weeks.

MRC trial: 1965. This involved 269 patients with operationally defined depression. At four weeks after random allocation of treatment it found:

- tricyclic antidepressant (imipramine) response rate of 53 per cent
- MAOI (phenelzine) response rate of 30 per cent
- placebo response rate of 39 per cent
- ECT response rate of 71 per cent

Antidepressants should be continued for four to six months after the amelioration of symptoms of the acute episode. Maintenance therapy usually with the same agent is used to treat the acute and continuation phases.

Lithium is efficacious in preventing recurrent depressive episodes, but less so than tricyclic antidepressants.

Patients maintained on the full effective treatment dose of antidepressants have proportionately fewer relapses than those whose dose is cut down to a lower maintenance level.

ATYPICAL DEPRESSION   This responds better to monoamine oxidase inhibitors than to tricyclic antidepressants.

PSYCHOTIC DEPRESSION   Spiker et al. (1985) found a superior response when antidepressant and antipychotic were used in combination in delusional depression.

- 41 per cent responded to amitriptyline alone
- 19 per cent responded to perphenazine alone
- 78 per cent responded to a combination of amitriptyline and perphenazine

RESISTANT MAJOR DEPRESSION   Up to 20 per cent of patients may be resistant to first line treatment with antidepressant medication, and another 20–30 per cent may have only a partial response. Patients with a partial response have a significantly higher rate of relapse during the first six months following response.

Those patients not showing response to adequate first line treatment may respond to augmentation with various agents including lithium, T3 or tryptophan. ECT should be tried if these measures fail.

BIPOLAR AFFECTIVE DISORDER   The treatment of acute mania is with neuroleptic medication. Lithium carbonate and citrate are used in the prophylaxis of bipolar disorder. They can also be used in the treatment of acute mania, but neuroleptics are preferred in the first instance.

A maintenance strategy consisting of lithium carbonate monotherapy in bipolar disorder is likely to result in sustained remission in approximately 50 per cent of cases.

The premature withdrawal of lithium in bipolar patients results in more than 80 per cent of recurrences within 36 months, a 28-fold increase compared to those left on lithium. Low-dose maintenance strategies (less than the usual acute anti-manic range of (0.8–1.2 mmol/L) lead to an increased risk of relapse.

In cases of bipolar disorder which are resistant to or intolerant of lithium, alternative prophylactic treatment with **carbamazepine** or **sodium valproate** are effective, both as acute anti-manic treatment and as prophylaxis.

ELECTROCONVULSIVE THERAPY (ECT)   Double-blind placebo-controlled trials have shown ECT to be superior to placebo, especially in delusional depression. It is considered the gold standard of antidepressant therapy and is often given to patients who have not responded to antidepressants. ECT is also used in the treatment of resistant mania or manic stupor.

Psychosocial treatments

PSYCHOTHERAPIES   This includes interpersonal therapy, cognitive therapy and behavioural therapy. Most progress has been made with psychotherapies for the acute treatment of major depression. Numerous trials have demonstrated the efficacy of psychotherapy in reducing the acute symptoms of depression, with greatest efficacy in more mildly ill patients. They are associated with a longer lag period for response than drug treatment. They may be a promising alternative to drugs during long-term maintenance treatment.

PROGNOSIS

Depression is a chronic and recurrent condition. It has become increasingly clear that a significant proportion of patients followed-up long term after suffering from depression remain chronically ill, despite the previously held belief that patients tended to recover fully between depressive episodes. Factors predicting a prolonged time to recovery are the longer duration and the increased severity of the index episode, a history of non-affective psychiatric disorder, lower family income and married status during the index episode.

It has been found that 15–20 per cent of depressed patients develop a chronic course of illness and 75–80 per cent of patients with depression suffer multiple episodes. The risk of relapse decreases the longer the patient remains well. For a first episode depression, an older age and a history of previous non-affective psychiatric illness predicts a shorter time to relapse. Continuing high levels of medication in the first few months is associated with a higher chance of remaining well. Overall, there is a suicide rate of around 15 per cent.

The time to recovery from the index episode of major depression in patients suffering from double depression is shorter than in patients suffering major depression alone, but they tend to relapse more frequently and rapidly.

PERSISTENT MOOD DISORDERS

ICD-10: persistent and usually fluctuating disorders of mood in which individual episodes are rarely sufficiently severe to warrant being described as hypomanic or mild depressive episodes. They may last for years at a time, sometimes for the greater part of adult life and involve considerable subjective distress and disability.

Two most important persistent mood disorders are cyclothymia and dysthymia. In ICD-10 the persistent mood disorders are classed with the mood disorders rather than with the personality disorders because of evidence from family studies which suggests that the persistent mood disorders are genetically related to other mood disorders.

CYCLOTHYMIA

Cyclothymia is defined in ICD-10 as:

> A persistent instability of mood, involving numerous periods of mild depression and mild elation. This instability usually develops early in adult life and pursues a chronic course, although at times the mood may be normal and stable for months at a time. The lifetime risk of cyclothymia is between 0.4 and 3.5 per cent, sex ratio equal. First-degree relatives of patients with cyclothymia are more likely than the general population to suffer from depressive episodes and bipolar disorder.

Some are treated successfully with lithium and/or with individual or group psychotherapy.

DYSTHYMIA

Dysthymia, also called depressive neurosis, is defined in ICD-10 as:

> A chronic depression of mood which does not fulfil the criteria for recurrent depressive disorder . . . The balance between individual phases of mild depression and intervening periods of comparative normality is very variable. Sufferers usually have periods of days or weeks when they describe themselves as well, but most of the time . . . they feel tired and depressed; everything is an effort and nothing is enjoyed. They brood and complain, sleep badly and feel inadequate, but are usually able to cope with the basic demands of everyday life.

It is probably more common in women than in men. It is more common in first-degree relatives of patients with a history of depressive episodes than in the general population.

Treatment with antidepressants, individual psychotherapy or cognitive therapy may be helpful.

SUICIDE AND PARASUICIDE (DELIBERATE SELF-HARM)

SUICIDE

Epidemiology
Incidence in England and Wales of approximately 1: 10 000 of the population per year.

It is more common in men than women and also more common in those aged over 45 years. Highest rates are in those who are divorced, single or widowed. Highest rates are in social classes I and V.

Suicide is associated with unemployment and retirement. Suicide rates fell in England and Wales during the First and Second World Wars.

There is a seasonal variation in suicide rates. In the northern hemisphere, suicide rates are highest during the months of spring and early summer. In the southern hemisphere, rates are highest in the months corresponding to spring and early summer.

There is evidence that the availability of method affects gross suicide rates as well as the choice of method. Suicide rates by hanging were constant until the 1960s when there was a rise after the abolition of capital punishment. A massive reduction in the number of deaths caused by gassing followed the switch from coal gas to the safer North Sea gas in the 1960s. A marked rise in poisoning in the early 1960s was because of the increased availability of medicines such as barbiturates.

Aetiology
Ninety per cent of people who commit suicide suffer from a psychiatric disorder. Of these approximately 50 per cent suffer depression, 25 per cent alcoholism, 5 per cent schizophrenia and 20 per cent other e.g. personality disorder, chronic neuroses, and psychoactive substance abuse disorders. The rate of suicide is increased by 50 times the population rate among psychiatric inpatients. There is also an association with physical illnesses, particularly chronic painful illnesses, epilepsy, especially temporal lobe epilepsy, cancer, peptic ulcer and gastric ulcer disease.

Following an act of deliberate self-harm the risk of completing suicide in the subsequent year is approximately 100 times that in the general population, and remains high in subsequent years.

Positive associations with suicide in the general population include being male, elderly, having suffered loss or bereavement, being unemployed or retired, childlessness, living alone in a big, densely populated town, a broken home in childhood, mental and physical illness, bereavement, loss of role, social disorganization including overcrowding, criminality, drug and alcohol misuse.

Negative associations include religious devoutness, lots of children and times of war.

RISK FACTORS BY PSYCHIATRIC DIAGNOSIS

- Schizophrenia: 10 per cent mortality from suicide. Roy (1982) characterized schizophrenics who commit suicide as young, male, and unemployed with chronic relapsing illness. Fewer schizophrenic patients give warning of their intention to commit suicide than patients in other diagnostic groups (23 per cent vs 50 per cent). Usually after recent discharge, good insight.

- Affective psychosis: 15 per cent mortality from suicide. Men are older, separated, widowed or divorced, living alone and not working. Women are middle-aged, middle-class, with a history of parasuicide and threats made in the last month. Those with obsessive compulsive symptoms are about six times less likely to commit suicide than those without.
- Neuroses: nearly 90 per cent have a history of parasuicide, and a high proportion have threatened suicide in the preceding month. There is a tendency after a failed attempt to resort to more violent means. There is a high risk in depressive neurosis and panic disorder, but a lower risk in obsessive compulsive disorder.
- Alcoholism: 15 per cent mortality from suicide. Tends to occur later in the course of their illness, and they are often also depressed. Associated with completed suicide is poor physical health, a poor work record, previous parasuicide and a recent loss of a close relationship.
- Personality disorder: lability of mood, aggressiveness, impulsivity, alienation from peers and associated alcohol and substance misuse are high-risk factors.

LIFE EVENTS AND SUICIDE   Risk of suicide increases, more among males than females, during the five years following the bereavement of a parent or a spouse.

Compared to psychiatric patient controls, suicides have experienced interpersonal losses more frequently, although schizophrenic suicides have experienced fewer losses than non-schizophrenic controls.

Age-related variations of stressors have been described, with conflict-separation-rejection more common in younger age groups, economic problems in middle-aged groups and medical illness among the older age groups.

BIOCHEMICAL DISTURBANCES   Low 5-HIAA concentration in cerebral spinal fluid is associated with increased suicidal behaviour and aggression. Irrespective of the clinical diagnosis, the group in which CSF concentration of 5-HIAA is low often includes persons who have attempted a violent method of suicide. Serotonin may play an important role in the biology of aggression and the control of impulsive behaviour.

Post-mortem ligand binding studies have found increased numbers of 5HT2 receptors in the prefrontal cortex of suicide victims, particularly those who used violent means. Low concentrations of serum cholesterol have been found to be prospectively associated with an increase in the risk of violent death or suicide. Biological mechanisms linking low serum cholesterol concentration and suicide have been hypothesized.

SOCIOLOGICAL THEORY   Durkheim in 1897 used the phenomenon of suicide to describe society. He described four types of suicide:

- altruistic: the individual sets no value on life, renounces their personal being in order to be engulfed into something wider e.g. religious or terrorist suicides
- egoistic: suicide springs from excessive individuation of the individual from society
- anomic: relates to how society regulates the individual. Suicide results from the fact that man's activities lack regulation
- fatalistic: a rare type of suicide, the opposite of anomic, deriving from excessive regulation by oppressive regimes

Assessment

Suicidal ideation should be explored in every patient and forms a part of the routine mental state examination. There is no evidence that asking patients about suicidal thoughts increases the risk of suicide.

The majority of people who commit suicide have told somebody beforehand of their thoughts. Two-thirds have seen their GP in the previous month. One-quarter have been psychiatric out-patients at the time of death; half of them will have seen a psychiatrist in the previous week.

Management

Once the need for treatment has been identified it should be provided quickly. The interval between GP referral to psychiatric services and consultation has been identified as a danger period and should be minimized.

If there is a serious risk of suicide the patient should be admitted to hospital. Any psychiatric disorder from which the patient suffers should be treated appropriately. If the patient is suffering from severe depression, electroconvulsive therapy may be required. Patients with manic depression have a mortality up to three times that of the general population, with suicide and cardiovascular disease being primarily responsible. In patients treated with lithium prophylaxis, cumulative mortality does not differ from that of the general population. A minimum length of two years' lithium treatment is needed to reduce the high mortality resulting from manic depression. It is proposed that lithium exerts its anti-suicide effect as a result of improved serotonergic transmission.

PARASUICIDE

Epidemiology

An incidence of about 3/1000, but this is probably an underestimate, however. It is commoner in females and in those aged below 35 years. The highest rates are in those who are divorced and single, among the lower social classes, unemployed, and living in overcrowded urban areas in which there are high rates of juvenile delinquency.

Ninety per cent of cases involve deliberate self-poisoning with drugs. Forty per cent use minor tranquillisers and a further 30 per cent use salicylates and paracetamol.

Aetiology

Compared with the general population, life events are more common in the six months before an act of parasuicide. These include the break-up of a relationship, trouble with the law, physical illness and the illness of a loved one.

Predisposing factors include marital difficulties, unemployment, physical illness particularly epilepsy, mental retardation, and parental neglect or abuse.

Motives include interruption, attention, communication and a true wish to die.

Assessment

A high degree of suicidal intent is indicated by the following:

- the act was **planned** and **prepared**
- **precautions** were taken to avoid discovery
- the patient **did not seek help** after the act
- the act involved a **dangerous method**
- there were **final acts** such as making a will or leaving a suicide note

In interviewing the parasuicidal:

- establish rapport
- try to understand the attempt
- enquire about current problems
- elicit background information
- implement a mental state examination

The presence of psychiatric disorders should be looked for, and any previous history of suicide attempts should be asked about. Social and financial support should also be detailed. Do not avoid asking about suicidal intent.

ASSESSMENT OF RISK FACTORS FOR SUBSEQUENT COMPLETION OF SUICIDE (TUCKMAN AND YOUNGMAN)   One point is awarded for each: age > 45, male, unemployed, not married, living alone, poor physical health, recent medical treatment, psychiatric disorder, violent attempt, suicide note, previous attempt.

Score 2–5: subsequent suicide rate 7/1000
>10: subsequent suicide rate 60/1000

Management

Treat medically as appropriate. Assess fully. Identify the risk factors. Reduce the immediate risk and treat the causes. If the patient suffers from a psychiatric disorder this should be treated appropriately.

MANAGEMENT OF SUICIDAL FEELINGS

- Allow ventilation: talking out avoids acting out
- Strike a bargain on medication: ask if they can cope with the responsibility of a bottle of tablets. If 'no', admit to hospital
- Agree a list of problems
- Establish possible practical help
- Allow for an underestimate of the true risk

PREVENTION

- Recognize high-risk cases and take them seriously
- Ask patients about their suicidal ideas
- Do not remove hope
- Prescribe safer drugs
- Treat underlying illness adequately

BIBLIOGRAPHY

Ahrens, B., Müller-Oerlinghausen, B. and Grof P. 1993: Length of lithium treatment needed to eliminate the high mortality of affective disorders. *British Journal of Psychiatry* 163 (suppl. 21), 27–9.

Beck, A.T., Rush, A.J., Shaw, B.F. and Emery, G. 1979: *Cognitive therapy of depression*, ed. M.J. Mahony. New York: The Guildford Press. The Guildford clinical psychology and psychotherapy series..

Bertelson, A. Harvald, B. and Hauge, M. 1977: A Danish twin study of manic–depressive disorders. *British Journal of Psychiatry* 130, 330.

Brown, G.W. and Harris, T. 1978: *Social origins of depression*. London: Tavistock Publications.

Cassano, G.B., Tundo, A. and Micheli, C. 1994: Bipolar and psychotic depressions. *Current Opinion in Psychiatry* 7, 5–8.

Egeland, J.A., Gerhard, D.S., Paus, D.L. *et al.* 1987: Bipolar affective disorders linked to markers on chromosome 11. *Nature* 325, 783–7.

Frank, E., Prien, R.F., Jarrett, D.B. et al. 1991: Conceptualization and rationale for consensus definitions of terms in major depressive disorder; response, remission, recovery, relapse, and recurrence. *Archives of General Psychiatry* 48, 851–5.

Gallerani, M., Manfredini, R., Caracciolo, S. *et al.* 1995: Serum cholesterol concentrations in parasuicide. *British Medical Journal* 310, 1632–6.

Heikkinen, M., Aro, H. and Lönnqvist, J. 1994: Recent life events, social support and suicide. *Acta Psychiatrica Scandinavica* (suppl. 377), 65–72.

Hirschfield, R.M.A. 1994: Major depression, dysthymia and depressive personality disorder. *British Journal of Psychiatry* 165 (suppl. 26), 23–30.

Keller, M.B. 1994: Depression: A long term illness. *British Journal of Psychiatry* 165 (suppl. 26), 9–15.

Kendler, K.S., Kessler, R., Walters, E.E. *et al.* 1995: Stressful life events, genetic liability and onset of an episode of major depression in women. *American Journal of Psychiatry* 152, 833–42.

King, E. 1994: Suicide in the mentally ill. An epidemiological sample and implications for clinicians. *British Journal of Psychiatry* 165, 658–63.

Kraepelin, E. 1921: *Manic depressive insanity and paranoia* (ed. G.M. Robertson, trans. R.M. Barclay). Edinburgh: Churchill Livingstone.

Medical Research Council 1965: Clinical trial of the treatment of depressive illness. *British Medical Journal* i, 881.

Nemeroff, C.B., Knight, D.L., Franks, J. *et al.* 1994: Further studies on platelet binding in depression. *American Journal of Psychiatry* 151, 1623–5.

Parkes, C.M. 1985: Bereavement. *British Journal of Psychiatry* 146, 11–17.

Roy, A. 1982: Suicide in chronic schizophrenia. *British Journal of Psychiatry* 141, 171–7.

Spiker, D.G., Cofskyweiss, J., Dealy, R.S. *et al.* 1985: The pharmacological treatment of delusional depression. *American Journal of Psychiatry* 142, 430–6.

Symonds, R.L. 1991: Books reconsidered. Suicide, a study in sociology: Emile Durkheim. *British Journal of Psychiatry* 159, 739–41.

Syvälahti, E.K.G. 1994: Biological aspects of depression. *Acta Psychiatrica Scandinavica* (suppl. 377), 11–15.

Thase, M.E. 1993: Maintenance treatments of recurrent affective disorder. *Current Opinion in Psychiatry* 6, 16–21.

Tuckman and Youngman, W.F. 1968: A scale for assessing risk of attempted suicides. *Journal of clinical Psychology* 24, 17–19.

Vaughn, C.E. and Leff J.P. (1976) The influence of family and social factors on the course of psychiatric illness. A comparison of schizophrenic and depressed neurotic patients. *British Journal of Psychiatry* 129: 125–137.

29
Neurotic, stress-related and somatoform disorders

HISTORY

CLASSIFICATION

1900   Freud distinguished between:

- **actual neuroses**: somatic causation, comprising neurasthenia, anxiety neurosis (generalized anxiety, panic disorder and agoraphobia) and hypochondriasis
- **psychoneuroses**: psychological causation, comprising hysteria and obsessions (simple phobia, social phobia and obsessive compulsive disorder)

Libidinous impulses reaching the ego generate anxiety; repression and symptom formation follow.

Fright neurosis, not related to repressed libido, was also described, similar to current post-traumatic stress disorder.

Neurosis is increasingly split into categories. There is debate as to the validity of this.

Tyrer *et al.* (1993) favour a **general neurotic syndrome**, supported by the following:

- A lifetime experience of more than one neurosis is more common, while frequency of a single neurotic diagnosis is less common than expected.
- Tyrer randomly assigned various neurotic groups to diazepam, dothiepin, cognitive–behavioural therapy, placebo and a self-help treatment programme. No difference in treatment response between diagnostic groups was found. Diazepam was less effective than dothiepin, cognitive-behavioural therapy or self-help, which were of similar efficacy in all groups.

- The effects of treatment were independent of neurotic subtype, thus division of the neuroses into subtypes was not supported.

Major psychiatric classifications continue to divide the neuroses into subtypes.

ICD-10

The traditional division between neurosis and psychosis is not used in ICD-10. The following are delineated:

- **Phobic anxiety disorders**: agoraphobia, with and without panic disorder; social phobias and specific phobias
- **Other anxiety disorders**: panic disorder, generalized anxiety disorder and mixed anxiety and depressive disorder
- **Obsessive–compulsive disorder**
- **Reaction to severe stress, and adjustment disorders**: acute stress reaction, post-traumatic stress disorder, and adjustment disorders
- **Dissociative (conversion) disorders**: dissociative amnesia, fugue and stupor; trance and possession disorders; dissociative motor disorders, convulsions, anaesthesia and sensory loss; Ganser's syndrome, and multiple personality disorder
- **Somatoform disorders**: somatization disorder; hypochondriacal disorder; somatoform autonomic dysfunction and persistent pain disorder
- **Other neurotic disorders**: neurasthenia and depersonalization-derealization syndrome.

GENERAL POINTS

EFFECT OF CHILDHOOD NEUROSIS   Robins (1966) found that most children with neurotic disorders do not suffer neurosis in adulthood. Adult neurotics develop neurosis in adult life.

In childhood there is excess neurosis in males. After puberty there is excess in females.

EFFECT OF PERSONALITY DISORDER   The prevalence of personality disorder in neurosis is 12 per cent in primary care and 40 per cent in psychiatric outpatients. Psychological treatment, particularly self-help, is more effective in neurotic patients without personality disorder. Neurotic patients with personality disorder respond better to antidepressant drug treatment.

MORTALITY   There is increased mortality in severe neurotic disorder. The relative risk of death in the decade following treatment for neurosis is 1.7. The biggest cause of increased risk is accidental death, particularly suicide (relative risk 6.1). There is also a major excess of deaths from nervous, circulatory and respiratory disease.

Suicide is most likely in the first year after discharge.

PHOBIC ANXIETY DISORDERS

The Greek word *phobos* means panic or terror.

In phobic anxiety disorders anxiety is evoked predominantly by certain well-defined situations, characteristically avoided. Contemplation of a feared situation generates anticipatory anxiety.

In defining fear as phobic the following are considered:

- out of proportion to objective risks
- cannot be reasoned or explained away
- beyond voluntary control
- leads to avoidance

Marks *et al.* (1993) classify adult fears as:

1   normal
2   abnormal fears

   (a) phobias of external stimuli

      - agoraphobia
      - social phobia
      - animal phobia
      - miscellaneous specific phobias

   (b) Phobias of internal stimuli

      - illness phobia
      - obsessive phobias

Epidemiology

The Epidemiological Catchment Areas study found:

- lifetime prevalence for all phobias ranged from 7.8 to 23.3 per cent between sites
- Six-month prevalence for agoraphobia: 2.8 to 5.8 per cent
- Six-month prevalence for simple phobia: 4.5 to 11.8 per cent
- Six-month prevalence for social phobia: 1.2 to 2.2 per cent

THE EDMONTON STUDY   (Dick *et al.* 1994) found:

- lifetime prevalence for all phobias 8.9 per cent (females 11.7 per cent, males 6.1 per cent)
- age of first symptoms 6 in females, 12 in males
- high rates of comorbidity with depression, alcohol abuse, drug abuse and obsessive compulsive disorder in all types of phobia

Phobic anxiety disorders affect females more than males (agoraphobia 75 per cent, simple phobia 95 per cent), except social phobia where the sex ratio is equal.

Aetiology

GENETIC   Phobic disorders or other psychiatric illnesses (neurosis, alcoholism, depressive illness) are more prevalent in families of phobic probands.
Kendler *et al.* (1993) using the twin registry demonstrated that familial aggregation of phobia resulted from genetic liability, not from shared environmental factors.
   The relatives of socially phobic probands have a threefold elevated risk of social phobia.

PSYCHOLOGICAL

Pavlovian classical conditioning: Watson in the 'Little Albert' experiment on an 18-month-old child, produced fear of a toy white rat by presenting it repeatedly with a loud noise. Fear is later generalized to all furry objects (see Chapter 1).
Operant conditioning: avoidance of a phobic situation is rewarded by a reduction in anxiety which reinforces avoidance.
Seligman's preparedness theory: anxiety is easily conditioned to certain stimuli e.g. heights, snakes, spiders, and is resistant to extinction. Prepared stimuli were dangerous to primitive man and may have been acquired by natural selection.

Freudian psychoanalytic theory: phobias represent a conflict leading to avoidance of situations symbolic of that conflict. 'Little Hans' developed a phobia of horses after seeing a male horse urinate. Freud believed that fear of castration by his father was displaced on to horses after this viewing.

COMORBIDITY   There is overlap between anxiety disorders e.g. 55 per cent of agoraphobics have social phobia and 30 per cent of social phobics also have agoraphobia.

Persons with major depression have 15 times the risk of having agoraphobia and nine times the risk of simple phobia as controls.

Twenty-five per cent of phobics report alcohol abuse/dependence; there are higher rates in agoraphobics and social phobics than in simple phobias.

Management

PSYCHOLOGICAL   Behaviour therapy is the treatment of choice. Exposure techniques are most widely used.

Wolpes' **systematic desensitization** combines relaxation with graded exposure.

Reciprocal inhibition prevents anxiety from being maintained when exposed to the phobic stimulus while relaxed.

Flooding entails maximal exposure to feared stimulus until anxiety reduction occurs. This is not more effective than other exposure techniques.

Modelling requires the patient to observe the therapist engaging in non-avoidant behaviour when exposed to a feared stimulus.

Psychoanalytic psychotherapy has proved to be ineffective.

Patients with agoraphobia/panic disorder are much improved following exposure therapy; these gains are maintained after 4–7 years.

Exposure, cognitive and cognitive-behavioural therapy result in similar improvement in social phobia.

PHARMACOLOGICAL   Monoamine oxidase inhibitors are effective in agoraphobics and social phobics. Eighty to ninety per cent of pure social phobics are almost asymptomatic at week 16; patients withdrawn from active drug relapse (Versiani *et al.* 1992).

Using fluoxetine, buspirone, phenelzine or moclobemide, two-thirds of socially phobic patients show significant improvement.

Benzodiazepines may help prevent the reinforcement of fear through avoidance.

AGORAPHOBIA

1871: Westphal first used the term to describe patients who experienced intense anxiety when walking across open spaces.

ICD-10

- Symptoms are manifestations of anxiety and are not secondary to other symptoms such as delusions or obsessional thoughts
- Anxiety is restricted to at least two of the following: crowds, public places, travelling away from home and travelling alone
- Avoidance of the phobic situation prominent

Course

Symptoms fluctuate, course prolonged. Eighty per cent of agoraphobics are never free of symptoms after five years of follow-up.

SOCIAL PHOBIAS

Fear of scrutiny by others in small groups. May progress to panic attacks. Avoidance is often marked.

ICD-10

- Symptoms are manifestations of anxiety and not secondary to other symptoms
- Anxiety restricted to or predominates in particular social situations
- Phobic situation avoided whenever possible.

Course
The course is continuous. It may improve gradually. Alcohol and drug abuse are common.

SPECIFIC (ISOLATED) PHOBIAS

Phobias are restricted to highly specific situations. The seriousness of the handicap depends on how easily a feared situation can be avoided.

ICD-10

- Symptoms are manifestations of anxiety and not secondary to other symptoms
- Anxiety restricted to the particular phobic situation
- Phobic situation avoided whenever possible.

Course
Childhood phobias are always improved after five years. Adult phobias: 20 per cent are unchanged, 40 per cent are better, 40 per cent are worse over five years.

OTHER ANXIETY DISORDERS

Manifestations of anxiety are the major symptoms, not restricted to any particular situation.

PANIC DISORDER

This involves recurrent unpredictable attacks of severe anxiety lasting usually for a few minutes only. There can be a sudden onset of palpitations, chest pain, choking, dizziness, depersonalization and derealization, together with a secondary fear of dying, losing control or going mad. It often results in a hurried exit and a subsequent avoidance of similar situations; it may be followed by persistent fear of another attack.

ICD-10
Absence of phobias and depressive disorder.
  Several attacks within one month:

- where there is no objective danger
- not confined to predictable situations
- with freedom from anxiety symptoms between attacks

Epidemiology
The Epidemiological Catchment Areas study found:

- three per cent of the population had experienced a panic attack in the previous six months

- Maximum period of onset from mid-teens to mid-thirties, rarely after the age of 40
- More common in females than males (2:1)
- Prevalence of strictly defined panic disorder 0.1 to 0.4 per cent
- One year prevalence 0.2 to 1.2 per cent
- Lifetime prevalence 1.4 to 1.5 per cent
- Women aged 25 to 44 years, with a family history of panic disorder, divorced or separated are at highest risk
- All socioeconomic groups are affected. There is no relationship with race or education

Aetiology

GENETIC   The morbid risk for panic disorder in relatives of probands is 15 per cent to 30 per cent, much higher than the general population (2 per cent). Female relatives are at higher risk than male relatives. There is an increased risk of alcoholism in the relatives of probands.

Kendler *et al.* (1993) estimate heritability for panic disorder with or without phobic avoidance is 35–40 per cent.

COMORBIDITY   One-third develop secondary depression following the onset of panic disorder. If depression does occur, the course is poorer.

Major controversy surrounds the relationship between anxiety disorders and depression.

There is evidence supporting the unitary position, that anxiety and depression lie along the same continuum:

- high overlap of symptoms (65 per cent of anxious patients have depressive symptoms) (Roth *et al.* 1972)
- difficulty separating primary disorder in patients experiencing both panic attacks and depression
- no differences in family history for anxiety and mixed anxiety depression groups

Evidence supporting separation:

- Family studies show no excess of depression in the relatives of probands suffering from pure panic disorder (Leckman *et al.* 1985)
- Children of probands with major depression show increased rates of major depression but not anxiety disorders
- Children of probands with major depression and panic disorder have higher rates of major depression and anxiety disorders
- Increased rate of panic disorder but not major depression or other anxiety disorders in the relatives of panic disorder probands

Agoraphobia usually occurs with panic disorder, but can occur separately.

There is an increased lifetime prevalence of alcohol abuse/dependence (54 per cent) and drug abuse/dependence (43 per cent) in persons with panic disorder. Some use substances as a complication of panic disorder; others develop panic disorder as a result of withdrawal from substances.

LIFE EVENTS   Excess of life events in the year prior to the onset of panic disorder, especially illness or death of a cohabitant or relative.

PHYSIOLOGICAL FACTORS   Pitts and McClure (1967) provoked panic attacks in patients with anxiety neurosis but not controls, by the intravenous infusion of sodium lactate.

There were higher levels of autonomic arousal in preinfusion panickers compared to non-panickers.

No single biochemical or neuroendocrine finding explains lactate-induced panic.

Yohimbine, a presynaptic $\alpha2$ adrenergic autoreceptor blocker induces panic attacks in a subgroup of individuals. This group show increased noradrenergic activity and blunted growth hormone response to clonidine, supporting the hypothesis of a dysregulation of the noradrenergic system and possibly the hypothalamus–pituitary–adrenal axis in a subgroup of panic-disorder patients. Very low rates of non-suppression during dexamethasone suppression test in panic disorder.

Panic attacks are associated with a reduced blood flow in the frontal lobes. Panic-disorder patients not having a panic attack have reduced perfusion of the hippocampus bilaterally and an increase in blood flow to the right inferior frontal cortex.

Mitral valve prolapse occurs in 40 per cent of panic-disorder patients compared to 9 per cent of controls. Patients suffering from mitral valve prolapse do not suffer more panic disorder than controls. An aetiological role for mitral valve prolapse in panic disorder is unlikely.

Panic-disorder patients have abnormal sleep breathing with increased irregularity in tidal volume during REM sleep and an increased rate of microapnoeas. One aetiological theory of panic disorder proposes that patients have a hypersensitive respiratory control system operating at the level of brainstem chemoreceptors. Their 'suffocation' alarm is thus at a pathologically low set point. Enhanced CO_2 sensitivity results in more frequent sighing to reduce CO_2 levels, which results in breathing pauses because CO_2 stimulus for breathing is withdrawn.

Management
DRUG TREATMENT   Tricyclic antidepressants imipramine and clomipramine, MAOIs and SSRIs are efficacious in the treatment of panic disorder.

The down-regulation of 5HT2 receptors may be responsible for therapeutic effects, which take up to four weeks. Increased anxiety or panic may occur in the first week of treatment.

Maprotiline, a specific noradrenaline reuptake inhibitor, is ineffective in the treatment of panic disorder.

Seventy-five per cent of patients with panic disorder and agoraphobia are responsive to treatment with imipramine relapse within six months of drug discontinuation, compared to none maintained on treatment. There is superior resistance to relapse in patients treated for longer periods, suggesting that treatment may alter subsequent course in an enduring manner.

Benzodiazepines e.g. alprazolam in high dosage reduce the frequency of panic attacks in the short term. There is the need to maintain treatment in the long term, and risks of dependency.

The re-emergence of symptoms following discontinuation of therapy is problematic.

PSYCHOLOGICAL TREATMENT   Cognitive behavioural therapy involving the **cognitive restructuring** of catastrophic interpretations of bodily experience, and **exposure techniques** which generate bodily sensations of fear during therapy with the aim of habituating the subject to them is efficacious in panic disorder.

Agoraphobic avoidance is treated by situational exposure and relaxation techniques.

Marks *et al.* (1993) comparing alprazolam and exposure therapy in patients suffering from panic disorder and agoraphobia found the effect size of exposure was twice that of alprazolam; during follow-up gains from alprazolam disappeared, but exposure gains were maintained. Treatment with a combination of exposure and alprazolam impaired improvement seen in the exposure alone group.

Course
Highly variable. Sixty per cent suffer mild impairment. Ten per cent suffer severe disability. Poor outcome predicted by lower social class and long duration of illness.

GENERALIZED ANXIETY DISORDER

The diagnostic reliability of generalized anxiety disorder (GAD) is lower than that of other anxiety disorders. Patients report uncontrollable worry. A negative response to the question 'Do you worry excessively over minor matters?' virtually rules out GAD as a diagnosis (negative predictive power 0.94). Symptoms of muscle and psychic tension are the most frequently reported by patients with GAD.

GAD is associated with the highest rates of comorbidity of all anxiety disorders.

ICD-10
There is generalized, persistent, free-floating anxiety. Continuous feelings of nervousness, trembling, muscular tension, sweating, light-headedness, palpitations, dizziness, and epigastric discomfort are common.

Anxiety presents most days for several weeks. Symptoms include:

- apprehension
- motor tension
- autonomic overactivity

Epidemiology
The Epidemiological Catchment Areas study found:

- six month prevalence of GAD 2.5–6.4 per cent.
- Age of onset earlier (majority before age 20) and more gradual than other anxiety disorders
- Early onset GAD is more likely to be female, have a history of childhood fears and have marital or sexual disturbance. Later onset is more likely to develop after stressful life event

Aetiology
GENETIC   Some studies show familial aggregation of GAD, others do not.

Kendler *et al.* (1993) concluded that GAD is a moderately familial disorder with a heritability of 30 per cent.

ENVIRONMENTAL FACTORS   Torgersen (1983): Probands with GAD had lost their parents by death far more often than probands with panic disorder, suggesting that environmental factors contribute a higher vulnerability for the development of GAD.

Management
DRUG TREATMENT   Benzodiazepines were effective in 40 per cent, although the effect was weak and short-lived.

Response to buspirone is slower than benzodiazepines. There is appreciable anxiolytic effect with no increase in psychopathology upon withdrawal.

PSYCHOLOGICAL THERAPIES   Patients respond less favourably to conventional cognitive-behavioural treatments than in other anxiety disorders. Treatments tend to be non-specific e.g. relaxation training. Interventions specifically targeting the worry associated with GAD may be more effective.

Course
Follow-up after six years reveals stability of diagnosis; the most common change of diagnosis is to alcoholism.

Sixty-eight per cent have mild or no impairment, 9 per cent have severe impairment.

OBSESSIVE–COMPULSIVE DISORDER

ICD-10
Obsessional symptoms or compulsive acts are present most days for at least two successive weeks causing distress or interfering with activities. Obsessional symptoms have the following characteristics:

- recognized as the individuals own
- at least one thought or act is resisted unsuccessfully
- the thought of carrying out the act must not in itself be pleasurable
- thoughts, images or impulses are unpleasantly repetitive

Obsessional symptoms developing in the presence of schizophrenia, Tourette's syndrome or organic mental disorder are regarded as part of these conditions.

Epidemiology
The Epidemiological Catchment Areas study found:

- Six month prevalence: 1.3–2.0 per cent
- Lifetime prevalence: 1.9–3.0 per cent
- *ECA* study findings were consistently higher than earlier accepted estimates
- Obsessive–compulsive disorder (OCD) is very rare in children. Rutter found no cases among 2000 10- and 11-year olds on the Isle of Wight
- Sex ratio equal
- Bimodal age of onset with peaks occurring age 12–14 and 20–22 years. Decline in onset after the age of 35

Aetiology
GENETIC   First degree relatives of OCD patients have a higher than normal incidence of psychiatric disorders, most commonly anxiety, phobias, depression and schizophrenia.

First degree relatives of OCD patients have higher than normal obsessional traits; the risk of OCD among relatives is higher in early onset OCD proband, suggesting aetiological heterogeneity.

Twin studies suggest that monozygotic twins are more likely to be concordant than dizygotic twins for OCD, but the literature conflicts.

Gilles de la Tourette's syndrome is a familial condition with a substantial genetic basis. Twin and family studies find high rates of OCD and obsessive compulsive symptoms among Tourette's families. This suggests that some forms of OCD may be related to Tourette's syndrome.

OCD is equally frequent in families of Tourette's proband regardless of whether proband has OCD. The rate of OCD alone is higher in female relatives and the rate of Tourette's and tics is higher in male relatives of Tourette's proband. These findings suggest that some forms of OCD are familial.

Probands with no relatives affected by OCD may represent a sporadic form of OCD which is aetiologically distinct from the familial form.

NEUROLOGICAL   The reported numbers of OCD cases increased following the 1915 and 1926 outbreaks of encephalitis lethargica.

OCD patients have more abnormal births than expected and more neurological disorders including Sydenham's chorea and encephalitis, suggestive of basal ganglia dysfunction. Flor-Henry observed neuropsychological deficits implicating left frontal lobe dysfunction.

Brain-imaging techniques show morphological changes of basal ganglia structures in OCD. Fronto-striatal abnormality is present. Functional neuroimaging studies show **increased** blood flow in the basal ganglia, orbital, prefrontal and anterior cingulate cortex. Caudate metabolic rate is reduced after treatment with drugs or behaviour therapy in those patients responsive to treatment, with the percentage change in symptom ratings correlating significantly with right caudate change.

PSYCHOLOGICAL   In learning theory, obsessions are thoughts with which anxiety has become associated. Rituals or neutralizing thoughts terminate exposure to the stimulus; thus anxiety is reduced and the rituals are negatively reinforced. The use of rituals prevents the natural reduction in anxiety that would occur if exposure to the stimulus was not cut short by the ritual or neutralizing thought.

In cognitive model obsessional distortion concerns exaggerated the responsibility for thoughts, with a tendency to neutralize thoughts with rituals.

In psychoanalysis OCD symptoms are seen as defensive responses to unconscious impulses. Obsessional symptoms arise from intrapsychic anxiety because of the conflicts being expressed by the defence mechanisms of displacement, undoing and reaction formation. The origin of obsessional personality is located at the anal-training stage of development; OCD is thought to represent regression to this stage.

Neuropsychological tests suggest the presence of amnestic deficits with respect to non-verbal memory and memory for actions. OCD patients also perform poorly on tests of frontal lobe function, particularly tests of shifting set.

Management

DRUG TREATMENT   Antidepressants are effective in the short-term treatment of OCD. Clomipramine and SSRIs have greater efficacy than antidepressants with no selective serotonergic properties. Concomitant depression is not necessary for serotonergic antidepressants to improve symptoms.

Relapse often follows discontinuation of treatment.

There are success rates of 50–79 per cent.

PSYCHOLOGICAL   Behavioural methods e.g. modelling, exposure and response prevention, are the most widely accepted psychological treatments; there are success rates of 60–85 per cent.

The value of cognitive therapy in the treatment of OCD is not conclusive.

Psychoanalytic therapy is not effective in the treatment of OCD.

PHYSICAL   Psychosurgery may be indicated in the chronic unremitting OCD of at least two years duration with severe life disruption, unresponsive to all recognized forms of therapy. Open, uncontrolled studies show that 65 per cent of patients with OCD are improved or greatly improved with cingulotomy plus bifrontal operations.

Course

Favourable prognostic factors include:

- mild symptoms
- predominance of phobic ruminative ideas, absence of compulsions
- short duration of symptoms
- no childhood symptoms or abnormal personality traits

Poor prognostic factors include:

- males with early onset
- symptoms involving the need for symmetry and exactness
- the presence of hopelessness, hallucinations or delusions
- a family history of OCD

Continuous, episodic or deteriorating course.

REACTION TO SEVERE STRESS AND ADJUSTMENT DISORDERS

ICD-10

Disorders are identifiable on the basis of symptomatology and causative influences. These disorders always arise as a direct consequence of acute severe stress or continued trauma without which the disorder would not have occurred.

ACUTE STRESS REACTION

This is a transient disorder developing in an individual without other mental disorder in response to exceptional stress; it usually subsides within hours or days. The risk is increased if physical exhaustion or organic factors are present.

ICD-10

Immediate temporal connection between impact of exceptional stressor and onset of symptoms. Onset within minutes. In addition symptoms:

- show a mixed and changing picture; initial state of daze, depression, anxiety, anger, despair, overactivity, and withdrawal may all be seen. No symptom predominates for long
- resolve rapidly, within a few hours if removal from the stressful environment is possible. If stress continues, symptoms diminish after 24–48 hours.

POST-TRAUMATIC STRESS DISORDER

ICD-10

- Arises within six months as delayed and/or protracted response to a stressful event of an exceptionally threatening nature
- Symptoms include repeated reliving of the trauma. Repetitive, intrusive memories (flashbacks), daytime imagery, or dreams of the event must be present
- Emotional detachment, persisting background numbness, avoidance of stimuli reminiscent of original event often present, but are not essential

- Autonomic disturbances (hyperarousal with hypervigilance, enhanced startle reaction, and insomnia), and mood disorder contribute to diagnosis but are not essential. Anxiety, depression and suicidal ideation are not uncommon. The excessive use of alcohol or drugs may complicate matters.

Aetiology

- About 25 per cent exposed to a potentially traumatic event develop PTSD
- Low education and social class, pre-existing psychiatric problems and female gender are vulnerability factors
- Viewing the dead body of a relative after the disaster is predictive of lower PTSD

PERSONALITY   Psychopathic traits are protective.

Sufferers of PTSD report childhood physical sexual abuse more often than expected.

BIOLOGICAL   PTSD patients have exaggerated physiologic responses (heart rate, skin conductance, electromyographic response) to traumatic imagery. They have a heightened physiological state specific to PTSD and are difficult to simulate. This may be mediated by noradrenergic and dopaminergic neurotransmitter systems, and HPA axis.

Initial mobilization and the subsequent depletion of noradrenaline following inescapable shock in animals indicates a possible catecholaminergic mediation of PTSD symptoms. Drugs effective in PTSD (MAOIs, tricyclics, benzodiazepines and clonidine) are also effective in preventing development of learned helplessness in animals when infused into the locus coeruleus.

There are similarities between PTSD symptoms and opioid withdrawal, leading to speculation that opioid function is disturbed in PTSD. Stress-induced analgesia is reversible by nalaxone in PTSD veterans exposed to traumatic stimulus.

Management

A flexible, staged approach using several techniques is advocated.

PSYCHOLOGICAL THERAPY   Exposure to aversive memories are central, irrespective of the specific therapy used.

Exposure to anxiety-producing stimuli in a supportive setting results in arousal, attenuation and symptom reduction or habituation. Another common element is some form of cognitive restructuring.

Behavioural techniques are most effective in relation to PTSD following simple trauma.

For more complicated traumas, such as torture, these should be combined with cognitive methods.

PHARMACOTHERAPY   MAOIs and tricyclic antidepressants are beneficial in PTSD, particularly for intrusive symptoms. SSRIs are helpful with avoidant symptoms.

Carbamazepine, propranolol and clonidine reduce hyperarousal and intrusive symptoms; fluoxetine and lithium reduce explosiveness and improve mood.

Buspirone may lessen fear-induced startle; it may play an adjunctive role.

Alprazolam is no more effective than placebo; there have been some positive reports with clonazepam.

There is an almost total lack of response to placebo in chronic PTSD.

The drugs require at least eight weeks duration before the effects are evident. The magnitude of the drug effect is limited. Progressive and continued improvement has been noted over several months in chronic PTSD treated with tricyclics.

EYE MOVEMENT DESENSITIZATION   Involuntary multi-saccadic eye movements occur during disturbing thoughts. It is claimed that inducing these eye movements while experiencing intrusive thoughts stops symptoms of PTSD.

Course

Half of the patients still have PTSD decades later. A dose–response relationship exists between the severity of the stressor and the degree of consequent psychological distress.

Most PTSD patients also have depression, anxiety disorders, substance abuse and/or sexual dysfunction.

ADJUSTMENT DISORDERS

ICD-10

There are states of distress and emotional disturbance arising in the period after a stressful life event.

Individual predisposition plays a greater role than in other conditions in this section, but the condition would not have arisen without a stressor.

Manifestations vary: they include depressed mood, anxiety, worry, an inability to cope and some inability to manage the daily routine. Conduct disorders may be associated, especially in adolescents. Regressive phenomena in children is frequently seen.

Onset is within one month of stressor; duration is usually less than six months, except for prolonged depressive reaction.

Grief reactions considered abnormal because of their form or content are included in this category.

The following adjustment disorders are outlined in ICD-10:

- brief depressive reaction: less than one month
- prolonged depressive reaction: less than two years
- mixed anxiety and depressive reaction
- predominant disturbance of emotions, and/or conduct

DISSOCIATIVE (CONVERSION) DISORDERS

ICD-10

This is presumed to be psychogenic in origin; it is associated with traumatic events, insoluble problems or disturbed relationships. The unpleasant affect associated with these conflicts is transformed (converted) into symptoms.

DIAGNOSTIC GUIDELINES

- no evidence of physical disorder that may explain symptoms
- evidence for psychological causation; clear association in time with stressful events.

DISSOCIATIVE AMNESIA

- Loss of memory of important event is not due to organic disorder, fatigue or ordinary forgetfulness
- Partial and selective amnesia is usually centred on traumatic events
- Extent varies from day to day; persistent core cannot be recalled while awake
- Perplexity, distress or calm acceptance may accompany
- Begins and ends suddenly, following stress

- More common in young adults; rare in the elderly
- Recovery complete, rarely lasts more than a couple of days; recurrence unusual

DISSOCIATIVE FUGUE

- All features of dissociative amnesia plus apparently purposeful journey away from home. New identity may be assumed
- Precipitated by severe stress
- Amnesia for period of fugue, but self-care and social interaction is maintained
- Lasts hours to days
- Recovery abrupt and complete

DISSOCIATIVE STUPOR

- Stuporose; no evidence of a physical or other psychiatric cause
- Onset sudden and stress-related
- Sits motionless for long periods, speech and movement absent; muscle tone, posture, breathing and eye movements indicate that the individual is neither asleep nor unconscious

TRANCE AND POSSESSION DISORDERS

- Temporary loss of personal identity and awareness of surroundings
- Attention and awareness limited to one or two aspects of the immediate environment
- Repeated movements, postures or utterances
- Only includes involuntary or unwanted trance, occurring outside culturally accepted situation

DISSOCIATIVE DISORDERS OF MOVEMENT AND SENSATION

- Loss of movement or sensations, usually cutaneous
- No physical cause
- Symptoms often reflect patient's concept of disorder, which may be at variance with physiological or anatomical principles e.g. glove and stocking anaesthesia
- Resulting disability helps patient to escape conflict, or express dependency or resentment indirectly
- Calm acceptance (*la belle indifférence*) not common and not diagnostic; also seen in normal people facing serious illness
- Premorbid personality and relationships often abnormal

DISSOCIATIVE CONVULSIONS

Pseudoseizures mimic epileptic seizures but tongue biting, serious bruising and incontinence of urine are uncommon. Loss of consciousness is absent or replaced by stupor or trance.

DISSOCIATIVE ANAESTHESIA AND SENSORY LOSS

- Patches of sensory loss that do not correspond to anatomical dermatomes
- Visual loss rarely total; general mobility well preserved
- Dissociative deafness and anosmia far less common

OTHER DISSOCIATIVE DISORDERS

GANSER'S SYNDROME   This is a complex disorder described by Ganser, characterized by approximate answers and usually accompanied by several dissociative symptoms, often in circumstances that suggest psychogenic aetiology.

The five main features of Ganser syndrome are:

1   approximate answers (*Vorbeireden*)
2   clouding of consciousness
3   somatic conversion
4   pseudohallucinations (often)
5   subsequent amnesia.

MULTIPLE PERSONALITY DISORDER (MPD)   Controversy exists about whether it is iatrogenic or culture specific.

There is an apparent existence of two or more distinct personalities within an individual, of which only one is evident at any time. Each personality is complete, with its own memories, behaviour and preferences.

One is personality dominant. It does not have access to memories of the other, and is unaware of the existence of others. The change from one personality to another is sudden and associated with stress.

Psychoanalysis views MPD as a complex, chronic developmental dissociative disorder related to severe, repetitive childhood abuse or trauma, usually beginning before the age of five. Dissociative defences are used to handle subsequent traumatic experience.

Additionally **mass hysteria** presents with abnormal illness behaviour transmitted in close communities spreading from individuals of high status down the hierarchy. Affected individuals are suggestible. **Couvade syndrome** presents in males whose partners are pregnant, with symptoms of morning sickness, abdominal pain and anxiety.

Epidemiology

Relatively high frequencies of dissociative experiences are reported in patients with PTSD, women with chronic pelvic pain, substance abusers (40 per cent), patients with eating disorders and those with a history of childhood abuse.

IQ is negatively correlated.

Aetiology

Freud introduced the term conversion to describe the unconscious rendering innocuous of threatening ideas by conversion into physical symptoms, which have symbolic significance. This results in the relief of emotional conflict (primary gain) and the direct advantages of assuming a sick role (secondary gain).

The spectrum of dissociation (multiple personality disorder is most extreme) with increasingly complex and symptomatic forms is related to increasingly severe childhood trauma.

Levels of psychological distress are highly correlated with dissociative experiences.

Of 100 substance-dependent subjects, 39 had dissociative disorder and 43 reported childhood abuse. Patients with dissociative disorder may use substances to block out more severe abuse memories and suppress dissociative symptoms.

Management

Do not confront. Complete physical investigations; emphasize that serious illness is excluded. Minimize the advantages of a sick role, and praise healthy behaviour. Allow the patient to discard symptoms without losing face.

The main treatment of MPD is long-term psychoanalytic psychotherapy aimed at the unification of divided mental processes.

Course

Dissociative states tend to remit after a few weeks or months. Chronic states of more than one to two years are often resistant to therapy. Those with acute, recent onset, a good premorbid personality and resolvable conflict have a better prognosis.

Slater in a classic paper (1965) conducted a nine-year follow-up study of 85 patients who were diagnosed hysterics by senior psychiatrists and neurologists. He found 33 per cent developed definite organic illness; 15 per cent had a major mental illness; 12 patients died, four from suicide of whom two had demyelinating neurological conditions, and eight from natural causes which could have accounted for their original presentations. Of the original sample of 85, he was left with seven young patients who had experienced acute psychogenic reactions in the form of a conversion syndrome, and 14 who were suffering from lasting personality disorders. Slater concluded that the diagnosis of hysteria should not be made.

SOMATOFORM DISORDERS

ICD-10

Repeated presentation of physical symptoms with persistent requests for medical investigations; no physical basis found. Attempts to discuss possible psychological causation resisted.

SOMATIZATION DISORDER

There are multiple, recurrent, frequently changing physical symptoms. Most patients have multiple contacts with primary and specialist medical services; many negative investigations. Gastrointestinal and skin symptoms are most common. Sexual and menstrual complaints are also common.

ICD-10 requires the presence of all the following:

- two years of multiple and variable physical symptoms; no physical explanation found
- persistent refusal to accept the advice of several doctors
- impairment of functioning attributable to symptoms and resulting behaviour

The possibility of developing an independent physical disorder should be considered.

Onset after the age of 40 may indicate the onset of affective disorder.

Emphasis on symptoms and their effects, distinguishes this from hypochondriacal disorder where emphasis of concern is on possible underlying disease.

Briquet's syndrome or St Louis hysteria is multiple somatization disorder.

Epidemiology

- 0.2–0.5 per cent prevalence in the UK
- 3 per cent of repeated gut clinic attenders have somatization disorder
- prevalence using abridged criteria (four unexplained symptoms in males, six in females):

  - community: 4.4 per cent
  - patients with medically unexplained symptoms: 32 per cent

- far more common in women than men
- usually starts in early adult life

Aetiology

GENETIC   Torgersen 1986 MZ:DZ concordance in somatoform disorder 29:10. This suggests that somatoform disorder has a familial transmission.

ENVIRONMENTAL   *The South London somatisation study*: Craig *et al*. 1993

This longitudinal study in primary care compared somatizers with those with pure emotional disorder and those with pure physical disorder. The physical symptoms of somatizers are less likely to improve; one-third went on to develop chronic somatoform disorders.

Changes in physical symptoms mirrored changes in emotional arousal. Somatizers were more likely to report parental physical illness and to have had more physical illness themselves in childhood; emotionally disordered subjects reported more parental lack of care.

Hypothesize that physical illness in childhood lessened the distress of lack of care, resulting in somatic rather than emotional responses as a means of attracting care or lessening hostility, which endures into adult life.

Management

Engage patient and spouse; no more investigations; listen empathically; elicit childhood experience of illness and parental disability; link physical symptoms to relevant life events (reattribution model: Goldberg); reduce all medication apart from antidepressants for the depressed; limit the expectations of cure.

Alexithymia (limited ability to describe emotions verbally) is common in somatoform disorder. Traditional psychotherapy with alexithymic individuals is difficult. A more reality-based educational and supportive approach is better.

Course

Chronic and fluctuating course. Use disproportionate health resources. If engaged as above, this significantly reduces the use of resources.

Depression and anxiety often present, and may require treatment.

HYPOCHONDRIACAL DISORDER

Persistent preoccupation with the possibility of having serious disease. Attention is usually focused on one or two organ systems only.

Occurs in both men and women; no familial characteristics.

ICD-10

- persistent belief in the presence of at least one serious physical illness, despite repeated investigations revealing no physical explanation of presenting symptoms, or persistent preoccupation with presumed deformity
- persistent refusal to accept the advice of several different doctors that there is no physical illness underlying the symptoms

If depressive symptoms are prominent and precede the onset of hypochondriacal ideas, then depressive disorder may be primary.

SOMATOFORM AUTONOMIC DYSFUNCTION

Symptoms presented as if caused by a disorder of a system or organ largely under autonomic control e.g. cardiac neurosis, psychogenic hyperventilation, gastric neurosis, nervous diarrhoea.

ICD-10

- Persistent and troublesome symptoms of autonomic arousal
- Symptoms referred to specific organ system
- Distress about the possibility of disorder of the organ system, not responsive to repeated reassurance
- No evidence of organ pathology

PERSISTENT SOMATOFORM PAIN DISORDER

This presents with persistent, severe, distressing pain, not explained by physical disorder. Pain occurs in association with emotional conflict, and results in increased support and attention.

OTHER NEUROTIC DISORDERS

NEURASTHENIA

ICD-10

- Persistent, distressing complaints of increased fatigue after mental effort, or persistent, distressing complaints of bodily weakness and exhaustion after minimal effort
- At least two of the following: muscular aches; dizziness; headaches; sleep disturbance; inability to relax; irritability or dyspepsia

DEPERSONALIZATION–DEREALIZATION SYNDROME

It is uncommon to experience these in an isolated form.

ICD-10

- Depersonalization symptoms and/or derealization symptoms
- Insight
- Clear sensorium and absence of toxic confusional state or epilepsy

BIBLIOGRAPHY

Andrews, G., Stewart, G., Morris-Yates, A. *et al.* 1990: Evidence for a general neurotic syndrome. *British Journal of Psychiatry* 157, 6–12.

Boer, J.A. den 1988: Serotonergic mechanisms in anxiety disorders. An enquiry into serotonin function in panic disorder. PhD thesis, University of Utrecht.

Brown, T.A., Barlow, D.H. and Liebowitz, M.R. 1994: The empirical basis of generalised anxiety disorder. *American Journal of Psychiatry* 151, 1272–80.

Craig, T.K.J., Boardman, A.P., Mills, K. *et al.* 1993: The South London somatisation study I: Longitudinal course and the influence of early life experiences. *British Journal of Psychiatry* 163, 579–88.

Davidson, J. 1992: Drug therapy of post-traumatic stress disorder. *British Journal of Psychiatry* 160, 309–14.

Dick, C.L., Bland, R.C. and Newman, S.C. 1994: Panic disorder. *Acta Psychiatrica Scandinavica* (suppl 376), 45–53.

Dick, C.L., Sowa, B., Bland, R.C. and Newman, S.C. 1994: Phobic disorders. *Acta Psychiatrica Scandinavica* (suppl. 376), 36–44.

James, I.A. and Blackburn, I.-M. 1995: Cognitive therapy with obsessive-compulsive disorder. *British Journal of Psychiatry* 166, 444–50.

Kendler, K., Neale, M., Kessler, R. *et al.* 1993: Major depression and phobias: the genetic and environmental sources of comorbidity. *Psychological Medicine* 23, 361–71.

Kendler, K., Neale, M., Kessler, R. *et al.* 1993: Panic disorder in women: a population based twin study. *Psychological Medicine* 23, 397–406.

Klerman, G.L. 1986: The national institute of mental health: Epidemiologic catchment areas (NIMH-ECA) program. Background, preliminary findings and implications. *Soc. Psychiat* 21, 159–66.

Kolada, J.L., Bland, R.C. and Newman, S.C. 1994: Obsessive–compulsive disorder. *Acta Psychiatrica Scandinavica* (suppl. 376), 24–35.

Leckman, J.F., Weissman, M.M., Merikangas, K.R. *et al.* 1985: Major depression and panic disorder: a family study perspective. *Psychopharmacological Bulletin* 21, 543–5.

Loewenstein, R.J. and Ross, D.R. 1992: Multiple personality and psychoanalysis: an introduction. *Psychoanalytic Inquiry* 12, 3–48.

Marks, I.M. and Gelder, M.G. 1966: Different ages of onset in varieties of phobia. *American Journal of Psychiatry* 123, 218–21.

Marks, I.M., Swinson, R.P., Basoglu, M. *et al.* 1993: Alprazolam and exposure alone and combined in panic disorder with agoraphobia. *British Journal of Psychiatry* 162 776–87.

McIvor, R.J. and Turner, S.W. 1995: Assessment and treatment approaches for survivors of torture. *British Journal of Psychiatry* 166, 705–11.

Pauls, D.L., Alsobrook, J.P., Goodman, W. *et al.* 1995: A family study of obsessive compulsive disorder. *American Journal of Psychiatry* 152, 76–84.

Piccinelli, M., Pini, S., Bellantuono, C. *et al.* 1995: Efficacy of drug treatment in obsessive-compulsive disorder: a meta-analytic review. *British Journal of Psychiatry* 166: 424–43.

Pitts, F.N. and McClure, J.N. 1967: Lactate metabolism in anxiety neurosis. *New England Journal of Medicine* 1329–36.

Robins, L.N. 1966: *Deviant children grown up.* Baltimore: Williams & Wilkins.

Roth, M., Gurney, C., Garside, R.F. *et al.* 1972: Studies in the classification of affective disorders: the relationship between anxiety states and depressive illnesses. I. *British Journal of Psychiatry* 121, 147–61.

Sims, A. and Prior, P. 1978: The pattern of mortality in severe neuroses. *British Journal of Psychiatry* 133, 299–305.

Slater, E. 1965: Diagnosis of hysteria. *British Medical Journal* i, 1395–9.

Spector, J. and Huthwaite, M. 1993: Eye-movement desensitisation to overcome post-traumatic stress disorder. *British Journal of Psychiatry* 163, 106–8.

Stein, M.B., Millar, T.W., Larsen, D.K. *et al.* 1995: Irregular breathing during sleep in patients with panic disorder. *American Journal of Psychiatry* 152, 1168–73.

Tallis, F. 1995: Reading about obsessive–compulsive disorder. *British Journal of Psychiatry* 166, 546–50.

Torgersen, S. 1983: Genetic factors in anxiety disorders. *Archives of General Psychiatry* 40, 1085–9.

Torgersen, S. 1985: Hereditary differentiation of anxiety and affective neuroses. *British Journal of Psychiatry* 146, 530–4.

Torgersen, S. 1986: Genetics of somatoform disorders. *Archives of General Psychiatry* 43, 502–5.

Tyrer, P., Seivewright, N., Murphy, S. *et al.* 1988: The Nottingham study of neurotic disorder. Comparison of drug and psychological treatments. *Lancet* ii, 235–40.

Tyrer, P., Seivewright, N., Ferguson, B. *et al.* 1993: The Nottingham study of neurotic disorder. Effect of personality status on response to drug treatment, cognitive therapy and self-help over two years. *British Journal of Psychiatry* 162, 219–26.

Versiani, M., Nardi, A.E., Mundim, F.D. *et al.* 1992: Pharmacotherapy of social phobia: a controlled study with moclobemide and phenelzine. *British Journal of Psychiatry* 161, 353–60.

30
Disorders specific to women

MENSTRUATION

Premenstrual syndrome
This includes emotional and/or physical symptoms occurring premenstrually (late luteal phase) but remitting usually during the week before menstruation (follicular phase).

More than 150 symptoms have been implicated in PMS. There are considerable between-subject differences in the patterns of symptoms, but there is strong support for cycle-related variability in most subjects. The existence of PMS as a discrete entity has often been questioned; there is a lack of consensus about its definition.

The common symptoms experienced by those women suffering PMS are:

MOOD SYMPTOMS   Irritable, easily angry or upset without good reason, tension, emotional lability, depressed mood, violent feelings.

OTHER SYMPTOMS   Bloated abdomen, tender breasts, carbohydrate craving, disturbed sleep, poor concentration, clumsiness, headaches, muscle and joint pain, spots.

EPIDEMIOLOGY

Forty per cent of women experience some cyclical premenstrual symptoms; 2–10 per cent report severe symptoms.

There are associations with the following:

- higher prevalence in those around 30 years of age
- prevalence increases with increasing parity
- higher prevalence in those women who have experienced natural menstrual cycles (unmodified by oral contraceptives and uninterrupted by pregnancy) for longer periods of time
- women using oral contraceptives, especially if nulliparous have reduced rates of PMS
- prevalence increased in those experiencing higher levels of psychosocial stress

AETIOLOGY

Genetic

Highly significant correlations between mother and daughter have been reported on a variety of menstrual variables including premenstrual tension.

Condon (1993): concordances for global PMS scores:

- 0.28 in DZ twin pairs
- 0.55 in MZ twin pairs

Concordances for MZ twins exceed those of DZ twins on every subscale. The findings support the hypothesis that the familial aggregation of PMS symptoms is determined largely by genetic factors.

Neuroendocrine

β-ENDORPHIN   Anxiety, food cravings and physical discomfort in PMS subjects is associated with a significant decline in β-endorphin (these symptoms are also found in opiate withdrawal).

SEROTONIN   Post-synaptic serotonergic responsivity is altered during the late luteal phase of the menstrual cycle. It is thought that gonadal hormones cause changes in the levels of activity of serotonergic systems. Carbohydrate craving and depression are linked to serotonergic brain changes which are marked in the late luteal phase.

Plasma taken from subjects suffering from PMS inhibits serotonin uptake in rat brain synaptosomes to a greater degree than serum taken from controls.

NORADRENALINE   CSF MHPG (3-methoxy 4-hydroxyphenylglycol, a metabolite of noradrenaline) is elevated in PMS subjects premenstrually.

ANDROGENS   Serum androgens are higher in women with premenstrual irritability and dysphoria than in controls. Serum-free testosterone levels are significantly higher in PMS subjects than in matched controls around ovulation, and 17-hydroxyprogesterone levels are higher in PMS women in the luteal phase.

OTHER   Various hypotheses have been explored, particularly in relation to the balance between oestrogen and progesterone with a relative lack of progesterone, excessive production of prolactin, aldosterone or antidiuretic hormone. None are conclusive.

Neurophysiological

The following have been reported:

- consistent cycle-dependent changes in electroencephalographic recordings, most prominent in the α range
- alterations in response to dichotic auditory stimuli premenstrually in comparison with the follicular phase, most marked in sufferers of PMS
- alterations in skin conductance in response to auditory stimuli premenstrually in comparison with the follicular phase, most marked in sufferers of PMS

Personality

Neuroticism may be an important determinant of women's experiences and reports of their menstrual cycle, and is higher in those reporting PMS.

Women with coronary-prone type-A behaviour experience 50 per cent more PMS symptoms than women with non-coronary-prone type-B behaviour.

Psychological

Psychological views of PMS attribute it to an impoverishment of the ego in relation to feminine self-acceptance and identification with the mother. It is suggested that popular beliefs that derogate femininity are internalized and form part of the socialization of women.

Self-report of PMS is strongly related to psychosocial stress, particularly unusual stress and unhappy relationships.

MANAGEMENT

Treatment should be supportive and directed towards symptom relief, psychosocial support, stress reduction and dietary change. No single medication has proven effective in the treatment of PMS.

ANTIDEPRESSANTS   Favourable results are sometimes found particularly when a serotonergic antidepressant is used. Psychic, but not somatic, symptoms improve. A 70 per cent reduction in premenstrual irritability and depressed mood is found using clomipramine, compared to a 45 per cent reduction with placebo. Similar results have been obtained using fluoxetine, adding support to the hypothesis that a serotonergic imbalance is involved in premenstrual psychic symptoms.

ORAL CONTRACEPTIVE PILL   Somatic symptoms are improved but psychic symptoms are not. Oestrogenic effects are thought to exacerbate premenstrual irritability, and progestogenic effects exacerbate premenstrual depression.

Oral contraceptive users report significantly less menstrual pain and premenstrual breast tenderness than controls, but also show significantly less improvement in negative mood during the menstrual phase than non-users.

OTHER TREATMENTS USED FOR WHICH THERE ARE CONFLICTING REPORTS OF EFFICACY

- alprazolam: some reports of usefulness, but double-blind placebo-controlled trial showed absence of any therapeutic benefit
- hysterectomy: no change in cyclical mood changes following hysterectomy
- vitamin B6: produces a reduction in prolactin synthesis; use advocated, but little evidence of improvement in PMS symptoms
- progesterones: use advocated, but little evidence of improvement in PMS symptoms
- diuretics: produce some relief in symptoms of bloatedness, but no improvement in psychic symptoms
- bromocriptine: effective only in the relief of breast symptoms

Cyclic Psychosis

A few reports of cyclic psychoses related to menstruation exist in the literature. Psychotic symptoms appear suddenly a few days before menstruation, resolve with the onset of menstrual bleeding, and reappear with the next cycle. Between psychotic episodes the patient appears largely asymptomatic.

Most cases do not show familial psychiatric morbidity.

The psychiatric picture is non-specific, and changes with every menstruation. Some common features include psychomotor retardation, anxiety, perplexity, disorientation and amnestic features.

Transitory EEG abnormalities may occur, not amounting to epileptic activity.

The first psychotic episode usually occurs at a young age.

It has been suggested that in some cases menstrual psychoses should be regarded as a specific variant of PMS.

Recommended treatments for menstrual cyclic psychosis include:

- bromocriptine which reduces prolactin
- progesterone which inhibits ovulation

- clomiphene citrate
- acetazolamide, a diuretic
- psychotropic medications: results inconclusive

Prognosis is good, spontaneous remission is usual.

PREGNANCY

Miscarriage

Miscarriage occurs in 12–15 per cent of clinically recognized pregnancies. About one-half are associated with chromosomal abnormalities. Other recognized causes include uterine malformation, cervical incompetence, trauma, infection, endocrine disorder, toxins, irradiation and immune dysfunction.

Animal evidence shows that stress leads to abortion in a number of mammal species including baboons.

O'Hare and Creed (1995) studied the relationship between life events and miscarriage in 48 case-control pairs matched for known predictors of miscarriage. They found that the miscarriage group were more likely to have experienced:

- a severe life event in the three months preceding miscarriage
- a major social difficulty
- life events of severe short-term threat in the fortnight immediately beforehand

Fifty-four per cent of the miscarriage group had experienced some psychosocial stress, compared to only 15 per cent of controls.

Other factors significantly associated with miscarriage include childhood maternal separation, poor relationships with partners and few social contacts.

Stress-induced abortion may involve increased catecholamine levels and α-adrenergic stimulation of the myometrium. Serotonin, implicated in stress responses, promotes abortion. This may be mediated via reduced gonadotrophin output.

In the management of recurrent miscarriage a psychosocial history should be taken in order to ascertain any sources of stress amenable to social intervention.

CONSEQUENCES OF MISCARRIAGE   A high percentage of women experience profound loss following miscarriage, reporting symptoms typical of the grief that follows bereavement. Friedman and Gath (1989) found that at four weeks after miscarriage 48 per cent of women were psychiatric cases as measured on the PSE, all suffering depressive disorders. Many of the women were already recovering at this time.

Symptoms are increased in women who have experienced previous miscarriage. Many women are fearful of experiencing loss in a future pregnancy.

Other factors increasing women's vulnerability to developing depressive symptoms are lack of a supportive partner, childlessness, neuroticism and previous psychiatric consultation.

Psychiatric morbidity can persist for several months. Duration of bereavement reaction is appreciably shortened by support and counselling.

Termination of pregnancy

Psychological disturbance occurring in association with therapeutic abortion are severe or persistent in only a minority, about 10 per cent of women. Depression and anxiety are most common with psychosis reported very uncommonly, in 0.003 per cent of cases. Of the latter, most have a previous psychiatric history.

Women at greater risk of adverse psychological sequelae include:

- those with a previous psychiatric history
- younger women
- those with poor social support
- those from cultural groups opposed to abortion

About one-third of women experience feelings of loss, guilt and self-reproach at six months after abortion, particularly those ambivalent towards the termination of pregnancy. Those requiring therapeutic abortion because of foetal abnormalities or medical complications have poorer psychological outcomes.

Gilchrist *et al.* (1995) studied psychiatric morbidity following termination of pregnancy compared with other outcomes of unplanned pregnancy in a large prospective cohort study. They found:

- rates of total psychiatric disorder were no higher after termination of pregnancy than after childbirth
- women with a previous psychiatric history were most at risk of disorder after the end of their pregnancy, whatever its outcome
- women without a past history of psychosis had a lower risk of psychosis after termination than after childbirth
- in women without a past psychiatric history, deliberate self-harm was more common in those who were refused a termination (relative risk 2.9), or who had a termination (relative risk 1.7)
- no overall increase in psychiatric morbidity was found in those having a termination of pregnancy

Mental disorders in pregnancy

MINOR MENTAL ILLNESS   There is an increased risk of minor mental illness in the first trimester. This usually resolves spontaneously by the second trimester, therefore reassurance and psychological interventions are usually most appropriate.

Benzodiazepines should be avoided particularly in the first and third trimesters.

MAJOR MENTAL ILLNESS   New episodes in pregnancy are uncommon, but the risk in puerperium is much increased.

Women with established mental illness have no increased risk of episodes during pregnancy, but a substantially increased risk in puerperium.

It is always best to avoid drugs in pregnancy if possible. Stable patients may often be withdrawn from medication before conception. In those with great risks of relapse a judgement has to be made about the relative risk of relapse against the relative risk of taking medication.

Neuroleptics can be maintained at minimal doses during pregnancy if necessary. It is best to withdraw anticholinergics if possible since the risk of teratogenesis in humans is inconclusive.

Lithium is teratogenic and is contraindicated in pregnancy especially in the first and third trimesters. Women of child-bearing age started on lithium should be informed of its effects and the need to avoid pregnancy. Lithium should be withdrawn at least a month before conception and immediately if a woman is found to be pregnant.

PUERPERAL DISORDERS

There are associations between the puerperal mental conditions. Severe postnatal blues can progress to postnatal depression; there may also be an association between postnatal blues and puerperal psychosis, since there is an excess of onset of the latter towards the end of the first week post-partum.

ICD-10 does not categorize puerperal mental disorders separately unless they do not meet criteria for disorders classified elsewhere. Thus under the chapter *Behavioural syndromes associated with physiological disturbances and physical factors* is a section (F53) *Mental and behavioural disorders associated with the puerperium, not elsewhere classified* which includes mild, severe and other mental and behavioural disorders associated with the puerperium.

Postnatal blues

This is a brief psychological disturbance, characterized by tearfulness, emotional lability and confusion in mothers occurring in the first few days after childbirth.

EPIDEMIOLOGY   It occurs in about 50 per cent of women, peaking at the third to fifth day post-partum.

AETIOLOGY   There is some evidence of links with biological factors including:

- a history of premenstrual tension
- serum calcium levels
- monoamines, serum tryptophan, platelet α_2-adrenoceptors
- progesterone withdrawal post delivery: women experiencing severe blues have higher antenatal progesterone levels, a steeper rise in the last two weeks of pregnancy, a bigger decrement from antenatal levels to the day of peak blues score, and lower progesterone levels on the day of peak blues

Postnatal blues have also been positively associated with:

- poor social adjustment
- poor marital relationship
- high scores on EPI neuroticism scale
- fear of labour
- anxious and depressed mood during pregnancy

There is no association between the development of postnatal blues and life events, demographic and social factors or obstetric factors.

Postnatal women differ significantly from women undergoing elective gynaecological surgery in the frequencies of different symptoms at different times, suggesting that postnatal mood swings are characteristic of the puerperium and are not simply non-specific reactions to stress.

MANAGEMENT   Reassurance.

Postnatal depression

This is a depressive illness not qualitatively different from non-psychotic depression in other settings. It is characterized by low mood, reduced self-esteem, tearfulness, anxiety, particularly about the baby's health, and an inability to cope. Mothers may experience reduced affection for their baby, and may have difficulty breast-feeding.

EPIDEMIOLOGY   Occurs in 10–15 per cent of post-partum women usually within three months of childbirth. Those women who are emotionally unstable in the first week after childbirth are at an increased risk of developing postnatal depression.

Postnatal depression is not associated with social class or parity.

AETIOLOGY

ENVIRONMENTAL   Of the puerperal psychiatric conditions, postnatal depression has the least biological cause. Onset after childbirth is spread over a few months, and studies have repeatedly indicated the importance of social stress in its causation.

Paykel *et al.* (1980) found the strongest associated factor in mild post-partum depressives was the occurrence of recent stressful life events. Younger age, poor marital relationships and absent social supports were also notable. Early post-partum blues was associated with postnatal depression in the absence of life events suggesting a small subgroup of postnatal depression with a hormonal aetiology. A past psychiatric history was a strong risk factor with or without life events.

Murray *et al.* (1995) found that postnatal depression, but not control depression, was associated with a poor relationship with the woman's own mother.

Postnatal depression is more contingent upon the acute biopsychosocial stresses caused by the arrival of a child, whereas depression not associated with childbirth is more closely related to longer-term social adversity and deprivation.

HORMONAL   Despite the modest association between progesterone levels and post-partum blues, no direct association has been demonstrated between progesterone levels and postnatal depression.

Oestrogens affect dopaminergic transmission in the CNS; their precipitate drop after delivery may be responsible for psychosis, and possibly also depression in predisposed women.

Puerperal women, whether depressed or not, are non-suppressers in terms of the dexamethasone-suppression test. However, no associations have been found between postnatal depression and cortisol.

Transient hypothyroidism, sometimes preceded by hyperthyroidism, occurs in up to 5 per cent of women in the post-partum year, peaking at four to five months. Such post-partum thyroid dysfunction is associated with depression. It is estimated that 1 per cent of post-partum women in the general population will experience a depressive episode associated with thyroid dysfunction.

Management

The education of health visitors and midwives is necessary to identify cases early. The Edinburgh Postnatal Depression Scale is a 10-item self-report questionnaire, used by health visitors to identify postnatal depression during the course of their normal contacts with new mothers.

Non-directive counselling by health visitors individually or in groups is effective in one-third of cases. Self-help groups and mother-and-baby groups are useful to combat isolation.

In those with more severe symptomatology, or those non-responsive to counselling, antidepressants are required.

If depression is severe, admission, preferably with the baby to a mother-and-baby unit may be required. Suicidal mothers may have thoughts of taking their babies with them, so questions about the safety of the child should form part of the normal assessment of mothers of young children. ECT may be required, particularly if worthlessness, hopelessness and despair are present.

Breast-feeding should not be routinely suspended. Tricyclic antidepressants are transmitted in reduced quantities in breast milk. They are, however, safe. Lithium is transmitted and should not be given to a breast-feeding mother because of the risk of toxicity to the child.

Outcome

If undetected, postnatal depression may last up to two years with serious consequences for the marital relationship and the development of the child. There is good evidence for a link between depressive disorders in mothers and emotional disturbance in their children.

The following are more frequent in the children of mothers suffering postnatal depression:

- insecure attachment
- behaviour problems
- difficulties in expressive language
- fewer positive, and more negative facial expressions
- mild cognitive abnormalities
- less affective sharing
- less initial sociability.

Social and marital difficulties are often associated with reduced quality of mother–child interaction.

The relapse rate for subsequent non-psychotic depression is 1 in 6.

Cooper and Murray (1995) distinguished between those whose postnatal depression was a recurrence of previous affective disturbance, and those for whom postnatal depression had arisen *de novo*. Those who were suffering from a recurrence of depression were at raised risk of further non-post-partum episodes but not post-partum episodes. Those for whom the depression had arisen *de novo* were at raised risk for further episodes of postnatal depression but not for non-post-partum episodes.

Puerperal psychosis

The risk of developing a psychotic illness is increased twenty-fold in the first post-partum month.

Certain symptoms that are distinctive are:

- abrupt onset, within the first two weeks of childbirth
- marked perplexity, but no detectable cognitive impairment
- rapid fluctuations in mental state, sometimes from hour to hour
- marked restlessness, fear and insomnia
- delusions, hallucinations and disturbed behaviour develop rapidly

EPIDEMIOLOGY   Kendell *et al.* (1987) linked psychiatric and obstetric registers in Edinburgh and found the number of admissions for psychotic disorders to be substantially elevated in the puerperium:

Table 30.1 Number of admissions to mental hospitals per month in the pre- and post-partum periods

	Non-psychotic	Psychotic
15 months preconception	8	2
During pregnancy	5	2
1st post-partum month	17	51
2nd post-partum month	14	25
3rd post-partum month	10	13
4th post-partum month	8	9
5th post-partum month	6	6
Mean for next 18 months	9	4

Eighty per cent of puerperal psychoses are affective. Schizophreniform psychoses often have manic features. Those with a previous history of manic depressive illness have a substantially higher risk than those with a history of schizophrenia or depression.

The following factors are associated with women developing puerperal psychoses:

- increased rate of Caesarean section
- higher social class
- older age at birth of first child
- primiparae

Psychosis following childbirth is usually of an affective type with a particularly high proportion of manic episodes within the first two weeks.

Puerperal psychoses follow 20–30 per cent of births in those with pre-existing bipolar mood disorders.

AETIOLOGY

GENETIC   Family studies of puerperal psychosis point to a familial aggregation of psychiatric disorder, particularly affective illness.

Children of probands who have had puerperal psychosis have an increased psychiatric morbidity.

Female relatives of puerperal probands have a higher rate of puerperal illness than the general population, but the majority of illness in the relatives of probands is non-puerperal.

The weight of evidence from clinical and family studies suggests that most cases of puerperal psychosis of early onset are closely related to bipolar disorder.

ENVIRONMENTAL   There is no evidence of any excess of life events in puerperal psychotics compared to matched normal puerperal controls. The absence of social stress in this group contrasts with the findings for post-partum depression and disorders with onset in pregnancy. These findings suggest that the aetiology of severe puerperal psychosis is predominantly biological and interactive with previous vulnerability.

HORMONAL   The pathophysiology of puerperal psychosis is not well understood but it is likely that the precipitous fall in the levels of circulating sex steroid hormones such as oestrogen occurring at the time of parturition play an important role.

In animals the administration of oestrogen leads to increased striatal dopamine binding, and oestrogen withdrawal leads to dopamine receptor supersensitivity.

Wieck et al. (1991) have reported increased sensitivity of dopamine receptors in the hypothalamus associated with the onset of affective psychosis following childbirth. It is possible that these changes in sensitivity are mediated by changes in circulating oestrogen levels.

Supersensitivity of dopamine receptors is then thought to precipitate psychosis.

Management

The identification of high-risk patients during pregnancy is important in the planning of postnatal management.

Admission to a psychiatric hospital is usually essential.

It is usually preferable to admit mothers with their babies.

ADVANTAGES OF JOINT ADMISSION   Most psychotic mothers are capable of looking after their babies with supervision and support.

There is evidence suggesting that joint admission may reduce the duration of illness and relapse rates.

DISADVANTAGES OF JOINT ADMISSION   The risk of non-accidental injury to the child from the mother or fellow patients. A nurse should be dedicated to the care and supervision of the child and a lockable nursery should be provided.

Joint admission needs higher staffing levels.

The long-term effects of admission upon the development of the child are not known.

The woman's partner needs support and education.

Phenothiazines and lithium are effective in the treatment of manic episodes. Control of lithium levels in the immediate post-partum period can be difficult because of fluid and electrolyte changes.

ECT is particularly effective in the treatment of puerperal psychoses, and accelerates recovery in all diagnostic categories. Generally used if the drug treatment has failed.

In breast-feeding mothers lithium is contraindicated because it is excreted into breast milk and is toxic to the baby.

Neuroleptics can be administered to breast-feeding mothers, but high doses should be avoided and the baby should be observed for signs of drowsiness, such as a failure to feed adequately.

Neuroleptics should be maintained for at least three months following recovery. If there are further manic or depressive episodes, lithium should be considered.

Following discharge from hospital the mother will require close support and follow-up. An assessment of the mother–baby interaction should be made prior to discharge.

Outcome

The initial prognosis is quite good. Cases often settle within six weeks, and most are fully recovered by six months. A few, however, have a protracted course.

After one episode of puerperal psychosis the risk of a further episode in each subsequent pregnancy is between one in three and one in five. For those with a previous psychiatric history or a family history the risk is higher; for those whose puerperal episode was associated with life events or Caesarean section the subsequent risk is lower.

MENOPAUSE

General population surveys indicate no major effect of the menopause on a variety of common psychiatric symptoms. If anything, women in the post-menopausal years show less evidence of psychiatric disturbance than younger women. Anxiety and depression in post-menopausal women do not respond to oestrogen therapy, but may respond to antidepressants. Where sexual symptoms are present hormone replacement therapy may be effective. There is some evidence that hormone replacement therapy ameliorates psychological symptoms after surgical menopause.

BIBLIOGRAPHY

Ashby, C.R., Carr, L.A., Cook, C.L. *et al.* 1992: Inhibition of serotonin uptake in rat brain synaptosomes by plasma from patients with pre-menstrual syndrome. *Biological Psychiatry* 31, 1169–71.

Ballinger, C.B. 1990: Psychiatric aspects of the menopause. *British Journal of Psychiatry* 156, 773–87.

Bancroft, J. and Rennie, D. 1993: The impact of oral contraceptives on the experience of premenstrual mood, clumsiness, food craving and other symptoms. *Journal of Psychosomatic Research* 37, 195–202.

Condon, J.T. 1993: The pre-menstrual syndrome: a twin study. *British Journal of Psychiatry* 162, 481–6.

Cooper, P.J. and Murray, L. 1995: Course and recurrence of postnatal depression. Evidence for the specificity of the diagnostic concept. *British Journal of Psychiatry* 166, 191–5.

Craddock, N., Brockington, I., Mant, R. *et al.* 1994: Bipolar affective puerperal psychosis associated with consanguinity. *British Journal of Psychiatry* 164, 359–64.

Dowlatshahi, D. and Paykel, E.S. 1990: Life events and social stress in puerperal psychoses: absence of effect. *Psychological Medicine* 20, 655–62.

Eriksson, E., Sundblad, C., Lisjo, P. *et al.* 1992: Serum levels of androgens are higher in women with pre-menstrual irritability and dysphoria than in controls. *Psychoneuroendocrinology* 17, 195–204.

Friedman, T. and Gath, D. 1989: The psychiatric consequences of spontaneous abortion. *British Journal of Psychiatry* 155, 810–13.

Giannini, A.J., Melemis, S.M., Martin, D.M. *et al* 1994: Symptoms of pre-menstrual syndrome as a function of beta-endorphin: two subtypes. *Progress in Neuropsychopharmacology and Biological Psychiatry* 18, 321–7.

Gilchrist, A.C., Hannaford, P.C., Frank, P. *et al.* 1995: Termination of pregnancy and psychiatric morbidity. *British Journal of Psychiatry* 167, 243–8.

Hannah, P., Adams, D., Lee, A. *et al.* 1992: Links between early post-partum mood and post-natal depression. *British Journal of Psychiatry* 160, 777–80.

Harris, B. 1994: Biological and hormonal aspects of postpartum depressed mood. Working towards strategies for prophylaxis and treatment. *British Journal of Psychiatry* 164, 288–92.

Hicks, R.A., Olsen, C. and Smith Robinson, D. 1986: Type A-B behaviour and the premenstrual syndrome. *Psychological Reports* 59, 353–4.

Iles, S., Gath, D. and Kennerley, H. 1989: Maternity blues II. A comparison between post-operative women and post-natal women. *British Journal of Psychiatry* 155, 363–6.

Kantero, R. and Widholm, O. 1971: Correlations of menstrual traits between adolescent girls and their mothers. *Acta Obstetrica and Gynecologica Scandinavica* 14 (suppl. 14), 30–36.

Kendell, R.E., Chalmers, J.C. and Platz, C.L. 1987: Epidemiology of puerperal psychoses. *British Journal of Psychiatry* 150, 662–73.

Kennerley, H. and Gath, D. 1989: Maternity blues III. Associations with obstetric psychological and psychiatric factors. *British Journal of Psychiatry* 155, 367–73.

Logue, C.M. and Moos, R.H. 1986: Pre-menstrual symptoms: prevalence and risk factors. *Psychosomatic Medicine* 48, 388–414.

Murray, D., Cox, J.L. Chapman, G. *et al.* 1995: Childbirth: life event or start of a long term difficulty? Further data from the Stoke-on-Trent controlled study of postnatal depression. *British Journal of Psychiatry* 166, 595–600.

O'Hare, T. and Creed, F. 1995: Life events and miscarriage. *British Journal of Psychiatry* 167, 799–805.

Paykel, E.S., Emms, E.M., Fletcher, J. *et al.* 1980: Life events and social supports in puerperal depression. *British Journal of Psychiatry* 136, 339–46.

Pearce, J., Hawton, K. and Blake, F. 1995: Psychological and sexual symptoms associated with the menopause and the effects of hormone replacement therapy. *British Journal of Psychiatry* 167, 163–73.

Schmidt, P., Grover, G.N. and Rubinow, D.R. 1993: Alprazolam in the treatment of pre-menstrual syndrome: a double-blind placebo-controlled trial. *Archives of General Psychiatry* 50, 467–73.

Stein, A., Gath, D.H., Bucher, J. *et al.* 1991: The relationship between post-natal depression and mother-child interaction. *British Journal of Psychiatry* 158, 46–52.

Stein, D., Hanukoglu, S., Blank, S. *et al.* 1993: Cyclic psychosis associated with the menstrual cycle. *British Journal of Psychiatry* 163, 824–8.

Sundblad, C., Hedberg, M.A. and Eriksson, E. 1993: Clomipramine administered during the luteal phase reduces the symptoms of pre-menstrual syndrome: a placebo controlled trial. *Neuropsychopharmacology* 9, 133–45.

Warner, P. and Bancroft, J. 1990: Factors related to self-reporting of the pre-menstrual syndrome. *British Journal of Psychiatry* 157, 249–60.

Wieck, A., Kumar, R., Hirst, A.D. *et al.* 1991: Increased sensitivity of dopamine receptors and recurrence of affective psychosis after childbirth. *British Medical Journal* 303: 613–16.

Zolese, G. and Blacker, C.V.R. 1992: The psychological complications of therapeutic abortion. *British Journal of Psychiatry* 160, 742–9.

31
Sexual disorders

HISTORY

Havelock Ellis (1910)	British pioneer, the first to subject normal as well as pathological sexuality to scientific investigation.
Kinsey *et al.* (1948, 1953)	Conducted landmark research into human sexual experience in thousands of men and women. A wide range of human sexual expression was noted. Methodological problems included non-random sampling. Volunteers were recruited from a variety of sources, with a non-representative excess of college-educated people. Criminals and sex offenders were also over-represented. Despite these shortcomings, their findings have been generalized to the wider population and remained authoritative for decades in the absence of methodologically superior work.
1981	AIDS was first described in the USA. It was initially believed to be confined to a small group of promiscuous homosexual men. Subsequently a primarily heterosexual worldwide epidemic of major proportions has developed.

British sexual behaviour and attitudes in the 1990s

A major survey of British sexual attitudes and lifestyle (Johnson *et al.* 1994) has provided the most comprehensive evaluation of sexual behaviour in the British public to date. It was motivated largely by the emergence in 1980s of the lethal epidemic of sexually transmitted infection, HIV, and the lack of baseline measures of sexual behaviour. 18 876 British men and women in a random population sample aged 16–59 participated.

The following statistics were among many that emerged:

FIRST HETEROSEXUAL INTERCOURSE

- Age at occurrence is decreasing over time. In the past four decades the median age of first heterosexual intercourse has fallen from 21 to 17 for women, and 20 to 17 for men
- Proportion occurring before age 16 has increased over time. Fewer than 1 per cent of women aged 55 or over report heterosexual intercourse before the age of 16, compared to one in 5 of those in their teens
- Convergence in behaviour of men and women over time
- People today are more likely to use contraception (usually condoms) than those of a previous generation
- The earlier first intercourse occurs, the less likely it is that contraception is used

- Early intercourse is associated with lower social class and lower educational level
- Now there is more planning and less spontaneity than formerly
- Majority of intercourse occurs within established relationship.
- Young women initiated by older male partner; men's first partners tend to be age peers
- Very rare for men's first sexual intercourse to be with a prostitute

HETEROSEXUAL PARTNERSHIPS

- Age and marital status are associated with multiple partnerships. The young and those previously married or single (including cohabitees) are most likely to report high partner numbers
- Increasing partner change with increasing social class
- Increasing numbers of partners over historical time
- Proportion reporting multiple partnerships in the last five years declines with increasing age
- Serial monogamy is more common in those aged 16–24, concurrent partnerships are more common in those over the age of 35
- Sex with a prostitute in the last five years is most common in the 25–34 year age group
- Raised odds of ever using prostitute associated with age, previous marriage or current cohabitation, working away from home and a history of having a homosexual partner

HETEROSEXUAL PRACTICES

- Frequency of heterosexual sex (oral, vaginal or anal intercourse) shows wide variability with a small proportion of the population reporting a very high frequency of sexual contact
- Age closely related to number of acts, frequency peaking in mid-twenties, then gradually declining
- Frequency affected by partner availability; highest in married and cohabiting groups of all ages
- Strong association in all age groups between length of relationship and frequency of sex. Much lower frequency in longer relationships
- Vaginal intercourse predominates. Seventy-five per cent have experience of non-penetrative sex and 70 per cent have some experience of oral sex. Any experience of anal intercourse is reported by 14 per cent of men and 13 per cent of women
- Increase in practice of oral sex, but not as a substitute to vaginal intercourse
- Those not married have a wider repertoire of sexual practice. Prevalence of oral, anal and non-penetrative sex increases with increasing numbers of partners
- Those outside married or cohabiting relationships have less frequent sex overall, but are more likely to have multiple partners, a wider range of practices and recent experience of high-risk practices

SEXUAL DIVERSITY AND HOMOSEXUAL BEHAVIOUR

- No sexual attraction or experience of any kind is reported by 0.4 per cent of men and 0.5 per cent of women
- Exclusively heterosexual attraction and experience is reported by 90 per cent of men and 92 per cent of women

- Mostly or exclusively homosexual attraction and experience is reported by 1 per cent of men and 0.25 per cent of women
- Some form of homosexual experience is reported by 6 per cent of men and 3 per cent of women
- Lifetime experience of homosexual orientation is higher in higher social classes
- Recent homosexual experience is strongly associated with region. Greater London has more than twice the proportion of men reporting homosexual experience and current practice than anywhere else in Britain
- Those who had a boarding-school education are more likely to report any homosexual contact; this has little or no effect on homosexual practice in later life
- Exclusively homosexual behaviour is rare. The majority of those with homosexual experience have had sex with both men and women. Ninety per cent of men and 95 per cent of women reporting same gender sexual partners in their lifetime have also had an opposite gender partner
- Men reporting anal sex do so usually (60 per cent) as both the receptive and insertive partner
- Highest levels of homosexual activity reported by 25–34-year-olds, nearly a decade later than heterosexual partnerships, consistent with later age at first experience

SEXUAL ATTITUDES

- Acceptance of premarital sex is now nearly universal, as is its practice
- Disapproval of infidelity extends to all age groups, the young being marginally more tolerant than older people
- The British public show widespread condemnation of homosexual relationships. Women are more tolerant than men
- Sex is not considered the most important part of a relationship; a monogamous relationship is considered more likely to lead to greater sexual satisfaction

PHYSICAL HEALTH

- Multiple sexual partnerships are significantly associated with smoking and increasing levels of alcohol consumption
- Attendance at an STD clinic is strongly associated with the number of heterosexual partners and a history of homosexual partnership
- No relationship is detected between the numbers of heterosexual partners and experience of infertility or miscarriage
- Likelihood of termination of pregnancy increases markedly with the numbers of heterosexual partners
- Survey findings confirm a strong relationship between sexual behaviour and the probability of STD clinic attendance, abortion and HIV testing

PERCEIVED RISK

- Less than 10 per cent of the British public is at risk of unplanned pregnancy
- The use of oral contraception declines steeply with age; condom use is most prevalent in the young; sterilization increases with age
- The message to use condoms to prevent the risks of STD has been more acceptable than the message to restrict numbers of partners
- The perceived risk of HIV infection is higher among those reporting higher risk behaviours

- Despite the uptake of messages about condom use, there is little sign of the widespread adoption of other safer sex practices among those reporting heterosexual behaviour.

SEXUAL DYSFUNCTION

The individual is unable to participate in a sexual relationship as they would wish. Both psychological and somatic processes are usually involved in the causation of sexual dysfunction. Women present more commonly with complaints about the subjective quality of sexual experience; men present with a failure of specific sexual response.

ICD-10
Categorizes **Sexual dysfunction not caused by organic disorder or disease under Behavioural syndromes associated with physiological disturbances and physical factors** as follows:

LACK OR LOSS OF SEXUAL DESIRE   Not secondary to other sexual difficulties. Does not preclude sexual enjoyment or arousal, but makes initiation of sexual activity less likely.

SEXUAL AVERSION   Sexual interaction associated with strong negative feelings of sufficient intensity that sexual activity is avoided.

LACK OF SEXUAL ENJOYMENT   Sexual responses and orgasm occur normally but there is a lack of pleasure. Much more common in women.

FAILURE OF GENITAL RESPONSE   In men primarily erectile dysfunction.
   In women primarily vaginal dryness.

ORGASMIC DYSFUNCTION   Orgasm does not occur or is delayed. More common in women than men.

PREMATURE EJACULATION   The inability to control ejaculation sufficiently for both partners to enjoy sex.

NON-ORGANIC VAGINISMUS   Occlusion of the vaginal opening caused by spasm of the surrounding muscles. Penile entry is either impossible or painful.

NON-ORGANIC DYSPAREUNIA   Pain during intercourse may occur in both sexes. Only used if organic cause is not present, and if there is no other primary sexual dysfunction.

EXCESSIVE SEXUAL DRIVE   Usually occurs in men or women during late teenage or early adult years. If secondary to mental illness (e.g. mania) the underlying disorder is coded.

Sexual response cycle

- desire
- arousal, mediated by parasympathetic nervous system
- plateau
- orgasm, mediated by sympathetic and central nervous system
- resolution, longer in male and increases with age

Sensate Focus: Masters and Johnson (1970)
Behavioural psychotherapy involving the couple in graded assignments which may be modified according to the particular problem presenting. Used extensively in the treatment of sexual disorders affecting both men and women. A combination of specified homework tasks together with setting specific limits to the extent of sexual contact allowed.

STAGE ONE   Touching partner without genital contact for subject's own pleasure.
STAGE TWO   Touching partner without genital contact for subject's and partner's pleasure.
STAGE THREE   Touching partner with genital contact, but intercourse not permitted.
STAGE FOUR   Simultaneous touching of partner and being touched by partner with genital contact, but intercourse not permitted.
STAGE FIVE   If both feel ready, the female invites the male to put his penis into her vagina. Female on top position heightens female control and allows male to relax. No thrusting. Initial containment brief, lengthening period of containment with each session.
STAGE SIX   Vaginal containment with movement. Different positions are encouraged. Does not inevitably lead to climax. Couple practice stopping before climax. Provided physical contact is pleasurable orgasm is not necessary.

Erectile dysfunction

Erection is a neurovascular phenomenon requiring intact arterial supply and intact venous valves, allowing cavernosal pressures to rise to those approaching systolic blood pressures. Vascular changes brought about by the parasympathetic autonomic nervous system (S2, 3, 4) influenced by tactile stimuli and central limbic and cognitive mechanisms. Psychic erections are mediated by thoracic sympathetic outflow, whereas reflex erections result from sacral parasympathetic outflow. Androgens also influence erection, particularly those occurring in sleep, via the limbic system.

EPIDEMIOLOGY   Studies with community samples indicate the prevalence of male erectile disorder of 4–9 per cent.

Comprises about 50 per cent of male cases presenting to psychosexual disorders service. Incidence rises with age, from about 1.3 per cent at 35 years, to 55 per cent at 75 years.

AETIOLOGY   Organic (in about 50 per cent), psychological or a combination.
ORGANIC
Local

- Peyronie's disease. Progressive fibrosis in tunica albuginea and sometimes also in cavernosa, resulting in curvature of the penis on erection. Cause unknown
- Congenital deformities e.g. hypospadias and epispadias, absence of suspensory ligaments
- Priapism, although rare, may result in impotence if not treated adequately within 24 hours

Endocrine

- Diabetes causes a combination of arteriopathy and neuropathy. Two-thirds of diabetic males have erectile impotence. Of these it is complete in two-thirds and partial in the remaining third. A few also complain of other difficulties such as premature ejaculation. Onset insidious, course progressive with marked decline in sexual activity and desire
- Hypogonadism. Nocturnal erections are androgen dependent. Studies are conflicting on the role of androgens in erectile disorders. Effects are probably mediated through lowered sexual interest
- Hyperprolactinaemia secondary to hypothalamic/pituitary disease, those on phenothiazines, sometimes in alcoholics
- Endorphins. Naltrexone therapy significantly improves impotence in males

with apparent non-organic cause. Alteration in central opioid tone may be responsible

Neurological

- Peripheral or autonomic neuropathy e.g. diabetes, alcoholism
- Radical pelvic surgery causing autonomic neurological disruption
- Spinal cord lesion e.g. transection, multiple sclerosis.

Vascular

- Arterial disease interfering with blood supply to pelvic organs
- Incompetent venous valves

Pharmacological

- **Alcohol** has complex effects, including neuropathy and indirect effects on sex steroids and gonadotrophins. Oestrogen levels are raised causing gynacomastia and testicular atrophy in advanced liver disease. Raised blood alcohol levels inhibit sexual responses through central inhibitory effects. Psychosocial factors are also prominent in these patients
- **Antihypertensives** Ganglion blockers interfere with both sympathetic and parasympathetic postganglionic transmission and cause both impotence and ejaculatory failure. Propranolol crosses blood-brain barrier and may exert its effect centrally. Alpha adrenergic blockers are not associated with erectile failure, but cause ejaculatory failure

PSYCHOLOGICAL   Classical history suggestive of psychological cause comprises lack of sexual interest, but continued morning erections.

PSYCHOANALYTIC CONCEPTS   Sexual physiological changes result from the interplay between conscious and unconscious thoughts and feelings, and interpersonal relationships. Anxiety and fear, whether conscious or unconscious, can interfere with vascular changes required for erection. Arousal phase disorders of erectile dysfunction in men are common. Interference with abandonment to erotic feelings can impair arousal in men and lead to difficulties with erection.

Psychoanalytic formulations of erectile disorders recognize anxiety about the persecutory object and unresolved Oedipal conflicts. Deep ambivalence about intimate involvement leading to fear of sexual failure are common.

In younger men with primary impotence Oedipal conflicts are said to predominate, whereas in secondary impotence, neurotic partnership conflicts at a pre-Oedipal level, and narcissistic crises in middle age are said to predominate.

COGNITIVE CONCEPTS   Erectile disorder is considered to be a sign of negative self-image within a depressive view of the relationship, and is linked to abandonment fear.

Subjects with psychogenic erectile impotence have a situational sexual disorder in which sexual anxiety plays an important role. Compared to those with organic impotence or to controls they view themselves as more insecure and tend to over-idealize their partners and their mothers.

Consider also fear of hurting female; fear of pregnancy; distaste for female genitalia; placing partner on a pedestal; non-sexual stress; unsympathetic or angry partner; trying too hard.

Management

ASSESSMENT

- Full history including the nature of the problem, detailed sexual history, medical and psychiatric histories, medication and substance use
- Assessment of couples' relationship is essential. Difficulties such as hostility, lack of communication, unresponsive or unerotic partner may be important
- Physical examination including external genitalia; laboratory investigations including blood glucose, tests of renal and hepatic function
- Penile-brachial artery pressure index of less than 0.6 is indicative of arterial disease to penis. Angiography may be necessary, especially in younger patients
- Nocturnal penile tumescence monitoring used to measure circumference change in sleep erections. This can help distinguish organic from psychogenic cause; if cause is organic, erections at night are abolished
- Dynamic cavernometry in which normal saline is infused into corpus cavernosum may detect venous incompetence
- Intracorporeal injection of papaverine or phentolamine can be diagnostic to establish the capacity for erection and hence reduce the likelihood of a primarily arterial cause

TREATMENT

Physical   Physical treatments are increasingly available which are efficacious for both physical and psychogenically induced erectile dysfunction. As a result the distinction is not always sought. Emotionally intensive sex therapy is often not considered, especially if it is managed by surgeons.

INTRA-CAVERNOSAL INJECTION OF VASOACTIVE DRUGS   Papaverine is commonly used to treat impotence. Self-injected, it gives an erection lasting about an hour, and may be used up to twice a week. Half those presenting to a sexual dysfunction clinic benefit from intracorporeal papaverine. Many decline the treatment because of the perception that injection is cumbersome and interrupts sexual foreplay, or because of objection to the use of needles. Intracorporeal pharmacotherapy provides a useful treatment option in the management of impotence but it is limited by the method of administration.

Complications include priapism which should be treated promptly by the withdrawal of 20–60 ml of blood and injection of an alpha adrenergic agent such as phenylephrine 1–5 mg, or metaraminol 2 mg. Fibrosis is associated with prolonged use and rises in proportion to the total numbers of injections given. Haematomas and bruising are relatively common but of little significance.

Alpha-adrenergic blocking agents phenoxybenzamine or phentolamine may also be used to give more prolonged erection.

SUCTION DEVICES   Vacuum tumescence constriction therapy is efficacious and useful in those with organic as well as psychogenic impotence. These devices provide a safe method of obtaining an erection adequate for penetration in up to 90 per cent of patients. Many couples derive substantial benefit from their use, but the disadvantages of a not fully rigid erection, lack of spontaneity, decreased sensation and delayed or absent ejaculation in some limit their acceptability.

VASCULAR SURGERY   Correction of venous leak may be successful if specific leak is detected. Arterial surgery is less successful. Large vessel reconstruction for proximal arterial obstruction generally give poor results, as most patients also have distal arterial disease.

PENILE PROSTHETIC IMPLANTS   Surgically implanted penile prostheses are inserted into the corpus cavernosa. Three types are available: malleable, constructed of silastic with a malleable metal core giving permanent rigidity; self-contained inflatable; and multipart inflatable prostheses.

The psychological outcome of penile prosthesis implantation appears to be mediated by the nature of the marital relationship. Follow-up of recipients of penile implants 2.5 years following surgery found that those with organogenic impotence had no adverse sequelae, but some of those with psychogenic impotence had an exacerbation of pre-existing relationship difficulties. Ideally couple therapy should be offered as well as mechanical treatments, especially in those with psychogenic cause.

Psychological

COUNSELLING   Practical advice about sexual technique is essential for all forms of treatment, even if the main treatment is physical.

PSYCHOTHERAPY   Cognitive behavioural methods report success rates of 70 per cent for erectile impotence. Couple therapy appears to be superior to surrogate or individual therapies. Factors associated with successful outcome include the state of the marriage, better pre-treatment communication, better general sexual adjustment, female partners interest and enjoyment of sex, absence of psychiatric history in female partner and early engagement in homework assignments.

Sensate focus therapy may need to be combined with other methods, such as improvement in communication skills. Once erections are starting to occur a form of 'paradoxical intent' may be used, in which the couple is instructed to get rid of the erection as soon as it occurs, and then to resume touching. The purpose is to demonstrate that erections do not need to be used as soon as they arise.

Psychodynamic therapists challenge disturbing fantasies, and prevent their re-enactment. The patient is offered a psychotherapeutic 'holding' to counteract the unsafe internal world. Gradually he becomes freed from his sexually disempowering psychic reality to respond to the external reality of erotic stimulation. Behavioural interventions may also be incorporated into the treatment.

Premature ejaculation

Orgasm, seminal emission and ejaculation are physiologically distinct processes, and are potentially separable.

Ejaculation is the forceful expulsion of semen from the urethra. If semen is released from the urethra without force it is emission. Before orgasm the male becomes aware that ejaculation is imminent and it follows within 1–3 seconds, 'ejaculatory inevitability'. Ejaculation and emission are mediated by the alpha-adrenergic sympathetic nervous system. Androgens have a role, since the first sexual consequence of castration is the inability to ejaculate, which is rapidly restored with androgen replacement.

In severe premature ejaculation, emission alone may occur with no ejaculatory component, minimal or absent orgasm and a long refractory period.

In youth males have a tendency to ejaculate quickly. This usually diminishes with increasing age bacause of increasing control with experience, an ability to recognize the approach of ejaculatory inevitability, the dampening in responsiveness with age and the lessening of novelty which arises in a stable relationship.

Epidemiology

Studies with community samples indicate the prevalence of 36–38 per cent for premature ejaculation. Thirteen per cent of attendees at a sexual disorders' clinic present primarily with this problem.

Aetiology

PSYCHOLOGICAL   Anxiety promotes emission but inhibits orgasm, and thus plays a crucial role in premature ejaculation.

Primary premature ejaculation is always present. Secondary premature ejaculation develops after a period of satisfactory sexual functioning.

Those with primary premature ejaculation are more impaired in sexual functioning, and are more anxious. Those with secondary premature ejaculation are more likely to have coexisting erectile disorder, a reduction in sex drive and a reduction in arousal.

In psychological terms whereas erectile disorder seems to belong to a depressive organization, premature ejaculation belongs to a phobic one.

LEARNING   A variety of psychological factors may interfere with the learning process, impairing the ability to identify the point of impending ejaculation.

PHYSICAL   There are few physical causes. Drugs do not cause premature ejaculation. It is possible that the autonomic control of ejaculation is very sensitive and therefore more difficult to control in some individuals.

Those with premature ejaculation do not have penile hypersensitivity compared to controls.

No differences in the pituitary gonadal system are found between those with erectile impotence, premature ejaculation and normal controls.

Management

Education in ejaculatory control using the 'pause' technique is the treatment of choice. During Sensate Focus exercises, the male, when he predicts that he will ejaculate shortly, asks his partner to stop, allow his arousal level to subside slightly and then return to being caressed, repeating the process again when arousal increases.

If difficulty is experienced using this method, then the 'squeeze technique' is used. Just before ejaculation becomes inevitable, stimulation is stopped and the tip of the penis is grasped firmly for about 10 seconds, reducing the reflex ejaculatory response.

At therapeutic doses some antidepressants (e.g. fluoxetine) have a beneficial effect in men with premature ejaculation.

Anorgasmia

The final stage of sexual excitement may be orgasm. In both sexes if no orgasm occurs, there is a slow resolution of physical and psychological changes associated with sexual excitement. Apart from ejaculation for which there is no female counterpart, the correlates of orgasm are similar in the sexes. Heart rate and blood pressure increase, there is a sudden increase in skeletal muscle activity involving almost all parts of the body. Rhythmic muscle contractions in the male genital tract expel semen; in females there is transient rhythmical contraction of the uterus and vagina. Psychologically there is an instant sense of relief; at its most extreme there can be a virtual loss of consciousness, and relaxation ensues.

The exact mechanism of orgasm not known. In addition to local spinal mechanisms, the central nervous activity is also involved. EEG recordings during intense orgasm show changes which have been likened to those occurring during epileptic fits.

Epidemiology

Prevalence in community samples of 5–10 per cent for inhibited female orgasm, and 4–10 per cent for inhibited male orgasm. Among attendees at a sexual disorders' clinic, 5 per cent of males and 7 per cent of females present primarily with orgasmic dysfunction. In females the prevalence of anorgasmia reduces with increasing age.

Aetiology
Little is known.

PHYSICAL   In primary complete anorgasmia in both sexes, the bulbocavernosus reflex has been reported to be absent in a proportion; this is strongly correlated with the failure of treatment.

Sometimes local pain, possibly secondary to muscle spasm, or in local viscera (uterus, rectum) can create fear of orgasm.

Opiates appear to have a direct inhibitory effect, and antiserotonergic drugs inhibit orgasm.

Female anorgasmia has been reported in association with tricyclic, MAOI, and SSRI antidepressants, and neuroleptic drugs.

PSYCHOLOGICAL   Usually psychological.

Anxiety inhibits orgasm in women but can hasten emission in men. Sex may be viewed as bad, disgusting or threatening the need to remain in control at all times. There may be a fear of pregnancy or venereal disease.

Management
Sociocultural expectations and deficits in skills and sexual techniques are the two most important factors present in most cases. Direct masturbation training is the treatment of choice.

Treatment may take place in individual, couple or group settings. Tasks include relaxation, fantasizing and masturbation. Treatment is often successful, but the generalization of orgasm induced by masturbation to that induced by intercourse does not always occur.

Vaginismus
When sexually aroused the upper two-thirds of the vagina are lax and capacious, whereas the lower third is closely invested by the surrounding musculature of the pelvic floor. The strongest of these muscles is levator ani which forms a 'u' shaped sling around the posterior and lateral vaginal wall. Intense spasm in a nulliparous woman can virtually occlude the vagina. If these muscles are too tense, vaginal entry is impaired and painful: a condition known as vaginismus. A vicious circle ensues; pain or anticipation of pain causes further muscle contraction thereby increasing the likelihood of experiencing pain.

Epidemiology
Ten per cent of women presenting to a sexual disorders' clinic have a primary presentation of vaginismus.

Aetiology
Majority are primary. The problem was evident at first attempt at intercourse, and usually the woman has been reluctant to introduce anything to her vagina previously.

Occasionally onset can be related to a traumatic episode such as a painful vaginal examination or rape.

Sometimes vaginismus results from ambivalence about the relationship, or it may be secondary to reluctance to assume the mature adult's role. Irrational fears may also underlie the condition.

Management
Emphasis upon helping the woman to gain comfort in exploring her own genitalia and inserting her finger. Finger insertion may be all that is required, combined

with Sensate Focus techniques. Additional dilatation may be required using graded dilators. Initially carried out on her own, the partner is included when her confidence has increased.

DISORDERS OF GENDER IDENTITY

ICD-10 Codes **Gender identity disorders** under **Disorders of adult personality and behaviour.**

TRANSEXUALISM   There is the desire to live as a member of the opposite sex; discomfort with anatomic sex; a wish to change body into that of the preferred sex.

It must have been persistently present for two years; it must not be a symptom of another mental disorder such as schizophrenia, or be associated with an intersex, genetic or sex-chromosomal abnormality.

DUAL ROLE TRANSVESTISM   This includes the wearing of clothes of the opposite sex for part of the time to enjoy the temporary experience of membership of the opposite sex, without the desire for a more permanent sex change. No sexual excitement accompanies this cross-dressing, distinguishing it from fetishistic transvestism.

GENDER IDENTITY DISORDER OF CHILDHOOD   This is persistent, intense distress about assigned sex, together with desire to be of the other sex, usually manifest during early childhood, and always before puberty. It is relatively uncommon. There is a profound disturbance of the sense of maleness or femaleness.

Between one- and two-thirds of boys with gender identity disorder of childhood show homosexual orientation during and after adolescence. However, very few exhibit transsexualism in later life, although most adults with transsexualism report having had a gender identity problem in childhood. Some girls retain male gender identification in adolescence and some go on to homosexual orientation. Most, however, do not.

It is more common in boys than girls in clinic samples.

Treatment

Sex-reassignment treatment for transsexuals is a process of active rehabilitation into the new gender role, the provision and monitoring of opposite-sex hormones, and after a reasonable period of successful cross-gender living, sex-reassignment surgery is performed. The majority of transsexuals do experience a successful outcome in terms of subjective wellbeing and personal happiness.

SEXUAL DEVIATION

ICD-10

Coded as **Disorders of sexual preference** under **Disorders of adult personality and behaviour.**

FETISHISM   The reliance on some non-living object as a stimulus for sexual arousal and gratification. It is often an extension of the human body such as clothing or footwear. It is often characterized by texture such as plastic, rubber or leather.

Fetishism is diagnosed only if the fetish is the most important source of sexual stimulation. Fantasies are common but do not amount to disorder unless they are so compelling that they interfere with sexual intercourse and lead to distress.

FETISHISTIC TRANSVESTISM   This is wearing of clothes of the opposite sex to obtain sexual excitement.

More than a single item is worn, often an entire outfit. It is clearly associated with sexual arousal; there is no wish to continue cross-dressing once orgasm occurs, distinguishing this from transsexual transvestism.

EXHIBITIONISM   This is the recurrent or persistent tendency to expose the genitalia to strangers or people usually of the opposite sex in public places. There is usually sexual excitement at the time, often followed by masturbation. The tendency may only manifest at times of emotional stress or crisis, without such behaviour between.

It is almost entirely limited to heterosexual males, exhibiting to adult or adolescent females, usually from a safe distance in a public place. For some it is their only sexual outlet; for others they may also continue a normal sex life.

A reaction in the victim heightens the excitement in the perpetrator.

VOYEURISM   This is the persistent tendency to look at people engaging in sexual behaviour or undressing. It usually leads to sexual excitement and masturbation. The victim is usually unaware.

PAEDOPHILIA   This is the sexual preference for children, usually prepubertal or pubertal. Some are attracted to either one or both sexes.

It is rare in women. Included in this diagnosis are those men who retain a preference for adult sex partners, but when frustrated in their efforts turn to children as substitutes.

SADOMASOCHISM   This is the preference for sexual activity that involves the infliction of pain or humiliation. It is only diagnosed if this is the most important source of sexual stimulation.

MULTIPLE DISORDERS OF SEXUAL PREFERENCE   This is when more than one disorder of sexual preference occurs in one person and none is predominant.

OTHER DISORDERS OF SEXUAL PREFERENCE   This includes obscene telephone calls (telephone scatologia), frotteurism, sexual activity with animals (bestiality), the use of anoxia to heighten sexual pleasure (anoxophilia), and necrophilia.

SEXUAL ORIENTATION

Sexual orientation alone is not a disorder. ICD-10 allows for variations of sexual development or orientation that are **problematic for the individual:**

- heterosexual
- homosexual
- bisexual
- other including prepubertal.

Evidence suggestive of a genetic basis to sexual orientation is provided in twin studies with 52 per cent MZ: 22 per cent DZ concordance in homosexual males, and 48 per cent MZ: 16 per cent DZ concordance in female homosexuals. Hamer *et al.* (1993) carried out a family pedigree study in which the distribution of homosexuality in the male relatives suggested a sex-linked inheritance. They found convincing evidence in this family of a correlation between homosexual orientation and the inheritance of polymorphous markers at the Xq28 region of the X chromosome.

ANTISOCIAL SEXUAL BEHAVIOUR

The acceptability of sexual behaviour is determined by society and is incorporated into the law. What constitutes unacceptable behaviour varies largely between cultures and within the same culture over time.

Antisocial sexual behaviours can be divided into two groups:

1. 'Normal' activities carried out inappropriately, without consent or with the wrong age group.
2. Sexual activity which is morally perverse.

Rape

This is unlawful sexual intercourse with a woman by force or against her will. Rapists are not a homogeneous group.

Classification of rapists (Trick and Tennant 1981):

SITUATIONAL STRESS RAPIST   Otherwise sexually normal, these individuals commit rape when under extreme situational stress. There is much guilt and remorse afterwards.

SOCIOPATHIC RAPIST   These have poor social adjustment with criminality, a poor work record, involve substance abuse, and have unstable relationships. Rape is often impulsive, with immediate gratification and little regard to the consequences. Threats of violence are common.

SEXUALLY INADEQUATE RAPIST   These are shy, timid and insecure, lacking social skills. They often plan a rape against an attractive or sexually threatening woman.

SADISTIC RAPIST   These have a deep-rooted hatred of women arising from early relationships. The object of the rape is the infliction of humiliation and suffering; intercourse may be trivial in comparison to humiliating acts and the serious injuries inflicted. The rape is often carefully planned; precautions are taken to avoid detection.

PSYCHOTIC RAPIST   These constitute a very small proportion of rapists. The rape is often bizarre, violent and terrifying for the victim.

Paedophilia

This is the sexual attraction and preference for partners who are physically immature. Offenders are mostly men. Some prefer child victims of the opposite sex, some of the same sex. About 10 per cent are bisexual in their preference.

Adolescent offenders have a better prognosis than older offenders.

The mentally immature offender with poor social skills may prefer child sexual partners because they are the only people with whom they can relate at a general level.

The persistent middle-aged offender often has evidence of personality problems with poor relationships and unstable work patterns. These offenders usually have low rather than high sex drives. There is often an emotional bond between them and their child victim.

Some paedophiles are more dangerous than those described above. This offender has evidence of a serious personality disturbance affecting more aspects of their lives than their choice of sexual outlet.

Killing a child as part of a sexual offence is rare. It usually results from a state of panic, or from a desire to dispose of the evidence.

Incest

This is generally forbidden across cultures. In law it is an offence for a man to have sexual intercourse with a woman he knows to be his daughter, granddaughter, mother, sister or half-sister, and for a woman over 16 to allow a man whom she knows to be her son, father, grandfather, brother or half-brother to have sexual intercourse with her.

Sibling incest relationships are the most common, but father–daughter relationships are most commonly seen in court. They often reflect some breakdown in the marital relationship.

Incestuous families are characterized by alienation, disorganization and disintegration. They are rarely reported to the police.

Sibling incest is often the result of experimentation. It is more likely if there is a lack of parental control. Youngest sisters are the most vulnerable.

Indecent exposure

This is an offence under the 1824 Vagrancy Act: 'openly, lewdly and obscenely exposing his person with intent to insult any female'.

It is one of the most common sexual offences.

Exhibitionism, the exposing of genitals to the opposite sex, is categorized in two main groups:

Type I: Inhibited young men of relatively normal personality and good character who struggle against the impulse but find it irresistible. They expose with a flaccid penis and do not masturbate. They expose to individuals, not seeking a particular response. The frequency of exposure is often related to other sexual stresses and anxieties, such as marital conflict, pregnancy in spouse.

Type II: Less inhibited, more sociopathic. Expose with erect penis in a state of excitement, and may masturbate. Obtain pleasure and show little guilt. More likely to expose to a group of women or girls, and may return repeatedly to the same place. Seeks a response from the victim, either shock or disgust. There are fewer attempts to resist the urge to expose. Associated with other psychosexual disorders and other types of offences. May lead on to more serious sexual offences.

Eighty per cent do not reoffend if they are charged with first offence. The chances of reconviction rise dramatically with the second offence. There is a small group of recidivists who persist, but these tend to reduce in their forties. It is generally a harmless non-violent offence, except in a minority who may progress to more violent offences.

There is a good prognosis associated with married, good social relationships and work record.

Treatment for the recidivist includes antilibidinal drugs temporarily, with psychotherapy particularly cognitive and behavioural.

Other

Fetishism may come to the attention of the police if articles used are stolen e.g. women's underwear.

Sadomasochism may result in conviction for assault if extreme injury results, even if both parties consent.

Transvestites may be charged with behaviour likely to cause a breach of the peace if they cross-dress in public.

Frotteurism is the practice of rubbing the penis against another person in a clandestine way in a public place. It is liable to charges of either indecent assault or offence against public order.

Treatment

In a critical review of the literature, Marshall *et al.* (1991) concluded that some treatment programmes have been effective with paedophiles and exhibitionists but not with rapists.

In examining the value of the various treatment approaches they concluded that comprehensive cognitive–behavioural programmes were most likely to be effective with paedophiles and exhibitionists. There was also a clear value in the use of antiandrogens in those offenders who engage in excessively high rates of sexual activity.

BIBLIOGRAPHY

Bancroft, J. 1983: *Human sexuality and its problems*. Edinburgh: Churchill Livingstone.

Bancroft, J. 1994: Homosexual orientation: the search for a biological basis. *British Journal of Psychiatry* 164, 437–40.

Bancroft, J. 1995: Sexual disorders. In Kendell, R.E. and Zealley, A.K. (eds), *Companion to psychiatric studies*, 5th edn. Edinburgh: Churchill Livingstone.

Brindley, G.S. and Gillian, P. 1982: Men and women who do not have orgasms. *British Journal of Psychiatry* 140, 351–6.

Cooper, A.J., Cernovsky, Z.Z. Colussi, K. 1993: Some clinical and psychometric characteristics of primary and secondary premature ejaculators. *Journal of Sex and Marital Therapy* 19, 276–88.

Derogatis, L.R., Schmidt, C.W., Fagan, P.J. *et al.* 1989: Subtypes of anorgasmia via mathematical taxonomy. *Psychosomatics* 30, 166–73.

Fabbri, A., Jannini, E.A., Gnessi, L. *et al.* 1989: Endorphins in male impotence: evidence for naltrexone stimulation of erectile activity in patient therapy. *Psychoneuroendocrinology* 14, 103–11.

Gilbert, H.W. and Gingell, J.C. 1991: The results of an intracorporeal papaverine clinic. *Sex and Marital Therapy* 6, 49–56.

Gregoire, A. 1992: New treatments for erectile impotence. *British Journal of Psychiatry* 160, 315–26.

Hamer, D.H., Hu, S., Magnuson, V.L. *et al.* 1993: A linkage between DNA markers on the X chromosome and male sexual orientation. *Science* 261, 321–7.

Hawton, K., Catalan, J. and Fagg, J. 1992: Sex therapy for erectile dysfunction: characteristics of couples, treatment outcome and prognostic factors. *Archives of Sexual Behaviour* 21, 161–75.

Hiller, J. 1993: Psychoanalytic concepts and psychosexual therapy: a suggested integration. *Sex and Marital Therapy* 8, 9–26.

Janssen, P.L. 1985: Psychodynamic study of male potency disorders: an overview. *Psychotherapy and Psychosomatics* 44, 6–17.

Johnson, A.M., Wadsworth, J., Wellings, K. *et al.* 1994: *Sexual attitudes and lifestyles*. Oxford: Blackwell Scientific Publications.

Kinsey, A.C., Pomeroy, W.B. and Martin, C.E. 1948: *Sexual behaviour in the human male*. Philadelphia: W.B. Saunders.

Kinsey, A.C., Pomeroy, W.B., Martin, C.E. *et al.* 1953: *Sexual behaviour in the human female*. Philadelphia: W.B. Saunders.

Kockett, G. 1980: Symptomatology and psychological aspects of male sexual inadequacy: results of an experimental study. *Archives of Sexual Behaviour* 9, 457–75.

Marshall, W.L., Jones, R., Ward, T. *et al.* 1991: Treatment outcome with sex offenders. *Clinical Psychology Review* 11, 465–85.

Masters, W.H. and Johnson, V.E. 1970: *Human sexual inadequacy*. London: Churchill Livingstone.

Mishra, D.N. and Shulka, G.D. 1988: Sexual disturbances in male diabetics: phenomenological and clinical aspects. *Indian Journal of Psychiatry* 30, 135–43.

Pena, L.E. 1987: An analysis of female primary orgasmic dysfunction. *Revista de Analisis del Comportamiento* 3, 151–63.

Pirke, K.M. *et al.* 1979: Pituitary gonadal system function in patients with erectile impotence and premature ejaculation. *Archives of Sexual Behaviour* 8, 41–8.

Rowland, D.L., Haensel, S.M., Blom, J.H. *et al.* 1993: Penile sensitivity in men with premature ejaculation and erectile dysfunction. *Journal of Sex and Marital Therapy* 19, 189–97.

Segraves, R.T., Taylor, R., Schoenberg, H.W. *et al.* 1982: Psychosexual adjustment after penile prosthesis surgery. *Sexuality and Disability* 5, 222–9.

Snaith, P., Tarsh, M.J. and Reid, R. 1993: Sex reassignment surgery. *British Journal of Psychiatry* 162, 681–5.

Spector, I.P. and Carey, M.P. 1990: Incidence and prevalence of the sexual dysfunctions: A critical review of the empirical literature. *Archives of Sexual Behaviour* 19, 389–408.

Tondo, L., Cantone, M., Carta, M. *et al.* 1991: An MMPI evaluation of male sexual dysfunction. *Journal of Clinical Psychology* 47, 391–6.

Trick, R.L. and Tennant, T.G. 1981: *Forensic psychiatry: an introductory text.* London: Pitman Medical.

32
Sleep disorders

CLASSIFICATION

The ICD-10 classification of non-organic sleep disorders is:

F51.0   Nonorganic insomnia
F51.1   Nonorganic hypersomnia
F51.2   Nonorganic disorder of the sleep–wake schedule
F51.3   Sleepwalking
F51.4   Sleep terrors
F51.5   Nightmares

INSOMNIA

Definition
This is a disorder characterized by an insufficient quantity or quality of sleep.

Epidemiology
The estimated prevalence in adults ranges from 15 per cent to over 40 per cent. It is particularly high in the elderly.

Clinical features
The main result of true insomnia is daytime tiredness.

Differential diagnosis
Important disorders that may cause insomnia, and that should therefore be excluded, include:

- depressive disorders
- mania
- anxiety disorders
- organic disorders (see Table 32.1)

Aetiology
Table 32.1 gives the main causes of insomnia.

Management
Aspects of the management of insomnia include:

- sleep hygiene
  - ↓ lighting
  - regular exercise
  - a familiar and acceptable level of noise
  - a comfortable bed
  - progressive muscle relaxation techniques for any associated anxiety
  - a moderate intake of easily digested warm food
  - sleep conditioning

Table 32.1 Causes of insomnia

Environmental	Poor sleep hygiene Change in time zone Change in sleeping habits Shiftwork
Physiological	Natural short sleeper Pregnancy Middle age
Life stress	Bereavement Exams House move etc.
Psychiatric	Acute anxiety Depression Mania Organic brain syndrome
Physical	Pain Cardiorespiratory distress Arthritis Nocturia GI disorders Thyrotoxicosis
Pharmacological	Caffeine Alcohol Stimulants Chronic hypnotic use
Parasomnias	Sleep apnoea Sleep myoclonus
Primary sleep disorders	

Reproduced with permission from Puri, B.K., Laking, P.J. and Treasaden, I.H. 1996: *Textbook of psychiatry*. Edinburgh: Churchill Livingstone.

- hypnotics: note the CSM guidelines on the prescription of benzodiazepines
- behavioural approaches: particularly with children

Course and prognosis
Chronic insomnia may last through to old age.

HYPERSOMNIA

Clinical features
Excessive daytime sleepiness and sleep attacks occur regularly or recurrently for short periods, causing a disturbance of social or occupational functioning.

Epidemiology
Daytime drowsiness occurs in 0.3 to 4 per cent of the population.

Differential diagnosis
Important differential diagnoses include:

- narcolepsy
- sleep apnoea
- organic disorders
- fatigue states
- Kleine–Levin syndrome

Aetiology
The common causes of hypersomnia are:

- as an early symptom of depressive disorder
- unknown cause: idiopathic

Management
Treat any identified underlying cause. In idiopathic hypersomnia, amphetamines and other stimulants are occasionally used.

Course and prognosis
These are that of the underlying disorder. Idiopathic hypersomnia may improve with age.

DISORDERS OF THE SLEEP-WAKE CYCLE

Definitions
Disorders of the sleep–wake cycle are characterized by sleep occurring out of phase with environmental and social cues (*Zeitgebers*).
ENTRAINMENT FAILURE   This refers to the independent running of the sleep-wake cycle.
DELAYED SLEEP-PHASE SYNDROME   In delayed sleep-phase syndrome the sleep length is normal, there are no other psychiatric symptoms, but sleep takes place later than usual.
ADVANCED SLEEP-PHASE SYNDROME   In advanced sleep-phase syndrome the sleep length is normal, there are no other psychiatric symptoms, but sleep takes place earlier than usual.

Epidemiology
Entrainment failure and primary delayed sleep-phase syndrome are rare.

Management
Treat any primary disorder. If entrainment failure is secondary to a lack of sleep–wake cues in a modality such as vision (because of poor vision, say) then cues from other modalities and a careful routine may be employed. Advancing sleep in small increments may help in cases of delayed sleep-phase syndrome.

PARASOMNIAS

Definition
The parasomnias are phenomena occurring as part of or alongside sleep; they are shown in Table 32.2

SOMNAMBULISM (SLEEP WALKING)

Clinical features
In this disorder there occurs a state of altered consciousness in which while asleep the individual arises and walks. The sufferer is difficult to awaken during an episode, and may suffer injury if sleeping in an unfamiliar setting. Although

Table 32.2 The parasomnias

Sleepwalking (somnambulism)

Night terrors (pavor nocturnus)

Nightmares or dream anxiety

Bruxism (teeth grinding)

Nocturnal enuresis

Headbanging (jacatio capitis nocturnus)

Sleep paralysis

Nocturnal painful erections

Cluster headache

Physical symptomatology occurring at night, e.g. paroxysmal nocturnal dyspnoea, sleep epilepsy

Sleep myoclonus

Reproduced with permission from Puri, B.K., Laking, P.J. and Treasaden, I.H. 1996: *Textbook of psychiatry*. Edinburgh: Churchill Livingstone.

complex behaviours, including attempted homicide, have been described as occurring during somnambulism, in general this is not common.

Epidemiology

SEX RATIO   male: female = 3: 4

PREVALENCE   It occurs at least once in 15 per cent of children aged five to 12 years, and in 0.5 per cent of adults.

Differential diagnosis

Important differential diagnoses to exclude include:

- psychomotor epilepsy during sleep
- fugue states
- sleep drunkenness

Aetiology

Somnambulism is familial in up to 20 per cent of cases. There are no characteristic EEG changes. Sleep laboratory studies do not lend credence to the view that somnambulism represents the acting out of dreams.

Management

The patient's night-time surroundings should be made safe in order to reduce the risk of injury during episodes. Reassurance and, sometimes, family work, anxiety reduction techniques and small doses of hypnotics, may help.

NIGHT TERRORS

Clinical features

Night terrors occur during stages 3–4 sleep, and therefore usually one to two hours after sleep starts. The affected patient, usually a child, awakes terrified and screaming, but little is recalled the following morning. Enuresis may occur during an episode.

Epidemiology
In children, night terrors are common and occur on a frequent basis in 1–4 per cent. They are far less common in adulthood.

Differential diagnosis
The main differential diagnosis is nightmares.

Aetiology
Aetiological factors that have been suggested include:

- stress
- previous loss of sleep
- familial in some cases
- can sometimes be induced by benzodiazepine antagonists: hence the theories about benzodiazepine receptor changes or endogenous substances acting on benzodiazepine receptors
- upper airway obstruction in children

Management
Methods that may be used include:

- reassurance: of the child and the parents
- changing the settling routine
- keeping a diary and then waking the child just before each episode is expected

Course and prognosis
These problems often resolve spontaneously.

NIGHTMARES

Clinical features
Nightmares tend to occur during middle and late sleep; they usually occur during REM sleep, but occasionally during stage 1–2. They cause awakening, when the dream is remembered.

Epidemiology
Nightmares occur universally.

Differential diagnosis
The main differential diagnosis is night terrors.

Aetiology
Aetiological factors that have been suggested include:

- negative dreams

  - daytime depression
  - daytime anxiety
  - daytime stress

- hypnotic withdrawal
- alcohol withdrawal
- medication

  - β-adrenoceptor antagonists
  - reserpine

Management
Any underlying disorder may require treating. The nightmares themselves do not need to be treated.

BIBLIOGRAPHY

Laking, P.J. 1996: Sleep disorders. In Puri, B.K. Laking P.J. and Treasaden, I.H. *Textbook of psychiatry.* Edinburgh: Churchill Livingstone.
Parkes, J.D. 1985: *Sleep and its disorders.* London: W.B. Saunders.

33
Personality disorders

HISTORY

Hippocrates described four temperaments: melancholic, sanguine, phlegmatic, and choleric.

1801 Pinel's **manie sans délire**.

1835 Prichard's **moral insanity**.

1906 Kraepelin's **psychopathic personality**: excitable, unstable, eccentric, liars, swindlers, antisocial and quarrelsome subtypes.

Schneider extended the concept of psychopathic personality to include suffering to the self as well as to society.

1939 Henderson's **psychopathic states** included three subtypes: aggressive, inadequate and creative psychopaths.

1955 Cleckley's sociopathy: unreliable, untruthful, lack remorse, poor motivation and antisocial behaviour.

1978 Eysenck called for a dimensional rather than a categorical approach to the description of personality.

PERSONALITY DEVELOPMENT

Normothetic theories are concerned with personality structure based on studies of populations.

Ideographic theories relate to individual uniqueness, based on the study of the individual.

Kelly's personal construct theory

Kelly considered every man to be a scientist, interpreting the world on the basis of past experience. Constructs are created and predictions are made accordingly. A system of constructs results, unique in each individual, existing at various levels of consciousness, those formed at earlier developmental stages being unconscious. Each construct has a range of convenience. Some are specific e.g. chewy versus tender; others have a wider range of convenience.

Constructs are arranged into hierarchies. Superordinate constructs are central to the individual's sense of identity; subordinate constructs are less so.

According to this theory anxiety results when the individual is presented with events outside their range of personal constructs. Hostility comprises the imposition of constructs upon another.

Bannister's repertory grid can be used to assess an individual's attitudes with respect to a series of bipolar constructs. (It can also be used to measure formal thought disorder.)

Roger's self-theory

Each individual has a drive to fulfil themselves and develop an **ideal self** within a **phenomenal field** of subjective experience. The most important aspect of personality is the congruence between the individual's view of themselves and reality and their view of themselves compared to the ideal self. If an individual acts at variance to their own self-image, anxiety, incongruence and denial result. The congruent individual is able to grow (self-actualization) and achieve their potential both internally and socially.

Psychoanalytic theory

Behaviour and feelings are explained by unconscious drives and conflicts.

The **id** is, derived from the libido. Irrational, impulsive instincts are unable to postpone gratification, and are present at birth.

The **ego** develops as the child grows. A conscious mind balances the demands of the id with the realities of the outside world. Anxiety results if the ego is unable to control the energies of the id.

The **superego** comprises the internalization of the views of parents and society, like a conscience.

The id, the ego and the superego are in balance with each other.

FREUD'S STAGES OF PSYCHOSEXUAL DEVELOPMENT

Oral stage

- Age 0–1
- Gratification through sucking, biting
- Failure to negotiate leads to oral personality traits: moodiness, generosity, depression and elation, talkativeness, greed, optimism, pessimism, wishful thinking, narcissism

Anal stage

- Age 1–3
- Anus and defaecation are sources of sensual pleasure
- Failure to negotiate leads to anal personality traits: obsessive-compulsive personality, tidiness, parsimony, rigidity and thoroughness

Phallic stage

- Age 3–5
- Genital interest, relates to own sexuality. Oedipus/Electra complex
- Failure to negotiate leads to hysterical personality traits: competitiveness and ambitiousness

Latency stage
Age 5–12

Genital stage

- Age 12–20
- Gratification from normal relations with people
- Able to relate to a partner

ERIKSON'S STAGES OF DEVELOPMENT

Age	*Sense of*
0–1	Trust/security
1–4	Autonomy
4–5	Initiative
5–11	Duty/accomplishment
11–15	Identity
15–adult	Intimacy
Adulthood	Generativity
Maturity	Integrity

Epigenesis is the process of development of the ego through these stages.

Situationist approach
External situation is considered the most powerful determinant of behaviour. Situationists maintain that traits *result* from differences in learning experiences. Behaviour changes according to the situation in which an individual finds themselves. Proponents dismiss the trait theory. Mischel (1983) argues against the existence of any stable personality dimension because of the poor correlation between behaviour or attitudes in one situation compared with another.

Interactionist model
Behaviour depends upon situation as well as personality traits.

CLASSIFICATION AND MEASUREMENT

Dimensional approach
Personality disorder differs from normal variation only in terms of degree. It assumes that universal traits are present in all people in differing degrees. Personality traits of some individuals are sufficiently maladaptive and abnormal as to constitute personality disorder.

CATTELL'S TRAIT THEORY   Cattell identified 20 000 words describing personality. Using factor analysis he derived 16 first order personality factors. Cattell's 16 PF test was devised on the basis of this work. Second order factor analysis resulted in three broad dimensions similar to Eysenck's dimensions:

- sociability (extra/intra)
- anxiety
- intelligence.

EYSENCK'S THEORY   Factor analysis of rating scale data yields orthogonal dimensions, assumed to be normally distributed:

- neuroticism/stability
- extroversion/introversion
- psychoticism/stability
- intelligence.

Personality inventories used to measure these traits:

- MPI (Maudsley Personality Inventory)

superseded by

- EPI (Eysenck Personality Inventory)

superseded by

■ EPQ (Eysenck Personality Questionnaire), measuring psychoticism and containing a lie scale.

MINNESOTA MULTIPHASIC PERSONALITY INVENTORY (MMPI)   Lengthy inventory, subject answers 'true', 'false' or 'cannot say'. It is empirically constructed; it measures traits; it is widely used.

RORSCHACH INK BLOT TEST   This is a projective test analysing fantasy material.

ROTTER'S INTERNAL–EXTERNAL LOCUS OF CONTROL.   Individuals vary along a continuum in their perception of the locus of control of events. Those attributing events to an internal source are more confident about changing their life and environment.

Categorical approach

This approach groups people into discreet categories. It is simple and widely used but most individuals do not conform to categories.

Kretschmer linked body-build with personality:

■ pyknic: sociable and relaxed
■ asthenic: self-conscious and solitary
■ athletic: robust and outgoing

Sheldon also linked build with personality:

■ endomorphic: viscerotonic personality
■ ectomorphic: cerebrotonic personality
■ mesomorphic: somatotonic personality

ICD-10 AND DSM-IV CLASSIFICATION

These are primarily categorical classifications, but they incorporate a dimensional approach, allowing the recording of personality traits subthreshold for a diagnosis of personality disorder.

ICD-10

Severe disturbance in characterological constitution and behavioural tendencies, involving several areas of the personality, is associated with personal and social disruption. Diagnosis usually inappropriate before the age of 16 or 17.

GENERAL DIAGNOSTIC GUIDELINES   Not attributable to brain damage, disease, or other psychiatric disorder.

(a) disharmonious attitudes and behaviours involving several areas of functioning
(b) enduring, long-standing, not limited to episodes of mental illness
(c) pervasive and maladaptive
(d) appears during childhood or adolescence, continues into adulthood
(e) personal distress
(f) problems in occupational and social performance usual

PARANOID PERSONALITY DISORDER

(a) excessive sensitiveness to setbacks and rebuffs
(b) bears grudges persistently
(c) suspicious, misconstrues actions as hostile
(d) combative, tenacious sense of personal rights
(e) suspicions regarding fidelity of partner

(f)   excessive self-importance
(g)   conspiratorial explanations of events

SCHIZOID PERSONALITY DISORDER

(a)   finds few activities pleasurable
(b)   emotional coldness, detachment or flattened affect
(c)   limited capacity to express feelings
(d)   apparent indifference to praise or criticism
(e)   little interest in sexual experiences with another person
(f)   preference for solitary activities
(g)   preoccupation with fantasy and introspection
(h)   lack of desire for close friends or confiding relationships
(i)   insensitivity to social norms and conventions

DISSOCIAL PERSONALITY DISORDER

(a)   callous unconcern for feelings of others
(b)   gross and persistent irresponsibility and disregard for social norms, rules and obligations
(c)   incapacity to maintain enduring relationships
(d)   low tolerance to frustration; low threshold for aggression and violence
(e)   incapacity to experience guilt or to profit from experience, especially punishment
(f)   blames others

Persistent irritability may be present. Conduct disorder during childhood and adolescence supports this diagnosis.

EMOTIONALLY UNSTABLE PERSONALITY DISORDER   Here the patient may act impulsively without consideration of consequences. There is affective instability. There is a minimal ability to plan ahead; outbursts of intense anger leading to violence are easily precipitated.
   There are two variants:
Impulsive type   Emotional instability and lack of control. Outbursts of violence or threatening behaviour are common, especially in response to criticism.
Borderline type   Emotional instability. Self-image, aims and internal preferences are often unclear or disturbed. Chronic feelings of emptiness. Intense unstable relationships cause repeated emotional crises; there are associated excessive efforts to avoid abandonment, suicidal threats or deliberate self-harm.

HISTRIONIC PERSONALITY DISORDER

(a)   self-dramatization, theatricality, exaggerated expression of emotions
(b)   suggestibility
(c)   shallow and labile affect
(d)   seeks excitement; centre of attention
(e)   inappropriate seductiveness
(f)   over-concern with physical attractiveness

Egocentric, self-indulgent, longing for appreciation, feelings easily hurt, manipulative.

ANANKASTIC PERSONALITY DISORDER

(a)   feelings of excessive doubt and caution
(b)   preoccupation with details, rules, lists, order, organization and schedule
(c)   perfectionism interferes with task completion

(d)   conscientiousness, scrupulousness, undue preoccupation with productivity to exclusion of pleasure and relationships
(e)   pedantic
(f)   rigid and stubborn
(g)   insist others submit to their way of doing things, reluctant to allow others to do things
(h)   intrusion of unwelcome, insistent thoughts or impulses

ANXIOUS (AVOIDANT) PERSONALITY DISORDER

(a)   persistent, pervasive tension and apprehension
(b)   believe they are socially inept, unappealing or inferior to others
(c)   preoccupation with being criticized or rejected in social situations
(d)   unwillingness to become involved unless certain of being liked
(e)   restrictions in lifestyle because of need for security
(f)   avoidance of activities involving interpersonal contact because of fear of criticism, disapproval or rejection

DEPENDENT PERSONALITY DISORDER

(a)   allows others to make important life decisions
(b)   subordination of own needs to those of others on whom they are dependent
(c)   unwillingness to make demands on people on whom they are dependent
(d)   uncomfortable or helpless when alone, fear inability to care for themselves
(e)   fear of being abandoned
(f)   unable to make decisions without excessive advice from others

DSM-IV

GENERAL DIAGNOSTIC CRITERIA

A. Enduring pattern of inner experience and behaviour, deviates markedly from expectations of individual's culture. Manifested in:

1   cognition
2   affectivity
3   interpersonal functioning
4   impulse control

B. Inflexible and pervasive across a range of situations.
C. Leads to significant distress or impairment in social, occupational, or other areas.
D. Stable, of long duration, onset can be traced back to adolescence or early adulthood.
E. Not a manifestation or consequence of another mental disorder.
F. Not caused by the effects of a substance or a general medical condition.
  Grouped into three clusters:

- **Cluster A**: paranoid, schizoid, and schizotypal personality disorders. Odd or eccentric
- **Cluster B**: antisocial, borderline, histrionic, and narcissistic personality disorders. Dramatic, emotional, or erratic
- **Cluster C**: avoidant, dependent, and obsessive–compulsive personality disorders. Anxious or fearful

Personality disorders are coded on Axis II, and listed in their order of importance. Specific maladaptive personality traits and the use of defence mechanisms may also be listed on Axis II.

PARANOID PERSONALITY DISORDER

A. Pervasive distrust and suspiciousness; beginning by early adulthood.
  Four (or more) of the following:

1   suspects others are exploiting, harming, or deceiving them
2   doubts about loyalty or trustworthiness of friends
3   reluctant to confide in others, fears that information will be used maliciously
4   reads hidden meanings into benign remarks or events
5   persistently bears grudges
6   perceives attacks on character not apparent to others; quick to react angrily
7   recurrent suspicions regarding fidelity of partner

B. Does not occur exclusively during the course of schizophrenia, mood disorder or other psychotic disorder; not caused by the direct effects of a general medical condition.

SCHIZOID PERSONALITY DISORDER

A. Pervasive detachment from social relationships; restricted expression of emotions; beginning by early adulthood.
  Four (or more) of the following:

1   neither desires nor enjoys close relationships, including being part of a family
2   chooses solitary activities
3   has little interest in sexual experience with another person
4   takes pleasure in few activities
5   lacks close friends or confidants
6   is indifferent to praise or criticism of others
7   shows emotional coldness, detachment, or flattened affect

B. Does not occur exclusively during the course of schizophrenia, mood disorder, other psychotic disorder, or pervasive developmental disorder; not caused by the effects of a general medical condition.

SCHIZOTYPAL PERSONALITY DISORDER

A. Pervasive social and interpersonal deficits; reduced capacity for close relationships; cognitive or perceptual distortions and eccentricities of behaviour; beginning by early adulthood
  Five (or more) of the following:

1   ideas of reference
2   odd beliefs or magical thinking inconsistent with subcultural norms
3   unusual perceptual experiences
4   odd thinking and speech
5   suspiciousness or paranoid ideation
6   inappropriate or constricted affect
7   behaviour or appearance odd, eccentric, or peculiar
8   lack of close friends or confidants
9   excessive social anxiety; does not diminish with familiarity

B. Does not occur exclusively during the course of schizophrenia, mood disorder, other psychotic disorder, or pervasive developmental disorder; not caused by the effects of a general medical condition.

ANTISOCIAL PERSONALITY DISORDER

A. Pervasive disregard for and violation of rights of others occurring since the age of 15 years.
  Three (or more) of the following:

1   failure to conform to social norms with respect to lawful behaviours
2   deceitfulness; repeated lying, use of aliases, conning others

3   impulsivity, failure to plan ahead
4   irritability and aggressiveness
5   reckless disregard for safety of self or others
6   consistent irresponsibility; repeated failure to sustain work or honour finan-
     cial obligations
7   lack of remorse

B. At least age 18 years.
C. Evidence of conduct disorder before the age of 15 years.
D. Not exclusively during the course of schizophrenia or mania.

BORDERLINE PERSONALITY DISORDER   Pervasive instability of interpersonal relationships, self-image and affects; marked impulsivity beginning by early adulthood.

   Five (or more) of the following:

1   frantic efforts to avoid real or imagined abandonment
2   unstable, intense relationships alternating between extremes of idealization
     and devaluation
3   identity disturbance: markedly and persistently unstable self-image
4   impulsivity in at least two areas that are potentially self-damaging
5   recurrent suicidal behaviour, gestures, or threats, or self-mutilating behaviour
6   affective instability caused by a marked reactivity of mood
7   chronic feelings of emptiness
8   inappropriate, intense anger
9   transient, stress-related paranoid ideation or severe dissociative symptoms

HISTRIONIC PERSONALITY DISORDER   Pervasive excessive emotionality and atten-tion-seeking, beginning by early adulthood.

   Five (or more) of the following:

1   uncomfortable if not centre of attention
2   inappropriate sexually seductive or provocative behaviour
3   rapidly shifting, shallow emotions
4   uses physical appearance to draw attention to self
5   style of speech is excessively impressionistic
6   self-dramatization, theatricality, exaggerated expression of emotion
7   suggestible
8   considers relationships more intimate than they are

NARCISSISTIC PERSONALITY DISORDER   Pervasive grandiosity, need for admiration, lack of empathy; beginning by early adulthood.

   Five (or more) of the following

1   grandiose sense of self-importance
2   fantasies of unlimited success, power, brilliance, beauty, or ideal love
3   believe they are 'special' and should associate with other special or high-
     status people
4   requires excessive admiration
5   sense of entitlement
6   interpersonally exploitative
7   lacks empathy
8   often envious of others
9   arrogant, haughty behaviours or attitudes

AVOIDANT PERSONALITY DISORDER   Pervasive social inhibition, feelings of inade-quacy, hypersensitivity to negative evaluation; beginning by early adulthood.

Four (or more) of the following:

1 avoids activities that involve interpersonal contact; fears of criticism, disapproval, or rejection
2 unwilling to get involved with people unless certain of being liked
3 shows restraint within intimate relationships because of the fear of being shamed or ridiculed
4 preoccupied with being criticized or rejected in social situations
5 inhibited in new interpersonal situations because of feelings of inadequacy
6 views self as socially inept, personally unappealing, or inferior to others
7 reluctant to take risks or engage in new activities because they may prove embarrassing

DEPENDENT PERSONALITY DISORDER Pervasive, excessive need to be taken care of; submissive, clinging behaviour and fears of separation; beginning by early adulthood.

Five (or more) of the following:

1 difficulty making everyday decisions
2 needs others to assume responsibility for most major areas of life
3 difficulty expressing disagreement; fear of loss of support
4 difficulty initiating projects or doing things on their own
5 goes to excessive lengths to obtain nurturance and support
6 feels uncomfortable or helpless when alone; fears of being unable to cope
7 urgently seeks another relationship as a source of care and support when a close relationship ends
8 preoccupied with fears of being left to take care of themselves

OBSESSIVE–COMPULSIVE PERSONALITY DISORDER Pervasive preoccupation with orderliness, perfectionism, and control, at the expense of flexibility, openness, and efficiency; beginning by early adulthood.

Four (or more) of the following:

1 preoccupied with details, rules, lists, order, organization or schedules to the extent that the point of the activity is lost
2 perfectionism interferes with task completion
3 excessively devoted to work and productivity to the exclusion of leisure activities and friendships
4 over-conscientious, scrupulous, inflexible
5 unable to discard worn-out or worthless objects
6 reluctant to delegate tasks
7 miserly
8 rigid and stubborn

PERSONALITY DISORDER NOT OTHERWISE SPECIFIED This does not meet criteria for any specific personality disorder, but that it causes distress or impairment in one or more important areas of functioning (e.g. social or occupational).

EPIDEMIOLOGY

Methodological problems encountered with prevalence studies:

- diagnosis of personality disorder during psychiatric illness
- lack of informants' account when making diagnosis

- 'either/or' approach to diagnosis
- diagnosis made by variously reliable methods
- inconsistent recording of the presence of more than one personality disorder

Gradient exists in the prevalence of personality disorder from community to inpatient setting.

Approximate prevalence of personality disorder in:

- community: 10 per cent
- general practice: 20 per cent
- psychiatric outpatients: 30 per cent
- psychiatric inpatients: 40 per cent

Generally more common in males than in females.

Certain personality disorders (e.g. antisocial personality disorder) are diagnosed more frequently in men, others (e.g. borderline, histrionic, and dependent personality disorders) in women.

The *American Epidemiologic Catchment Area* (ECA) study found, using a Diagnostic Interview Schedule, a prevalence of personality disorder in the community of 6 per cent.

SPECIFIC PERSONALITY DISORDERS
Antisocial personality disorder:

- Lifetime prevalence: 2.3–3.6 per cent
- Sex ratio: 7 male:1 female
- Twice as prevalent in inner cities compared to rural areas
- Antisocial behaviours usually start age 8–10. Do not develop after age 18
- Highest lifetime prevalence in 25–44-year-old group, followed by 18–24-year-old group
- Spontaneous remission may occur in middle age. Correlation between increasing age and remission rate
- Excess mortality
- Less likely to be married, less well educated
- Highly significant correlation between antisocial personality disorder and drug and alcohol dependence
- High proportion (90 per cent) have at least one lifetime psychiatric diagnosis

Table 33.1 The prevalence of personality disorders in different settings

Personality disorder	Prevalence %		
	Community	Outpatients	Inpatients
Paranoid	0.5%–2.5%	2%–10%	10%–30%
Schizoid		uncommon	
Schizotypal	3%		
Antisocial	3% in males; 1% in females	3%–30%	
Borderline	2%	10%	20%
Histrionic	2%–3%		10%–15%
Narcissistic	less than 1%		2%–16%
Avoidant	0.5%–1.0%	10%	
Dependent		The most frequently reported	
Obsessive–compulsive	1%	3%–10%	

AETIOLOGY

Environment

PSYCHODYNAMIC THEORY

Psychoanalytic The failure to negotiate stages of psychosexual development and the characteristic use of defence mechanisms are said to result in disorders of personality. For example:

- paranoid personality is the result of the projection of homosexual impulses. Later it was thought that excessive parental rage causing feelings of inadequacy resulted in projection on to others of hostility and rage
- borderline personality results from early traumatic experiences occurring within a context of sustained neglect resulting in enduring rage and self-hatred
- histrionic personality results from difficulties in the Oedipal phase of psychosexual development
- dependent personality results from fixation at the oral stage of psychosexual development
- obsessive–compulsive personality results from difficulties in the anal stage of psychosexual development

Object relations Personality is shaped by the child's early parental relationships. Dependent personality traits are thought to result from parental deprivation, obsessive–compulsive traits from the struggle with parents for control, and hysterical traits from parental seduction and competition.

For example, borderline personality is the result of a lack of stably involved attachment during development. This leads to an inability to maintain a stable sense of self or others without ongoing contact.

Neurological

Eighty per cent of children with minimal brain dysfunction syndrome suffer from various personality disorders in adult life.

EEG studies in antisocial personality disorders demonstrate abnormalities which have led to speculation that psychopathic behaviour reflects cortical immaturity. Abnormalities found in this group more often than in normals include:

- generalized widespread slow (theta) wave activity
- 'positive spike' abnormality over temporal lobes
- localized temporal slow wave activity

These abnormalities are more likely to occur in highly impulsive and aggressive psychopaths.

Psychopaths have lower cortical arousal, measured by slower cortical evoked potentials. Autonomic arousal is also lower, leading to speculation that sensation-seeking behaviour may be an attempt to increase cortical arousal.

Goyer *et al.* (1994) in a PET scanning study of personality disordered subjects found a significant inverse correlation between a history of aggressive impulse difficulties and regional cerebral metabolic rates in the frontal cortex. Those subjects with borderline personality disorders had significantly reduced frontal cortex metabolism.

Genetic

Normal personality appears to be at least moderately heritable:

- Breeding over generations of animals e.g. dogs, produces strains with more or less aggressive temperaments
- Psychophysiological characteristics are partly genetically inherited e.g. EEGs of monozygotic twins (MZ) are easily distinguished from those of dizygotic twins (DZ), even when reared apart; the habituation of galvanic skin response is largely genetically determined
- Large representative twin studies using model-fitting approaches consistently find a heritability of 35–50 per cent for traits measured by questionnaire. Although 50 per cent of the variance in personality traits is environmental, a shared family environment has consistently shown a negligible contribution to the variance
- Monozygotic twins reared apart are more alike on personality measures than those raised together. It is suggested that reared together twins react against one another in an attempt to establish individual identities

ANTISOCIAL PERSONALITY DISORDER   Most twin and adoption studies suggest that antisocial personality disorder has a partial genetic aetiology. The heritable form of criminality is associated with petty recidivism and property offences rather than violent crime.

Mednick *et al.* (1984) studied 14 427 adoptees and their biological and adoptive parents.

The effect is stronger when the biological mother is convicted than if the biological father is convicted. Association for property offences only, playing significant role in repeat offences; did not apply to violent offences.

Robins (1966) found that the father's criminal behaviour was the single best predictor of antisocial behaviour in a child.

MZ:DZ concordance rates for adult criminality 52 per cent: 22 per cent. Suggests definite genetic contribution. However, concordance rates of 87 per cent: 72 per cent for juvenile delinquency is suggestive of a familial but not a genetic component to aetiology.

Within a family that has a member with antisocial personality disorder, males more often have antisocial personality disorder and substance-related disorders, whereas females more often have somatization disorder. However, in such families, there is an increase in the prevalence of all of these disorders in both males and females compared with the general population.

It is suggested that family background plays a part in subsequent criminality, but only when there is already a genetic predisposition. The risk of criminality is increased in those with prolonged institutional care, multiple temporary placements and those where the socioeconomic status of their adoptive home is low.

SCHIZOTYPAL PERSONALITY DISORDERS   Kety *et al.* (1971) in an adoption study demonstrated that abnormalities were more common in the biological relatives of

Table 33.2   Percentages of convictions in male adoptees and the biological and adoptive parents

	Conviction rate %
Neither biological nor adoptive parent convicted	13.5
Adoptive parents convicted. Biological parents not convicted	14.7
Adoptive parents not convicted. Biological parents convicted	20.0
Adoptive and biological parents convicted	24.5

schizophrenics than in adoptive relatives or controls ('schizophrenia spectrum disorders'). From this derived the operational criteria for schizotypal personality disorder. Almost all studies of the families of schizophrenic probands have found an excess of both schizophrenia and schizotypal personality disorder among relatives (22 per cent in the biological relatives of schizophrenics versus 2 per cent of adoptive relatives and controls).

The heritability found in anxious personalities is probably related to trait anxiety, in obsessional personalities to a more general neurotic tendency as measured by the Eysenck Personality Inventory, and in hysterical personalities to extroversion.

Coccaro *et al.* (1993) examined the heritability of personality traits (impulsiveness, irritability and inhibition of assertive behaviour) in 500 healthy MZ and DZ twin pairs raised together and apart. The results showed substantial genetic influences, and were consistent with a genetic, but not a shared environmental influence.

MANAGEMENT

Most research focuses upon the management of the 'borderline' patient, partly because these are the patients commonly presenting in clinical practice.

Assessment
Assessment can be difficult. Personality traits are egosyntonic, such that patients are often not aware of them and will not complain of them. In the diagnosis of personality disorder multiple sources of information should be used, including an informant who has known the patient for a considerable time.

Personality traits should:

- be enduring, not transient
- be pervasive across situations
- be early in onset
- cause distress or impairment

Account should be taken of social and cultural norms when considering behaviour or symptoms.

Axis I symptom disorder and medical illness should be identified since they may complicate the diagnosis.

Many difficulties of adolescence resolve as the person matures. Personality disorder should be diagnosed with care in adolescence.

Psychotherapy
Psychoanalysis or intensive **psychoanalytic psychotherapy** is considered by many psychotherapists to be the treatment of choice for borderline individuals. The duration of therapy is between two and seven years. Treatment consists of interpretation of the transference and primitive defence mechanisms, the neutrality of the therapist and a consistent limit setting. Attention is particularly focused on the present rather than interpreting childhood experience.

An alternative is **supportive psychotherapy** which aims to strengthen a patient's adaptive functioning through education, suggestion and a facilitating interpersonal relationship. The interpretation of transference, defence mechanisms and regression and dependency are avoided, since they are considered likely to lead to suicide or other forms of acting out.

Group psychotherapy has been traditionally avoided because borderline patients are considered too demanding and disruptive. However, gentle confrontation delivered by a group is considered by some to be effective, rendering egosyntonic traits more egodystonic.

Most groups can contain no more than one or two borderline patients. Apart from the cost, there is no evidence to recommend group therapy over individual therapy.

FAMILY THERAPY   This is frequently offered to borderline adolescent patients, and is regarded by many as the treatment of choice for these patients.

INPATIENT TREATMENT AND THERAPEUTIC COMMUNITY   This is controversial. Currently there is a trend away from long-term admissions for borderline patients, probably driven by cost-containment. There is evidence to support the value of therapeutic communities such as the Henderson or the Cassel Hospitals. The therapeutic community approach is a multi-component treatment programme, incorporating individual therapy, ward groups, and patient participation in the maintenance of the community.

The risks of hospitalization to the patient include:

- stigma
- disruption of social and occupational roles
- loss of freedom
- hospital-induced behavioural regression

Some consider the drawing up of a contract between the patient and doctor essential to the success of inpatient care. Miller (1989) considers a good **treatment contract** to incorporate the following:

1   mutual agreement by all involved parties
2   specific, focused, achievable goals with strategies to achieve them
3   specific responsibilities of patient and staff
4   provision of the minimum degree of structure necessary
5   patient foregoes their usual means of managing intolerable feelings; alternative strategies are provided
6   positive reinforcement of desirable behaviour
7   not drawn up when staff have unresolved punitive wishes towards the patient
8   strictly enforced, but room for negotiated modification

The alternative approach of brief admissions at the time of crisis is increasingly popular.

COGNITIVE-BEHAVIOURAL THERAPY   Linehan *et al.* (1991) randomly allocated cognitive-behavioural therapy or 'treatment as usual' over a period of one year, to chronically parasuicidal borderline patients. During the year the cognitive-behavioural therapy group showed fewer and less severe incidents of parasuicide, and had fewer inpatient days.

Pharmacotherapy

Placebo-controlled drug trials among those with personality disorder show small specific drug effects as well as large placebo effects.

NEUROLEPTIC DRUGS   Low-dose neuroleptic treatment has been shown to be beneficial particularly in the management of borderline subjects in a majority of trials. Low-dose flupenthixol significantly reduced the number of suicide attempts by six months when compared to placebo and mianserin in a mixed group of parasuicidal personality-disordered subjects.

Low-dose neuroleptics improve a broad spectrum of neurotic symptoms as well as reducing behavioural dyscontrol and numbers of suicide attempts, compared to placebo.

ANTIDEPRESSANTS

Tricyclics   Some patients with borderline or schizotypal personality disorder improve with tricyclics on ratings of depressed mood, impulsive and manipulative behaviour, but there is significant potential for paradoxical effects and rage reactions. As a result they are not particularly recommended in the management of personality disorders unless major depression co-occurs. Depression complicated by personality disorder is only half as likely to respond to tricyclic drug treatment compared to pure major depression, however.

Monoamine oxidase inhibitors   Selected borderline subjects respond to MAOIs particularly where there is a history of childhood hyperactivity.

Selective serotonin re-uptake inhibitors   Serotonergic dysfunction has been implicated in key symptoms particularly depression, impulsivity and obsessive-compulsive phenomena. Fluoxetine at doses of 20–80 mg per day result in the improvement in depressed mood and impulsivity as well as reducing self-mutilation. Sertraline used in impulsive aggressive patients results in marked improvements in overt aggression and irritability, evident from the fourth week of treatment.

Electroconvulsive therapy   The immediate response is good in depressed borderline subjects, but the relapse rate is high.

Lithium   In male convicts with a pattern of recurring easily triggered violence a marked reduction in infractions resulted from treatment with lithium. The reduction in aggressive episodes requires lithium levels above 0.6 mmol/L. Major infractions such as assault or threatening behaviour are responsive to lithium in about 60 per cent; minor infractions are unresponsive.

Lithium is helpful in a small numbers of patients with diverse personality disorders. Affective features, a family history of affective disorder or alcoholism may help select subjects. A two-month trial of lithium may be necessary to establish responders.

Carbamazepine   Impulsive aggression is the most serious symptom of personality disorder. In patients with behavioural dyscontrol aggressive acts are reduced by about two-thirds and the severity of the outburst is improved. It is helpful even in the absence of epileptic, affective or organic features.

Benzodiazepines   These are contraindicated in personality disorder because of their propensity to disinhibit, induce rage reactions and states of dependence.

Psychostimulants   Psychostimulants such as dexamphetamine and pemoline may occasionally, sometimes dramatically, help personalities with aggression and hostility, particularly where there is an earlier history of drug-responsive attention-deficit disorder. However, because of their psychotogenic effects and addictive properties, extreme caution is used in prescribing.

It is usually the case that both drug therapy and psychotherapy would be used in a patient with personality disorder.

OUTCOME

The personality disorders have a high morbidity and mortality. The standardized mortality ratio for the 20–39-year-old age group is raised six-fold, similar to that rise reported for the major functional psychoses.

Patients with personality disorder have high rates of co-morbidity with both

Axis I and Axis II conditions. Response to treatment of Axis I disorder is almost always worse in the presence of personality disorder. Patients are at a high risk of suicide.

In those borderlines treated with psychotherapy the aim of supportive psychotherapy may be to diminish suicidal behaviour and impulsive acts while awaiting a remission since the long-term prognosis of this disorder is good. A 15 year follow-up of 100 borderline personality disordered patients found that 75 per cent were no longer diagnosed as borderline. All scales showed a reduction of symptomatic behaviour, with a clear functional improvement. However, there is a high risk of suicide, with 8.5 per cent completing suicide in the 15-year follow-up period. Those patients with chronic depression, good motivation, a psychological attitude, low impulsiveness and a stable environment are most responsive to treatment.

In those with antisocial personality disorders there is a significant association between the ability to form a relationship with the therapist and treatment outcome. In confined settings such as prison or in the military, confrontation by peers may bring changes in social behaviour. Prevalence seems to decrease with increasing age.

Schizotypal personality disorder has a relatively stable course, with only a small proportion of individuals going on to develop schizophrenia.

Some types of personality disorder (antisocial and borderline) tend to become less evident or to remit with age, whereas this appears to be less true for some other types (obsessive–compulsive and schizotypal).

BIBLIOGRAPHY

American Psychiatric Association 1994: *Diagnostic and statistical manual of mental disorders*, 4th edn. Washington DC: American Psychiatric Association.

Brennan, P.A. and Mednick, S.A. 1993: Genetic perspectives on crime. *Acta Psychiatrica Scandinavica* (suppl.) 370, 19–26.

Coccaro, E.F., Bergeman, C.S. and McClearn, G.E. 1993: Heritability of irritable impulsiveness: a study of twins reared together and apart. *Psychiatry Research* 48, 229–42.

DeBattista, C. and Glick, I.D. 1995: Pharmacotherapy of the personality disorders. *Current Opinion in Psychiatry* 8, 102–5.

Freeman, C.P.L. 1995: Personality disorders. In Kendell, R.E. and Zealley, A.K. (eds), *Companion to psychiatric studies*, 5th edn. Edinburgh: Churchill Livingstone.

Gelder, M., Gath, D. and Mayou, R. 1985: *Oxford textbook of psychiatry.* Oxford: Oxford University Press.

Goyer, P.F., Andreason, P.J., Semple, W.E. *et al.* 1994: Positron emission tomography and personality disorders. *Neuropsychopharmacology* 10, 21–8.

Higgitt, A. and Fonagy, P. 1992: Psychotherapy in borderline and narcissistic personality disorder. *British Journal of Psychiatry* 161, 23–43.

Kety, S.S., Rosenthal, D., Wender, P.H. *et al.* 1971: Mental illness in the biological and adoptive families of adopted schizophrenics. *American Journal of Psychiatry* 128, 302–6.

Linehan, M.M., Armstrong, H.E., Svarez, A. *et al.* 1991: Cognitive behavioural treatment of chronically parasuicidal borderline patients. *Archives of General Psychiatry* 48, 1060–4.

McGuffin, P. and Thapar, A. 1992: The genetics of personality disorder. *British Journal of Psychiatry* 160, 12–23.

Mednick, S.A., Gabrielli, W.F. and Hutchings, B. 1984: Genetic influences on criminal convictions: evidence from an adoption cohort. *Science* 224, 891–4.

Miller, L.J. 1989: Inpatient management of borderline personality disorder: a review and update. *Journal of Personality Disorders* 3, 122–34.

Mischel, W. 1983: Alterations on the pursuit of predictability and consistency of persons: stable data that yield unstable interpretations. *Journal of Personality* 51, 578–604.

Paris, J., Brown, R. and Nowis, D. 1987: Long term follow up of borderline patients in a general hospital. *Comprehensive Psychiatry* 28, 530–5.

Robins, L.N. 1966: *Deviant children grown up*. Baltimore: Williams & Wilkins.

Stein, G. 1992: Drug treatment of the personality disorders. *British Journal of Psychiatry* 161, 167–84.

Swanson, M.C.J., Bland, R.C. and Newman, S.C. 1994: Antisocial personality disorders. *Acta Psychiatrica Scandinavica* (suppl.) 376, 63–70.

Tyrer, P. and Ferguson, B. 1987: Problems in the classification of personality disorder. *Psychological Medicine* 17, 15–20.

WHO 1992: *Tenth revision of the international classification of diseases*. Geneva: World Health Organization.

34
Child and adolescent psychiatry

CHILD AND ADOLESCENT PSYCHIATRIC DISORDER

Classification
The ICD-10 classification of behavioural and emotional disorders with onset usually occurring in childhood and adolescence is shown in Table 34.1.

Epidemiology
PRESCHOOL   The main epidemiological study is the Waltham Forest Study (by Richman and colleagues) in the early 1970s of three-year-olds, carried out in the London borough of that name. The Vineyard study (Martha) essentially confirmed its findings. The main findings included:

- prevalence of moderate to severe behavioural and emotional problems = 7 per cent; boys slightly greater than girls
- prevalence of mild behavioural and emotional problems = 15 per cent
- strong associations were found with:

  - maternal depression
  - poor parental marriage
  - delayed development of language

- strong continuities of behaviour and language disorders over the early school years

MIDDLE CHILDHOOD   The main epidemiological studies are the Isle of Wight and Inner London Borough Studies (by Rutter and colleagues) in the 1960s of 10- and 11-year-olds. Recent studies in Norway and Puerto Rico essentially confirmed the findings. The main findings included:

- overall point prevalence of child psychiatric disorder in the Isle of Wight = 6.8 per cent

  - conduct disorder: 4 per cent
  - emotional disorder: 2.5 per cent
  - overall, boys:girls = 1.9:1

- overall point prevalence of child psychiatric disorder in inner London = twice that in the Isle of Wight

Table 34.1 F90-F98 Behavioural and emotional disorders with onset usually occurring in childhood and adolescence (ICD-10)

F90	**Hyperkinetic disorders**
	F90.0 Disturbance of activity and attention
	F90.1 Hyperkinetic conduct disorder
	F90.8 Other hyperkinetic disorders
	F90.9 Hyperkinetic disorder, unspecified
F91	**Conduct disorders**
	F91.0 Conduct disorder confined to the family context
	F91.1 Unsocialized conduct disorder
	F91.2 Socialized conduct disorder
	F91.3 Oppositional defiant disorder
	F91.8 Other conduct disorders
	F91.9 Conduct disorder, unspecified
F92	**Mixed disorders of conduct and emotions**
	F92.0 Depressive conduct disorder
	F92.8 Other mixed disorders of conduct and emotions
	F92.9 Mixed disorder of conduct and emotions, unspecified
F93	**Emotional disorders with onset specific to childhood**
	F93.0 Separation anxiety disorder of childhood
	F93.1 Phobic anxiety disorder of childhood
	F93.2 Social anxiety disorder of childhood
	F93.3 Sibling rivalry disorder
	F93.8 Other childhood emotional disorders
	F93.9 Childhood emotional disorder, unspecified
F94	**Disorders of social functioning with onset specific to childhood and adolescence**
	F94.0 Elective mutism
	F94.1 Reactive attachment disorder of childhood
	F94.2 Disinhibited attachment disorder of childhood
	F94.8 Other childhood disorders of social functioning
	F94.9 Childhood disorders of social functioning, unspecified
F95	**Tic disorders**
	F95.0 Transient tic disorder
	F95.1 Chronic motor or vocal tic disorder
	F95.2 Combined vocal and multiple motor tic disorder [Gilles de la Tourette's syndrome]
	F95.8 Other tic disorders
	F95.9 Tic disorder, unspecified
F98	**Other behavioural and emotional disorders with onset usually occurring in childhood and adolescence**
	F98.0 Nonorganic enuresis
	F98.1 Nonorganic encopresis
	F98.2 Feeding disorder of infancy and childhood
	F98.3 Pica of infancy and childhood
	F98.4 Stereotyped movement disorders
	F98.5 Stuttering [stammering]
	F98.6 Cluttering
	F98.8 Other specified behavioural and emotional disorders with onset usually occurring in childhood and adolescence
	F98.9 Unspecified behavioural and emotional disorders with onset usually occurring in childhood and adolescence

ADOLESCENCE

- Prevalence of psychiatric disorder = 10 to 20 per cent
- Male:female = approximately 1:1.5

Aetiology
In general the aetiology of psychiatric disorders in children and adolescents is multifactorial.

Assessment
The information to be obtained in a child psychiatric interview is shown in Table 34.2.

DEPRESSION

Depressive disorder occurs in 0.5 to 8 per cent of 14- to 15-year-olds. Compared with adults, depressive disorder in childhood and early adolescence is more likely to present with:

- running away from home
- ↓ school academic performance
- separation anxiety/school refusal
- somatic pain, particularly

    - head
    - abdominal
    - chest

- antisocial behaviour in males

SCHOOL REFUSAL

Definition
School refusal is refusal to attend or stay at school because of anxiety and in spite of parental or other pressure.

Epidemiology
SEX RATIO   Male = female.
INCIDENCE PEAKS   There are three main incidence peak ages:

- 5 years: separation anxiety
- 11 years: may be precipitated by the change from junior to secondary school
- 14–16 years: this may be a symptom of a psychiatric disorder

    - depressive disorder
    - a phobia (e.g. social phobia)

The most common presentation is the one at 11 years.

Differences from truancy
Truancy is an important differential diagnosis. Truancy differs from school refusal in that it is:

Table 34.2 Information to be amassed in a child psychiatric interview

Source and nature of referral
- Who made referral?
- Who initiated referral?
- Family attitudes to referral

Description of presenting complaints
- Onset, frequency, intensity, duration, location (home, school etc.)
- Antecedents and consequences
- Ameliorating and exacerbating factors
- Specific examples
- Parental and family beliefs about causation
- Past attempts to solve problem

Description of child's current general functioning
- School
    behaviour and emotions
    academic performance
    peer and staff relationships
- Peer relationships generally
- Family relationships

Personal/developmental history
- Pregnancy, labour, delivery
- Early developmental milestones
- Separations/disruptions
- Physical illnesses and their meaning for parents
- Reactions to school
- Puberty
- Temperamental style

Family history
- Personal and social histories of both parents especially
    history of mental illness
    their experience of being parented
- History of family development
    how parents came together
    history of pregnancies
    separations and effects on children
- Who lives at home currently
- Strengths/weaknesses of all at home
- Current social stresses and supports

Information from observation of family interaction:
structure, organization, communication, sensitivity

Information from observation of child at interview:
motor, sensory, speech, language, social relating skills

Mental state, concerns, and spontaneous account if age appropriate

Results of physical examination

Plan for future investigation and management

Reproduced with permission from Puri, B.K., Laking, P.J, and Treasaden, I.H. 1996: *Textbook of psychiatry.* Edinburgh: Churchill Livingstone.

- ego-syntonic and intended
- often accompanied by other antisocial symptoms
- more likely to be associated with a family history of antisocial behaviour
- more likely to be associated with poor academic school performance
- more likely to be associated with ↑ family size

Management

The mechanisms underlying the school refusal should be identified. If the condition is acute, a return to school should be arranged as soon as possible (the Kennedy approach), whereas, if the condition is chronic, a graded return to school should be arranged. Any specific problems (e.g. social phobia) should be treated. If the patient does not return to school, then inpatient treatment may be necessary.

Course and prognosis

Younger children have a better prognosis. Most children and adolescents do return to school, but approximately one-third of older patients seen in clinics develop neurotic difficulties or social impairment or social withdrawal in adulthood.

HYPERKINETIC DISORDERS

Diagnosis

The cardinal features are:

- impaired attention
- overactivity
- impulsivity

These should:

- occur in more than one environmental situation
- begin before the age of six years
- be of long duration

The diagnosis is made far more commonly in the United States than it is in Britain.

Differential diagnosis

The main differential diagnoses are:

- pervasive development disorders
- conduct disorder
- anxiety disorder

Epidemiology

POINT PREVALENCE 1.7 per cent
SEX RATIO   male > female
AGE   ↓ incidence with ↑ age
SOCIAL CIRCUMSTANCES   ↑ incidence with ↑ social adversity

Clinical features

In addition to impaired attention and overactivity, other associated features that may occur include:

- social disinhibition
- recklessness
- learning difficulties
- clumsiness

Aetiology

Possible causes that have been proposed include:

- brain abnormality
- genetic contribution
- dietary factors
- food allergy

Management
A full assessment, including psychometric testing, should be carried out. Behavioural managment approaches and pharmacotherapy with stimulants (methylphenidate or dexamphetamine) may be used (but beware side-effects). (Second-line drugs that are occasionally used include tricyclic antidepressants and haloperidol.)

Course and prognosis
With development, there is usually an improvement of restlessness and impaired attention. However, poor self-esteem may result from the disorder, leading in turn to the possibility of affecting the development of personality. The presence of other disorders, such as conduct disorder, leads to a worse prognosis.

CONDUCT DISORDERS

Diagnosis
According to ICD-10 conduct disorders are characterized by a repetitive and persistent pattern of dissocial, aggressive, or defiant conduct, which when at its most extreme, amounts to major violations of age-appropriate social expectations, and is therefore more severe than ordinary childish mischief of adolescent rebelliousness.

Differential diagnosis
Conduct disorder overlaps with hyperkinetic disorders and emotional disorders. In the former case, the diagnosis should be hyperkinetic disorder if the criteria for this are met, whereas in the latter case in ICD-10 a diagnosis should be made of mixed disorder of conduct and emotions.

Epidemiology
POINT PREVALENCE   Four per cent in 10- and 11-year-olds in the Isle of Wight study (higher in inner London); with aggressive components in 1.1 per cent.
SEX RATIO   male > female
AGE   Aggressive (rather than antisocial) symptoms are more common in younger children.

Clinical features
The antisocial behaviour may manifest in different ways, such as:

- temper tantrums: early and middle childhood
- oppositional defiant behaviour: older children

Aetiology
Possible causes that have been proposed include:

- life events
    - bereavement
    - parental divorce
    - separation from parents

- social

  - poor school
  - aberrant peer group
  - socially disadvantaged

- parental

  - rejection
  - inconsistency
  - punitiveness
  - negativism
  - modelling of aggression
  - failure to set rules
  - failure to monitor
  - maternal depression

- individual

  - anxiety
  - depression
  - difficult temperament
  - ↓ IQ
  - educational retardation
  - neurological impairment

Management

A full assessment should be carried out. Management strategies that may be employed include:

- behavioural management techniques
- cognitive therapy
- group therapy

Course and prognosis

Aggressive behaviour in middle childhood (but not that occurring in the pre-school years) is associated with later sociopathy, particularly if there is also poor academic achievement. Fifty per cent of highly antisocial children become anti-social adults. Of adult sociopaths:

- 60 per cent manifest highly antisocial behaviour as children
- another 30 per cent manifest moderately antisocial behaviour as children

ELECTIVE MUTISM

Diagnosis

According to ICD-10 elective mutism is characterized by a marked, emotionally determined selectivity in speaking, such that the child demonstrates their language competence in some situations but fails to speak in other (definable) ones.

Epidemiology

PREVALENCE   < 0.8 per 1000 children

SEX RATIO   male = female

AGE   Elective mutism usually manifests in early childhood.

Clinical features
In addition to the features given above, elective mutism tends to be associated with personality features such as:

- social anxiety
- withdrawal
- sensitivity
- resistance

Management
Management approaches include:

- exclude any speech abnormalities
- behavioural approaches
- use of tape recordings or the telephone
- play therapy
- art therapy
- family therapy

Prognosis
In general in the long-term the prognosis is good unless other disorders are also present.

TIC DISORDERS

Clinical features
Common simple motor tics include (ICD-10):

- eye-blinking
- neck-jerking
- shoulder-shrugging
- facial grimacing

Common simple vocal tics include (ICD-10):

- throat-clearing
- barking
- sniffing
- hissing

Common complex motor tics include (ICD-10):

- hitting one's self
- jumping
- hopping

Common compex vocal tics include (ICD-10):

- repeating certain words
- coprolalia
- palilalia

Epidemiology
GENERAL Ten to 24 per cent of children manifest tics during development.
TOURETTE'S SYNDROME (COMBINED VOCAL AND MULTIPLE MOTOR TIC DISORDER)

- Lifetime prevalence = 1.01–1.6 per cent

Table 34.3 Aetiology of tics

Family	Family clusters reported, especially Tourette's
	Prevalence of multiple tics in 14–24% of first-degree relatives of patients with Tourette's
	Increased family psychopathology in families of ticqueurs although may be cause or effect
Individual	No gross neurological abnormalities
	Increased incidence of 'soft' neurological signs and 'non-specific' EEG changes
	Some verbal – performance discrepancies in functioning
	Some neuroleptic medications effective in controlling tics
	Tics exacerbated by dopamine agonists
	Wide range of psychological mechanisms proposed for tic disorders, from the psychoanalytic to the classically behavioural
	Tic movement have been shown to mimic involuntary startle responses to sudden stimulus

Reproduced with permission from Puri, B.K., Laking, P.J. and Treasaden, I.H. 1996: *Textbook of psychiatry.* Edinburgh: Churchill Livingstone.

- Male: female $\simeq$ 2:1
- Average age of onset = 7 years (range 2 to 15 years)

Aetiology
The causes of tics are shown in Table 34.3

Management
Points in the management of tic disorders include:

- full assessment, including a physical and detailed neurological examination
- reassurance of the patient and family
- advise the family or other carers not to be annoyed or anxious at the occurrence of potentially embarrassing tics such as coprolalia
- liaise with the school
- psychological treatments

  - behavioural techniques such as massed practice
  - relaxation therapy
  - hypnotherapy

- pharmacotherapy (but beware side-effects)

  - haloperidol
  - pimozide
  - sulpiride
  - SSRIs

Course and prognosis
In most cases the tics disappear spontaneously within a few months. In a minority, however, there may be a progression from simple tics to Tourette's syndrome. One-third of cases of the latter present initially with vocal tics.

NONORGANIC ENURESIS

Diagnosis
According to ICD-10 nonorganic enuresis is characterized by the involuntary voiding of urine, by day and/or by night, which is abnormal in relation to the individual's mental age and which is not a consequence of a lack of bladder control resulting from any neurological disorder, epilepsy, or a structural urinary tract abnormality. It is generally not diagnosed before the age of five years, and may be subdivided into:

- primary: urinary continence never achieved
- secondary: urinary continence has been achieved in the past

Clinical features
Nonorganic enuresis may be associated with emotional problems, although it should be noted that the latter may be secondary to the enuresis itself.

Epidemiology
PREVALENCE   The prevalence at different ages has been found to be:

- 7 years: 6.7 per cent in boys and 3.3 per cent in girls
- 9–10 years: 2.9 per cent in boys and 2.2 per cent in girls
- 14 years: 1.1 per cent in boys and 0.5 per cent in girls

SEX RATIO

- Male:female = 1:1 at the age of five years; approximately 2:1 in adolescence
- Secondary enuresis is more common in boys

Aetiology
Possible causes that have been proposed include:

- genetic: 70 per cent have a first-degree relative with late attainment of continence
- stressful life events: doubling of frequency
- delayed toilet training
- developmental delay: twice as common in enuretic children as in controls
- bladder structure: enuretic children are more likely than non-enuretics to have a different shape of bladder baseplate and to have a reduced functional bladder volume

Management
Points in the management include:

- full assessment including a physical assessment to exclude a physical cause; look for evidence of

  - urinary frequency
  - haematuria
  - dysuria
  - urgency

- urinary microscopy and microbiological analysis
- observation period
- star chart: relapse rate of approximately 40 per cent
- pad and buzzer or, in older children, a pants alarm: relapse rate of approximately 40 per cent

- low-dose tricyclic antidepressants: but there are side-effects and there is a high rate of relapse on discontinuation; can be useful for short time periods, e.g. school trips
- nasal desmopressin: should not be continued for more than three months without stopping for a week for full reassessment
- exercises to increase the functional capacity of the bladder
- habit training

Prognosis
In general the prognosis is very good.

NONORGANIC ENCOPRESIS

Diagnosis
According to ICD-10 nonorganic encopresis is the repeated voluntary or non-voluntary passage of faeces, usually of normal or near-normal consistency, in places not appropriate for that purpose in the individual's own socioculture setting.
   It may be subdivided into:

- continuous encopresis: bowel control has never been achieved
- discontinuous encopresis: there has been a period of normal bowel control in the past

Clinical features
The presentation of this disorder is summarized in Table 34.4.

Table 34.4 Presentation of faecal soiling (encopresis)

Consistency of faeces	Normal, loose or constipated
Place deposited	In pants, hidden or in 'significant' places (e.g. in a particular person's cupboard)
Development	Never continent (continuous), after period of continence (discontinuous) or regression (in various contexts – see below)
Activity	Smearing, anal fingering, or masturbation
Context	Power battle, upsetting life events (e.g. sexual abuse, divorce) and/or other psychiatric disorder
Physical	With soreness, anal fissures etc., or with normal anus

Reproduced with permission from Puri, B.K., Laking, P.J. and Treasaden, I.H. 1996: *Textbook of psychiatry.* Edinburgh: Churchill Livingstone.

Epidemiology
PREVALENCE   At the age of five years, the prevalence is 1.5 per cent. In 12-year-olds, the Isle of Wight study found a prevalence of 1.3 per cent in boys and 0.3 per cent in girls.
SEX RATIO   Male: female = (3 to 4):1

Aetiology
Causes of nonorganic encopresis are shown in Table 34.5.

Table 34.5 Causes of encopresis

Congenital	Constitutional variability can include bowel control

Individual	Developmental delay
	Physical trigger
	  – anal fissure
	  – constipation (low-roughage diet)
	  – other bowel disorders

Parent–child	Coercive toilet training Emotional abuse or neglect 'Battleground' for relationship problems
Wider environment	Sexual abuse Family disharmony

Reproduced with permission from Puri, B.K., Laking, P.J. and Treasaden, I.H. 1996: *Textbook of psychiatry*. Edinburgh: Churchill Livingstone.

Management

Points in the management include:

- full assessment, but take care in carrying out an anal and rectal examination as informed consent is required from the child who may have been sexually abused (if there is evidence of sexual abuse, the appropriate procedures should be brought into play)
- assess famly relationships and the home circumstances
- educate the carers with respect to the mechanics of defaecation
- improve the child's self-esteem
- individual therapy
- family therapy
- pharmacotherapy to soften the stools or to promote gastrointestinal motility

If the above procedures fail, an intense behavioural programme in hospital may be required.

Prognosis

In general the prognosis is very good.

BIBLIOGRAPHY

Black, D. and Cottrell, D. (eds) 1993: *Seminars in child and adolescent psychiatry*. London: Gaskell.

Graham, P. 1986: *Child psychiatry: a development approach*. Oxford: Oxford University Press.

Hoare, P. 1993: *Essential child psychiatry*. Edinburgh: Churchill Livingstone.

Laking, P.J. 1996: Child and adolescent psychiatry. In Puri, B.K., Laking, P.J. and Treasaden, I.H. *Textbook of psychiatry*. Edinburgh: Churchill Livingstone.

35
Learning disability

CLASSIFICATION

Definition
ICD-10 defines mental retardation as being a condition of arrested or incomplete development of the mind, which is especially characterized by impairment of skills manifested during the developmental period, which contribute to the overall level of intelligence, i.e. cognitive, language, motor, and social abilities.

ICD-10 classification of mental retardation
Table 35.1 summarizes the ICD-10 classification of mental retardation:

Table 35.1 ICD-10 Diagnoses of mental retardation

F70	**Mild mental retardation** IQ range 50–69 Delayed understanding and use of language Possible difficulties in gaining independence Work in practical occupations Any behavioural, social and emotional difficulties are similar to the 'normal'
F71	**Moderate mental retardation** IQ range 35–49 Varying profiles of abilities Language use and development variable (may be absent) Often associated with epilepsy, neurological and other disability Delay in achievement of self-care Simple practical work Independent living rarely achieved
F72	**Severe mental retardation** IQ range 20–34 More marked motor impairment than F71 often found Achievements lower end of F71
F73	**Profound mental retardation** Severe limitation in ability to understand or comply with requests of instructions IQ difficult to measure but < 20 Little or no self-care Mostly severe mobility restriction Basic or simple tasks may be acquired (e.g. sorting and matching)

Disorder of psychological development

These disorders, which have an onset in infancy/childhood and a steady course, may cause disability in adulthood. The ICD-10 disorders of psychological development are:

Table 35.2 ICD-10 Diagnoses of Disorders of psychological development

---

F80 Specific developmental disorders of speech and language
  F80.0 Specific speech articulation disorder
  F80.1 Expressive language disorder
  F80.2 Receptive language disorder
  F80.3 Acquired aphasia with epilepsy [Landau–Kleffner syndrome]
  F80.8 Other developmental disorders of speech and language
  F80.9 Developmental disorder of speech and language, unspecified

F81 Specific developmental disorders of scholastic skills
  F81.0 Specific reading disorder
  F81.1 Specific spelling disorder
  F81.2 Specific disorder of arithmetical skills
  F81.3 Mixed disorder of scholastic skills
  F81.8 Other developmental disorders of scholastic skills
  F81.9 Developmental disorder of scholastic skills, unspecified

F82 Specific developmental disorder of motor function

F83 Mixed specific developmental disorders

F84 Pervasive developmental disorders
  F84.0 Childhood autism
  F84.1 Atypical autism
  F84.2 Rett's syndrome
  F84.3 Other childhood disintegrative disorder
  F84.4 Overactive disorder associated with mental retardation and stereotyped movements
  F84.5 Asperger's syndrome
  F84.8 Other pervasive developmental disorders
  F84.9 Pervasive developmental disorder, unspecified

F88 Other disorder of psychological development

F89 Unspecified disorder of psychological development

EPIDEMIOLOGY

Epidemiology of impairment

The prevalence of learning disability defined as having an IQ of less than 70 is 3.7 per cent, which is considerably higher than would be expected from the normal distribution of IQ. The levels of coexistence of different impairments is shown in Table 35.3:

Epidemiology of specific syndromes

The frequencies (per 1000 births) of common specific syndromes are:

- cerebral palsy: 2.2
- fetal alcohol syndrome: 1.6
- Down syndrome: 1.43
- fragile X syndrome: 0.92

Table 35.3 Levels of coexistence of different impairments

	Severe mental retardation (%)	Mild mental retardation (%)
Cerebral palsy	approx. 20	approx. 8
Epilepsy	30–37	12–18
Hydrocephalus	5–6	2
Severe visual impairment	6–10	1–9
Severe hearing impairment	3–15	2–7
One or more major impairments	40–52	24–30

- spina bifida: 0.6 to 3.0
- early infantile autism: 0.45
- phenylketonuria: 0.1
- Prader–Willi syndrome: 0.1
- Huntington's disease: 0.1

Psychiatric disorder
The Isle of Wight study (see Chapter 34) found the presence of:

- a physical disorder not affecting the brain → prevalence of psychiatric disorder ↑ 2×
- brain damage → prevalence of psychiatric disorder ↑ 5×
- brain damage + epilepsy → prevalence of psychiatric disorder ↑ 10×

CLINICAL FEATURES

Behavioural phenotypes
The associations of behaviour with specific syndromes are summarized in Table 35.4.

Challenging behaviours
Common challenging behaviours that occur are shown in Table 35.5.

Self-esteem
Low self-esteem is common in people with learning disabilities.

Family changes
Figure 35.1 shows the psychological processes that may occur in families having an impaired or disabled member.

Childhood autism (Kanner's syndrome)
This is characterized by the following triad:

- Poor or absent social interaction
- language and communication disorder
- restricted and repetitive behaviour

The abnormality is apparent before the age of three years, and there is a male to female ratio of 3–4 to 1. Clinical features include:

Table 35.4 Behavioural phenotypes: summary of associations of behaviour to specific syndromes

Angelman syndrome	Happy disposition; laughing at minimal provocation; handflapping; inquisitiveness
Down's syndrome	Common obsessionality and stubbornness; 25% have attention deficit disorder in childhood
Fragile X syndrome	Idiosyncratic linguistic and interpersonal styles; disagreement about whether close association with autism
Klinefelter's syndrome	Passive and compliant in childhood; aggressive and antisocial past puberty
Lesch–Nyhan syndrome	Compulsive severely mutilating self-injurious behaviour
Sanfilippo syndrome (a mucopolysaccharidosis)	Prominent sleep disorder
Noonan's syndrome	Common problems in peer-relations; stubbornness and perseverative behaviour
Prader–Willi syndrome	Insatiable appetite (diagnostic); sleep abnormalities; frequent temper tantrums; self-injury through skin picking
Rett syndrome	Reduced interest in play in early infancy followed by autistic-like symptoms; stereotypic hand movements; self-injury; anxiety and depression common
Tuberous sclerosis	75% autism, hyperactivity or both.

Table 35.5 Common challenging behaviours

Violence to self or others	Biting
	Hitting
	Spitting
	Headbanging
	Scratching
	Pinching
	Tantrums
	Property damage
Behaviours out of usual context	Shouting
	Undressing
	Running away
	Masturbation
	Urination
	Defecation
	Sexual behaviours towards others
	Vomiting
	Passivity and oppositional behaviour
Generally inappropriate behaviours	Rocking
	Flapping
	Stealing
	Kleptomania

- echolalia
- palilalia
- lack of social usage of language
- relative lack of creativity and fantasy in thoughts

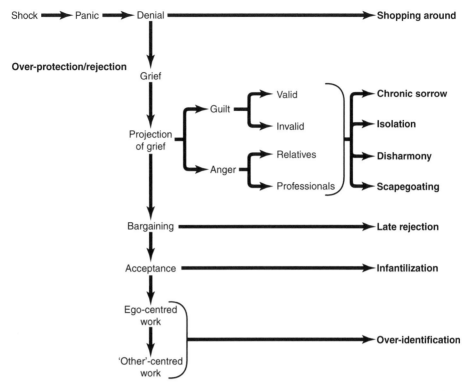

Figure 35.1 Psychological processes in families with an impaired or disabled member. (Reproduced, with permission, from Bicknell, J. 1983: The psychopathology of handicap. *British Journal of Medical Psychology* 56, 167–78.)

- poor eye contact
- lack of socioemotional reciprocity
- self-injury
- stereotyped behaviour
- epilepsy in adolescence
- resistance to change in routine
- attachments to unusual objects

Down syndrome

The clinical features of Down syndrome include:

- bradycephaly
- widely spaced eyes with epicanthic folds and oblique palpebral fissures
- Brushfield spots
- small nose and mouth
- horizontally furrowed tongue
- high arched palate
- malformed ears
- broadening and shortening of the neck and hands
- single transverse palmar crease
- curvature of the fifth finger
- an increased range of joint movements
- hypotonia
- ↑ incidence of cataract

- ↑ incidence of congenital cardiac disease
- ↑ incidence of umbilical herniae
- ↑ incidence of respiratory infections
- ↑ incidence of acute leukaemia
- IQ < 50 in approximately 85 per cent of cases

Fragile X syndrome

- elongated facies

  - oedema
  - tissue thickening
  - prognathism

- large everted ears
- single transverse palmar crease
- soft velvety skin
- large forehead
- blue eye colour
- high arched palate
- ↑ incidence of connective tissue disorders
- hyperextensible joints
- flat feet
- delay in language acquisition with cluttering speech
- learning disability
- mitral valve prolapse in 80 per cent
- macro-orchidism in 70 per cent postpubertally

AETIOLOGY

The causes of learning disability are summarized in Table 35.6.

Table 35.6 Aetiology of disability

Prenatal	Perinatal	Postnatal
Inborn errors of metabolism	Asphyxia/hypoxia at birth	Meningitis/encephalitis
Chromosomal abnormalities	Mechanical birth trauma	Head injury (accidental or inflicted)
Congenital infections (rubella, cytomegalavirus syphilis, HIV, toxoplasmosis)	Small babies Hyperbilirubinaemia (kernicterus)	Lead poisoning (and other heavy metals)
Irradiation	Hyperoxia (iatrogenic)	
	Hypoglycaemia	Malnutrition
Drugs (e.g. thalidomide)	Prematurity (intraventricular haemorrhage etc.)	Other infections (e.g. whooping cough)
Maternal alcohol intake		
Malnutrition, including vitamin deficiencies		Environmental chemicals

MANAGEMENT

The management of learning disability must be tailored to the individual case and may include:

- behavioural treatments
- family therapy
- modified individual psychotherapy
- modified group psychotherapy
- pharmacotherapy

    - for a diagnosed psychiatric disorder
    - for a challenging behaviour

BIBLIOGRAPHY

Clarke, A.M., Clarke, A.D.B and Berg, J.B. (eds) 1985: *Mental handicap: the changing outlook.* London: Methuen.
Laking, P.J. 1996: Psychiatry of disability. In Puri, B.K., Laking, P.J. and Treasaden, I.H. *Textbook of psychiatry.* Edinburgh: Churchill Livingstone.
Russell, O. 1985: *Mental handicap.* Edinburgh: Churchill Livingstone.

36
Eating disorders

ANOREXIA NERVOSA

ICD-10
This is characterized by deliberate weight loss resulting in undernutrition with secondary endocrine and metabolic disturbance.

It requires the presence of all the following:

(a) Body weight maintained at 15 per cent below expected; Quetelet's body mass index <17.5 kg m^{-2}.

Quetelet's body mass index $=$ mass(kg)/[height(m)]^2; age 16 or over

(b) Weight loss self-induced by the avoidance of fattening foods and one or more of the following: self-induced vomiting; self-induced purging; excessive exercise; the use of appetite suppressants and/or diuretics.

(c) Body-image distortion; a **specific psychopathology** comprising a dread of fatness which persists as an intrusive, over-valued idea. Low weight threshold is imposed on self.

(d) Amenorrhoea in women; loss of sexual interest and potency in men. Endocrine disorder of hypothalamus–pituitary–gonadal axis (HPA), elevated growth hormone and cortisol levels, abnormal peripheral metabolism of thyroid hormone and abnormalities of insulin secretion.

(e) If onset is prepubertal, the sequence of pubertal events delayed or arrested. Puberty is often completed with recovery, but menarche late.

DSM-IV
Diagnostic features

A. Individual refuses to maintain minimally normal body weight ($<$ 85 per cent normal weight)

B. Intense fear of gaining weight (loss of appetite rare)

C. Disturbance in perception of shape or size of body

D. Amenorrhoea i.e. absence of at least three consecutive menstrual cycles.

SUBTYPES Used to specify presence or absence of regular binge eating or purging during current episode.

RESTRICTING TYPE Weight loss accomplished through dieting, fasting, or excessive exercise.

BINGE EATING/PURGING TYPE Regular binge eating or purging (or both) during current episode. Most engage at least weekly. This group are more likely to have other impulse-control problems, abuse alcohol or drugs, exhibit mood lability, and be sexually active.

CLINICAL FEATURES OF ANOREXIA NERVOSA

- Morbid fear of fatness/excessive pursuit of thinness
- Denial of problem
- Distorted body image
- Fear of losing control of eating
- Problems with separation and independence
- Depressive feelings; insomnia, lack of concentration, irritability
- Suicidal ideas
- Obsessional thoughts and rituals which may improve with weight gain
- Preoccupation with thoughts of food. Enjoy cooking for others; do not like eating in public
- Withdrawn

PHYSICAL SIGNS AND COMPLICATIONS OF ANOREXIA NERVOSA

- Emaciation
- Slowed metabolic rate. Low blood pressure, slow pulse
- Lanugo
- Cardiac arrhythmias and failure
- Peripheral oedema
- Amenorrhoea/loss of libido
- Reproductive system atrophy, shrunken uterus and ovaries with cystic multi-follicular ovarian changes
- Osteoporosis from low calcium intake and absorption, reduced oestrogen and increased cortisol secretion. Bone pain and deformity. Bone density reduces with increasing years of amenorrhoea; pathological fractures after about 10 years
- Hypoglycemia
- Dehydration
- Hypothermia, cold intolerance
- Seizures
- Delayed gastric emptying
- Acute gastric dilatation
- Pancreatitis
- Tetany
- Degeneration of myenteric plexus of bowel. Cathartic colon. Constipation
- Reduced growth, delayed puberty
- Cardiac and skeletal muscle-wasting
- Purpura secondary to reduced collagen in skin and bone marrow suppression
- Mitral valve prolapse
- Proximal myopathy
- Impaired liver function
- Impaired renal function (caused by chronic dehydration and hypokalemia)
- Diffuse EEG abnormalities, reflecting metabolic encephalopathy, may result from fluid and electrolyte disturbances
- Brain imaging: increase in the ventricular: brain ratio secondary to starvation

SECONDARY TO REPEATED SELF-INDUCED VOMITING

- Erosion of tooth enamel
- Dental caries
- Parotid gland enlargement

COMMON BLOOD ABNORMALITIES

- Hypokalaemia (cardiac arrhythmias, cardiac arrest, renal damage)
- Hypoglycaemia
- Metabolic alkalosis
- Hypomagnaesemia
- Hypozincaemia
- Hypophosphataemia
- Raised serum amylase
- Hypercholesterolaemia
- Hypercarotaemia
- Leucopenia with relative lymphocytosis
- Normochromic normocytic anaemia
- Low T_3
- Raised cortisol and growth hormone
- Low plasma gonadotrophins and gonadal steroids; in females, low serum oestrogen, in males low serum testosterone
- 24–hour pattern of secretion of luteinizing hormone resembles that normally seen in the prepubertal

EPIDEMIOLOGY

Incidence and prevalence estimates vary depending on the diagnostic criteria used, and the population studied.

- Rare
- Prevalence about 1–2 per thousand women
- *Epidemiological Catchment Areas* study found only 11 cases in 20 000 persons studied
- Peak age 15–19 years
- Higher prevalence in higher socioeconomic classes; significant association with greater parental education; more common in Western Caucasians
- Rates in private schools 1 per cent much higher than in state schools 0.15 per cent; much higher again in ballet or modelling schools 7 per cent
- Suggestion of increasing prevalence over time probably not supported, although greater numbers are coming to the attention of services
- Incidence is 10 times higher in females compared to males

AETIOLOGY

Genetic
Family studies show increased incidence of eating disorders among first- and second-degree relatives of those suffering from anorexia nervosa.

Twin studies have shown higher concordance rates for monozygotic than for dizygotic twins. Holland *et al.* (1988) found MZ:DZ concordance ratio of 56:5.

Five per cent of first-degree relatives are affected. This suggests that genetic factors are significant in aetiology. This study suggested 80 per cent of variance in liability to anorexia nervosa was genetic.

Walters and Kendler (1995) in a population-based twin study found higher concordance rates among DZ twins than among MZ twins.

Data suggest a familial component to anorexia nervosa, but very low prevalence in the general population has prevented discrimination of whether this is genetic or environmental.

There is an increased risk of mood disorders among first-degree biological relatives, particularly of those with binge eating/purging type. The morbid risk of affective disorder in families of eating disordered is similar to that of families of bipolar probands, and is significantly greater than that in families of schizophrenics or the borderline personality disordered. This supports growing evidence that anorexia nervosa and bulimia nervosa are closely related to affective disorder.

Environmental

Non-genetic factors are thought to play a crucial role in the aetiology of anorexia nervosa.

FAMILY   Minuchin *et al.* (1978) found that relationships in families of anorexics are characterized by overprotection and enmeshment. Kendler found that a typical anorexic came from an inward, often overprotected and highly controlled family.

Higher rates of childhood sexual abuse are reported by eating disordered patients than controls. Childhood sexual abuse appears to be a vulnerability factor for psychiatric disorder in general, not for eating disorders in particular.

SOCIOCULTURAL   There is a cult of thinness.

Anorexic and bulimic women viewing fashion images of women show a 25 per cent increase in their body size estimation afterwards. The media presentation of idealized women are likely to have some effect upon eating disordered subjects, overestimation of their body size. Among 15-year-old schoolgirls the relative risk of developing anorexia nervosa was eight times greater in those who dieted compared to those who did not in a prospective study.

Immigrants from low-prevalence to high-prevalence cultures may develop anorexia nervosa as thin-body ideals are assimilated. Cultural factors influence the manifestation of the disorder: in some cultures, for example, body-image disturbance may not be prominent and the expressed motivation for food restriction may have a different content, such as epigastric discomfort or distaste for food.

PHYSICAL ILLNESS   An excess of physical illness in childhood has been found in those with anorexia nervosa. Physical illness may be a risk factor for the later development of anorexia nervosa, possibly by inducing pathology in the family dynamics.

Cases of anorexia nervosa have been reported with onset immediately related to a glandular fever-like illness. The disruption of the central CRH regulation has been suggested as the mediator of this.

Psychological

Psychodynamic theories: fantasies of oral impregnation. Dependent relationships with passive father, guilt over aggression toward ambivalently regarded mother.

Operant conditioning: phobic avoidance of food resulting from sexual and social tensions generated by physical changes associated with puberty.

Personality

Anorexics have a high prevalence of defined personality disorders and an excess of obsessive, inhibited and impulsive traits. It is suggested that in an environment that emphasizes thinness as a criterion for self-worth, vulnerable individuals cope with the challenges of adolescence by repetitive reward-seeking behaviour.

Braun *et al.* (1994) found that 69 per cent of eating disordered patients have at least one personality disorder; these are also more likely to have affective disorder or substance dependence than those without personality disorder.

Anorexics are more likely to suffer from anxious-avoidant personality disorders (cluster C) whereas dramatic-erratic personality disorders (cluster B) are more common in bulimics.

Neurotransmitters

Brain serotonin systems are implicated in the modulation of appetite, mood, personality variables and neuroendocrine function. An increase in intrasynaptic serotonin reduces food consumption; a reduction in serotonin activity increases food consumption and promotes weight gain.

Kaye et al. (1991) found increased CSF concentrations of major serotonin metabolite 5-HIAA in long-term weight-restored anorectics, which may indicate an increased serotonin activity contributing to pathological feeding behaviour.

It has been suggested that amenorrhoea is caused by primary hypothalamic dysfunction. This is supported by the fact that a return to normal menstruation lags behind the return of body weight, and amenorrhoea sometimes precedes weight loss. This, however, is not proven.

Amenorrhea is caused by abnormally low levels of estrogen, because of the diminished pituitary secretion of follicle-stimulating hormone [FSH] and luteinizing hormone [LH]. This is usually a consequence of weight loss but, in a minority of individuals, it may actually precede it. In prepubertal females, menarche may be delayed.

MANAGEMENT

Weight restoration and psychotherapy are the main treatments.

If very emaciated, inpatient care may be necessary because of physical danger. Full physical assessment is required, including electrolytes.

Nursing support is important.

There is slowed gastric emptying; meals must be introduced slowly to reduce the risks of gastric dilatation or rupture. If the patient is very emaciated, liquid feeds may be better initially. Gradually build up from 1000 to 3500 kcal per day.

Aim for one, and not more than two kilograms weight gain per week.

While emaciated the initial aim of therapy is weight gain. Psychotherapy at this stage is difficult; wait until the weight has ceased to be dangerously low.

Premorbid weight or weight at which periods stopped plus five kilograms are guides to healthy weight.

There may be reduced circulating oestrogens; shrunken uterus, small amorphous ovaries. As weight is gained, the uterus increases in size and the ovaries become multifollicular. At normal weight the ovaries become follicular; this is detected by pelvic ultrasound. It is used to indicate correct weight.

Psychotherapy

Family therapy is the treatment of choice particularly in young restricting anorexics (age < 22), with a duration of illness < 4 years. Therapy is directive, and parents are encouraged to take control of eating. Work also covers issues of individuation and separation.

Parental counselling also effective.

For older anorexics cognitive behavioural therapy is the treatment of choice.

Pharmacotherapy
Chlorpromazine is sometimes used to promote weight gain. Beware of postural hypotension, arrhythmias and hypothermia.

Differential diagnosis
Other causes of weight loss should be considered, especially when presenting features are atypical (e.g. an onset of illness after the age of 40).

In medical conditions (e.g. gastrointestinal disease, brain tumours, occult malignancies, and acquired immunodeficiency syndrome (AIDS), serious weight loss may occur; individuals do have a distorted body image or a desire for futher weight loss.

Superior mesenteric artery syndrome (postprandial vomiting is secondary to intermittent gastric outlet obstruction) should be distinguished from anorexia nervosa, although it may develop in anorexia nervosa because of emaciation.

Depressives do not have a desire for excessive weight loss or excessive fear of gaining weight.

Schizophrencies may exhibit odd eating behaviour and occasionally weight loss; they rarely fear weight gain or have body-image distrubance.

PROGNOSIS

The course and outcome are variable. Some patients recover fully after a single episode; some exhibit fluctuating patterns of weight gain followed by a relapse; others experience a chronically deteriorating course of the illness over many years.

It is a serious disorder with substantial mortality.

Hsu *et al.* (1979) in a four-to-eight-year follow-up of 100 cases of severe anorexia nervosa treated at a specialist centre found 48 had good outcome, 30 intermediate, 20 poor and two had died of inanition.

Poor outcome is associated with a longer duration of illness, an older age of onset and presentation, lower weight at onset and at presentation, the presence of bulimia, anxiety when eating with others, vomiting, poor childhood social adjustment and poor parental relationships. The more intractable the illness, the poorer the outcome.

Sullivan (1995) found that the aggregate mortality rate for anorexia nervosa is 5.6 per cent per decade. This is 12 times the annual death rate due to all causes for females aged 15–24. The aggregate mortality rate for anorexia nervosa is substantially greater than that reported for psychiatric inpatients and the general population.

The causes of death were complications of eating disorder in 54 per cent and suicide in 27 per cent. Suicide rates are 200 times greater than in the general population.

BULIMIA NERVOSA

ICD-10
This includes repeated bouts of overeating, excessive preoccupation with the control of body weight leading to extreme measures to mitigate against the fattening effects of food. It shares the same **specific psychopathology** of fear of fatness as anorexia nervosa.

ICD-10 requires all of the following:

(a) Persistent preoccupation with eating and an irresistable craving for food. Episodes of overeating in which large amounts of food are consumed in short periods of time

(b) Attempts to counteract the fattening effects of food by one or more of the following: self-induced vomiting; purgative abuse; alternating periods of starvation; use of drugs (appetite suppressants, thyroid preparations, diuretics). Diabetic bulimics may neglect insulin treatment

(c) Morbid dread of fatness. Patient sets weight threshold well below healthy weight. Often there is a history previously of anorexia nervosa.

DSM-IV
DIAGNOSTIC FEATURES

A. Recurrent episodes of binge eating, characterized by the following

   1   eating, in a discrete period of time (e.g. within any two-hour period), an amount of food that is definitely larger than most people would eat during a similar period of time and under similar circumstances
   2   a sense of lack of control over eating during the episode

B. Recurrent inappropriate behaviour to prevent weight gain e.g. self-induced vomiting; misuse of laxatives, diuretics, enemas, or other medications; fasting; or excessive exercise

C. Binge eating and inappropriate compensatory behaviours both occur, on average, at least twice a week for three months

D. Self-evaluation unduly influenced by body shape and weight

E. Disturbance does not occur exclusively during episodes of anorexia nervosa

SUB-TYPES

Purging type   Regularly self-induced vomiting or misuse of laxatives, diuretics, or enemas during current episode.

Nonpurging type   Has used inappropriate compensatory behaviours, such as fasting or excessive exercise, but has not regularly engaged in self-induced vomiting or the misuse of laxatives, diuretics, or enemas during the current episode.

Binge-eating disorder

Recurrent episodes of binge eating in the abscence of the regular use of inappropriate compensatory behaviours characteristic of bulimia nervosa.

CLINICAL FEATURES OF BULIMIA NERVOSA

- Morbid fear of fatness
- Distorted body image; overconcern with shape and weight
- Overwhelming urge to overeat with subsequent guilt and disgust
- Self-induced vomiting (90 per cent); use fingers, later reflex vomiting. Results in relief from physical discomfort and reduction of fear of gaining weight
- Laxative abuse (30 per cent), excessive exercise and food restriction
- Depression, irritability, poor concentration, suicidal ideas
- Older than the anorectic, more socially competent and sexually experienced
- May be normal weight, slightly underweight or overweight
- Menstrual abnormalities occur in < 50 per cent

- More insight than anorexia nervosa, often eager for help
- Majority have depressive symptoms, anxiety, impulsive and compulsive behaviours and problems with interpersonal relationships. Stealing and dependence upon substances is common

There is also a high prevalence of depression; self-mutilation; attempted suicide; substance abuse and low self-esteem.

PHYSICAL SIGNS AND COMPLICATIONS OF BULIMIA NERVOSA
Related to vomiting

- Dental erosion; toothache
- Parotid gland enlargement
- Callouses on backs of hands: **Russell's sign**
- Oedema
- Conjunctival haemorrhages caused by raised intrathoracic pressure
- Oesophageal tears
- Ipecacuanha intoxication causing cardiomyapathy and cardiac failure, usually fatal

Related to purgative abuse

- Rectal prolapse
- Constipation
- Diarrhoea
- Cathartic colon, damaged myenteric plexus.

Related to binges Acute dilatation of stomach (medical emergency).
Common biochemical abnormalities

- Hypokalaemic alkalosis
- Raised serum bicarbonate
- Hypokalaemia: direct potassium loss from vomiting, indirect renal loss in response to raised aldosterone secondary to volume depletion
- Hypochloraemia
- Hypomagnesaemia
- Metabolic acidosis with reduced serum bicarbonate in those abusing laxatives
- Raised serum amylase (salivary isoenzyme). Monitoring serum amylase can be used to monitor vomiting behaviour

Electrolyte disturbances can cause weakness, lethargy, arrhythmias and cardiac arrest.

EPIDEMIOLOGY

- Prevalence among adolescent and young adult females is approximately 1–3 per cent
- Lifetime prevalence for strictly defined bulimia nervosa is 1.1 per cent in females and 0.1 per cent in males
- MZ:DZ concordance rates 23:9. Kendler *et al.* (1991) estimates heritability of liability to bulimia nervosa of 50 per cent
- Social class distribution more even than anorexia nervosa
- Average age of onset 18, slightly older than anorectics
- Female to male ratio 10:1

- Reported more frequently in Caucasians in Western Europe, North America and Australasia
- Reports of increasing prevalence with time

AETIOLOGY

Genetic
MZ:DZ concordance for narrowly defined bulimia nervosa 23:9.

Neurotransmitters
Many abnormalities in eating disorders are secondary to dieting, weight loss, and binge/purge behaviour.

Serotonin is involved in the mediation of satiety responses to feeding as well as the regulation of mood, anxiety and impulsive behaviour. There is evidence in normal weight bulimics of altered **post-synaptic** $5HT_{1c}$ receptor sensitivity, depression associated with dysregulation of **pre-synaptic** 5HT function.

There is further support for the 5HT dysregulation hypothesis from findings that CSF concentrations of the serotonin metabolite 5HIAA and dopamine metabolite HVA are inversely correlated with a frequency of binge eating in the month prior to admission.

β-endorphin concentration in CSF of bulimics is significantly reduced, possibly related to the chronic activation of HPA axis secondary to dieting.

Cholecystokinin-8 (CCK-8) is involved in regulating satiety and anxiety. It is dependent upon an intact 5HT function. Bulimics have lower CSF CCK-8 concentrations than controls. A central, but not peripheral CCK dysfunction is implicated in bulimia nervosa.

Arginine-vasopressin (AVP) CSF concentrations are high in bulimics. An increased central AVP may be related to obsessive preoccupation with the aversive consequences of eating and weight gain. It also interacts with 5HT.

There is a general reduction of sympathetic responsivity and activation of HPA activity in bulimia nervosa, probably as a result of long-term neuroendocrine adaptation to caloric restriction.

Environment
Prior to onset bulimics are more likely to be overweight than their peers.

Rigid dieting is the most common precipitant of binge eating. Gross bingeing is the most common precipitant for self-induced vomiting. Dieting may affect appetite and satiety mechanisms. Second World War veterans who had been prisoners of war and suffered weight loss report more binge eating afterwards than veterans who had not been prisoners. Data is supportive of an aetiological role for eating restraint in promotion of bingeing.

Many normal weight bulimics are the eldest or only daughters. Lacey *et al.* (1991) postulates at times of parental marital discord the mother can use her daughter as an easily available therapist, burdening the child at an age when she cannot deal with the expressed emotions.

Bulimics report more sexual abuse in childhood than controls.

Personality
Personality disturbance is more common in patients with eating disorders than in the general population. On the Eysenck Personality Inventory bulimics score higher for psychoticism and neuroticism than anorexics and controls. On MMPI bulimics have elevated scores for psychopathic deviance.

Low self-esteem, low paternal care, external locus of control and high neuroticism scores are risk factors for bulimia.

Bulimics are more likely than anorexics to abuse substances (20 per cent). Lifetime rates of alcohol dependence are high.

The prevalence of social phobia in eating-disordered subjects, especially in bulimics, far exceeds the general population.

Bulimics have high rates (40 per cent) of major depression. There is significant comorbidity between anorexia and bulimia.

MANAGEMENT

Psychotherapy
Freeman *et al.* (1988) conducted a controlled trial of psychotherapy. The controls were significantly worse than all treatment groups at the end of the trial. Behavioural, cognitive-behavioural and group therapy were all effective; 77 per cent stop bingeing. Improvements are maintained at one year. Behavioural therapy is the most effective: lowest drop-out rate and earlier onset of action. There is no advantage in adding a cognitive element.

Psychotherapy produces a wider range of changes with more stable maintenance than drug therapy.

BEHAVIOURAL THERAPY   This aims to stop bingeing and purging by restricting exposure cues that trigger binge/purge behaviour, developing alternative behaviours and delaying vomiting.

COGNITIVE–BEHAVIOURAL THERAPY   This includes psychoeducation, self-monitoring and cognitive restructuring. Eating regular meals is very important.

Pharmacotherapy
Imipramine, phenelzine, amitriptyline, nortriptyline, desipramine and fluoxetine are all superior to placebo in double-blind controlled trials. The dose required is similar to the antidepressant dose. There is a 50–70 per cent reduction in bingeing. The magnitude of the change is smaller than with psychotherapy.

Lithium, anticonvulsants, serotonin promoters and opiate antagonists have all been used successfully.

Cognitive and/or behavioural therapies are the treatment of choice. Antidepressants alone are not adequate.

Differential diagnosis
In certain medical conditions, such as the Kleine–Levin syndrome, there is distrubed eating behaviour, but characteristic psychological features, such as overconcern with body shape and weight, are not present.

Overeating is common in atypical depression, but do not engage in inappropriate compensatory behaviour or exhibit overconcern with body shape and weight.

Binge eating is included in the impulsive behaviour criterion that is part of the DSM-IV definition of borderline personality disorder. If full criteria for both disorders are met, both diagnoses are given.

PROGNOSIS

The outcome for bulimia nervosa improves with time. The majority of patients make a full recovery or suffer only moderate abnormalities in eating attitudes after ten years.

There is comorbidity with depression, and prominent anoretic features increases the likelihood of a poor response.

In a 10-year follow-up of treated bulimics: 52 per cent recovered fully; 39 per cent continued to suffer some symptoms; 9 per cent continued to suffer full syndrome.

Predictors of favourable outcome:

- younger age at onset
- higher social class
- family history of alcohol abuse

Bulimics with multi-impulsive personality disorder do less well than those with bulimia alone.

BIBLIOGRAPHY

Braun, D.L., Sunday, S.R. and Halmi, K.A. 1994: Psychiatric comorbidity in patients with eating disorders. *Psychological Medicine* 24, 859–67.

Brewerton, T.D. and Ballenger, J.C. 1994: Biological correlates of eating disorders. *Current Opinion in Psychiatry* 7, 150–53.

Collings, S. and King, M. 1994: Ten-year follow-up of 50 patients with bulimia nervosa. *British Journal of Psychiatry* 164, 80–7.

Fahy, T.A., Eisler, I. and Russell, G.F.M. 1993: Personality disorder and treatment response in bulimia nervosa. *British Journal of Psychiatry* 162, 765–70.

Fairburn, C.G. 1993: Eating disorders. In Kendell, R.E. and Zealley, A.K. (eds), *Companion to psychiatric studies*. Edinburgh: Churchill Livingstone.

Fombonne, E. 1995: Anorexia nervosa: no evidence of an increase. *British Journal of Psychiatry* 166, 462–71.

Freeman, C.P.L., Barry, F., Dunkeld Turnbull, J. *et al.* 1988: Controlled trial of psychotherapy for bulimia nervosa. *British Medical Journal* 296, 521–5.

Garfinkel, P.E., Lin, E., Goering, P. *et al.* 1995: Bulimia nervosa in a Canadian community sample: prevalence and comparison of subgroups. *American Journal of Psychiatry* 152, 1052–8.

Hamilton, K. and Waller, G. 1993: Media influences on body size estimation in anorexia and bulimia: an experimental study. *British Journal of Psychiatry* 162, 837–40.

Holland, A.J., Sicotte, N. and Treasure, J.L. 1988: Anorexia nervosa: evidence for a genetic basis. *Journal of Psychosomatic Research* 32, 561–71.

Hsu, L.K.G., Crisp, A.H. and Harding, B. 1979: Outcome of anorexia nervosa. *The Lancet* i, 61–5.

Hudson, J., Pope, H.G., Jenas, J.M. *et al.* 1983: Family history of anorexia nervosa and bulimia nervosa. *British Journal of Psychiatry* 142, 133–8.

Kaye, W.H., Gwirtsman, H.E., George, D.T. *et al.* 1991: Altered serotonin activity in anorexia nervosa after long-term weight restoration. *Archives of General Psychiatry* 48, 556–62.

Kendler, K.S., Maclean, C., Neale, M. *et al.* 1991: The genetic epidemiology of bulimia nervosa. *American Journal of Psychiatry* 148 1627–37.

Lacey, H.J., Gowers, S.G. and Bhat, A.V. 1991: Bulimia nervosa: family size, sibling sex and birth order. A catchment area study. *British Journal of Psychiatry* 158, 491–4.

Minuchin, S., Rosman, B.C. and Baker, L. 1978: *Psychosomatic families: anorexia nervosa in context*. Cambridge, Mass.: Harvard University Press.

Palmer, R.L. and Robertson, D.N. 1995: Outcome in anorexia nervosa and bulimia nervosa. *Current Opinion in Psychiatry* 8, 90–2.

Park, R.J., Lawrie, S.M. and Freeman, C.P. 1995: Post-viral onset of anorexia nervosa. *British Journal of Psychiatry* 166, 386–9.

Patton, G.C., Johnson-Sabine, E., Wood, K. *et al.* 1990: Abnormal eating attitudes in London schoolgirls – a prospective epidemiological study: outcome at twelve months follow-up. *Psychological Medicine* 20, 383–94.

Patton, G.C., Wood, K. and Johnson-Sabine, E. 1986: Physical illness and anorexia nervosa. *British Journal of Psychiatry* 149, 756–9.

Robins, L.N. and Regier, D.A. (eds) 1991: *Psychiatric disorders in America: the Epidemiologic Catchment Area Study*. New York: The Free Press.

Sohlberg, S. and Strober, M. 1994: Personality in anorexia nervosa: An update and a theoretical integration. *Acta Psychiatrica Scandinavica* 89 (suppl. 378), 1–15.

Sullivan, P.F. 1995: Mortality in anorexia nervosa. *American Journal of Psychiatry* 152, 1073–4.

Vize, C.M. and Cooper, P.J. 1995: Sexual abuse in patients with eating disorders, patients with depression and normal controls: a comparative study. *British Journal of Psychiatry* 167, 80–5.

Walters, E.E. and Kendler, K.S. 1995: Anorexia nervosa and anorexia-like syndromes in a population-based female twin sample. *American Journal of Psychiatry* 152, 64–71.

37
Cross-cultural psychiatry

INTERNATIONAL

CULTURE   This is the learned way of life of a group of people bound together by a common social heritage. People of the same cultural group behave, think and give meaning to life in a similar way, and share a set of values and beliefs.

Schizophrenia

Kraepelin delineated dementia praecox and manic depression. In 1904 he visited the asylum of Buitenzorg in Java to examine the similarities and differences between European patients and those from another culture. He was satisfied that he could recognize cases of dementia praecox in Java, giving credence to his diagnostic distinction. This represents one of the first investigations in transcultural psychiatry.

THE *INTERNATIONAL PILOT STUDY OF SCHIZOPHRENIA* (IPSS): WHO 1973   This study was devised to determine whether schizophrenia could be recognized as the same condition in a wide variety of cultural settings. Nine centres (Columbia, Czechoslovakia, Denmark, India, Nigeria, Russia, Taiwan, the UK and the USA) participated. The Present State Examination was translated into seven languages, and psychiatrists trained in its use interviewed 1200 patients. Diagnoses were then generated using the computer program CATEGO.

Main findings:

- When narrow criteria of Schneider's first rank symptoms were applied, an incidence of schizophrenia was found which did not differ significantly across cultural settings. Therefore schizophrenia is recognizable as the same condition across a wide variety of cultures.
- Broadly defined, schizophrenia has an incidence which differs significantly from one country to another.
- The outcome of schizophrenia was found to vary inversely with the social development of the society. Those from developing countries had a better prognosis than those from the developed world.

DETERMINANTS OF OUTCOME STUDY (SARTORIUS *ET AL.* 1986)   This study extended its case-finding techniques to include rural primary healthcare centres, traditional healers, police stations, and prisons as well as the more conventional psychiatric settings. More than 1300 cases were interviewed in 12 centres across 10 countries.

Main findings:

- The incidence of narrowly defined schizophrenia was stable across a wide range of cultures, climates and ethnic groups, confirming findings of the IPSS.

The form of presentation of schizophrenia varied across cultures:

- Catatonic schizophrenia is a common form of presentation in the under-developed world, but has become much rarer in the West. Catatonia present in 10 per cent of cases in developing countries but in only a handful of those in developed countries.
- Hebephrenic schizophrenia was diagnosed in 13 per cent of cases from developed countries, but in only 4 per cent of cases from developing countries.
- In developing countries acute schizophrenia was diagnosed more often than in developed countries.

To identify the cause of the good prognosis for schizophrenia in the less-developed world, Leff *et al.* (1990) determined the levels of expressed emotion (EE) in a subsample of the Chandigarh cohort of first contact schizophrenic patients from the WHO determinants of the outcome study. At one-year follow-up a dramatic reduction had occurred in each of the EE components. No rural relative was rated as high EE at follow-up. It is concluded that the better outcome of this cohort of schizophrenic patients is partly attributable to tolerance and acceptance by family members.

Neurosis
Using standardized interviewing and case-finding techniques, the prevalence rates for neurosis in developing countries are comparable with or higher than those found in the West, contrary to what was previously believed.

In many Third World countries, hysteria represents a high proportion of psychiatric practice. In the West there has been a substantial decrease in the numbers of patients with hysteria, and a compensatory rise in the incidence of anxiety and depression. It is suggested that this can be seen as a shift from a somatic to a psychological mode of communication of emotional distress. The tendency to express distress in a psychological form is associated with higher social class and education. Catatonia could similarly be viewed as a non-verbal manifestation of schizophrenia.

Orley and Wing (1979) investigated the rates of psychiatric illness in two villages in East and West Africa. The rates of depression and anxiety showed large differences between East and West Africa (22 per cent and 10 per cent respectively). Compared to rates in Western countries (10–12 per cent) these rates are high. Communities in the developed and undeveloped world are heterogeneous, a point emphasized by the 'new cross-cultural psychiatry'.

In comparing the psychopathology of Jewish and gentile East London depressives, hypochondriasis and tension are much more common in the Jewish group, whereas guilt is more common in the gentiles. Guilt is culturally determined and more common in Christians.

Somatic symptoms of depression appear to be universal, but the concept of depression of mood is not recognized in all cultures; many cultures do not have the language to express the feeling of depression as described in the West. Instead such terms as 'sinking heart' or 'soul loss' are found. In China 87 per cent of people suffering from neurasthenia fulfil the criteria for major depression and respond to treatment with antidepressants.

THE 'NEW CROSS-CULTURAL PSYCHIATRY'   Kleinman (1977) described the 'new cross-cultural psychiatry'. He criticized as a **category fallacy** the assumption that Western diagnostic categories were themselves culture-free entities.

Anthropologists have criticized the older transcultural epidemiological research for imposing Western concepts of psychopathology on non-Western people.

These studies have also been criticized on the grounds of translation difficulties, the poor quality of questionnaire-generated diagnosis, a disregard for various understandings of the self, and for ignoring the cultural variation for broadly defined illness.

Beliefs about the mechanisms of illness among people in the underdeveloped world have been divided into three main ideas:

- **Object intrusion**: illness caused by a physical object being intruded into the patient's body
- **Spirit intrusion**: a spirit is believed to take possession of the patient's body
- **Soul loss**: the soul of the patient is believed to have been stolen by spirits

TRANSLATION AND VALIDITY OF RATING SCALES   In the translation of rating scales five kinds of problem in validity arise:

1   **Content validity**: the content of instruments must be relevant in the culture into which the instrument is translated. e.g. coca paste abuse is common in Peru, so the substance-abuse schedule should reflect this
2   **Semantic validity**: words used in the original and new instruments must have the same meaning
3   **Technical validity**: where languages are not written or illiteracy rates are high, answering a questionnaire may elicit answers that represent a misunderstanding of the intention
4   **Criterion validity**: whether responses to similar items measure the same concept in two cultures, e.g. in American Indians hallucinations normally occur during the course of bereavement, but this is not the case in North Americans generally; this must thus be accommodated
5   **Conceptual validity**: requires that responses relate to a theoretical construct within the culture

CLASSIFICATORY SYSTEMS   Europe and North America have greatly influenced the models of mental illness and the classification of mental illness over the last century. ICD-10 has been criticized in cross-cultural terms. The international group of psychiatrists involved in drawing up the first draft consisted of 47, only two of whom were from Africa. Thus conditions encountered in many other cultures which do not resemble Western categories have been assigned the title 'culture bound' conditions, or 'masked' representations of 'real' illness.

Culture-bound syndromes

Debate exists about what constitutes a culture-bound syndrome. The term is used to describe disorders which are considered unique to a given culture (cultural determinist view). However, the question of whether the classically described 'culture-bound syndromes' are actually unique to the given culture, or are in fact universal phenomena merely influenced by culture (universalist view), has not been settled.

The following syndromes are frequently cited:

AMOK   Occurring in Malays, it consists of a period of withdrawal, followed by a sudden outburst of homicidal aggression in which the sufferer will attack anyone within reach. The attack typically lasts for several hours until the sufferer is overwhelmed or killed. If alive, they typically pass into a deep sleep or stupor for several days, followed by amnesia for the event. It almost always occurs in men.

It was first described in Malays in the mid-16th century. It is believed to have originated in the cultural training for warfare among Malay warriors. Later it became a personal act by an isolated individual, apparently motiveless, but the motive could be understood as the restoration of self-esteem or 'face'.

It was very common in Malaya at the beginning of the nineteenth century, but the incidence was reduced when the British took over the administration of Malaya. Today it has virtually disappeared.

It is most common in Malays, but reports of amok from other countries exist, questioning its position as a culture-bound syndrome; it is clear, however, that there is a strong cultural element.

Among Malay cases in mental hospitals, the most common diagnosis is schizophrenia. Depression, acute brain syndrome and hysterical dissociation have also been found in some cases. The majority do not have a mental illness. Attacks are often preceded by interpersonal discord, insults or personal loss, and social drinking.

KORO This is common in south-east Asia and China; it may occur in epidemic form. It involves the belief of genital retraction with disappearance into the abdomen, accompanied by intense anxiety and the fear of impending death.

Cases of a similar condition have been described in non-Chinese subjects. In these cases the syndrome is often only partial, such as the belief of genital shrinkage, not necessarily with retraction into the abdomen; it usually occurs within the context of another psychiatric disorder and resolves once the underlying illness has been treated.

Debate about the cultural specificity of this disorder continues. Some argue that the culturally determined syndrome is clearly different to the symptom of genital retraction occurring in some non-Chinese psychotic subjects.

The development of koro has been associated with psychosexual conflicts, personality factors and cultural beliefs in the context of psychological stress.

DHAT This is commonly recognized in Indian culture, and is also widespread in Nepal, Sri Lanka, Bangladesh and Pakistan. It includes vague somatic symptoms (fatigue, weakness, anxiety, loss of appetite, guilt, etc.) and sometimes sexual dysfunction (impotence or premature ejaculation) which the subject attributes to the passing of semen in urine as a consequence of excessive indulgence in masturbation or intercourse.

Patients are typically from a rural area, from a family with conservative attitudes towards sex and of average or low socioeconomic status. Literacy and religion are unimportant.

Bhatia and Malik (1991) studied male patients attending a sexual problems clinic in New Delhi. They found that 65 per cent arrived with a primary complaint of Dhat syndrome. Twenty-three per cent of these also complained of impotence or premature ejaculation. The age of presentation is early twenties, with half unmarried. Most are literate. Although some suffered from depression and anxiety, those with Dhat syndrome differed from the others only in the relative absence of depression and anxiety. Treatment with anti-anxiety or antidepressant drugs resulted in significant improvement, however.

Dhat syndrome is considered by many to be a true culture-bound condition. The belief in the precious properties of semen is ingrained in Indian culture.

WINDIGO This is described in North American Indians, and ascribed to depression, schizophrenia, hysteria or anxiety. It is a disorder in which the subject believes they have undergone a transformation and become a monster who practises cannibalism. However, it has been suggested that windigo is in fact a local myth rather than an actual pattern of behaviour.

LATAH This usually begins after a sudden frightening experience in Malay women. It is characterized by a response to minimal stimuli with exaggerated startles, coprolalia, echolalia, echopraxia and automatic obedience. It has been suggested that this is merely one form of what is known to psychologists as the 'hyperstartle reaction' and is universally found.

PIBLOKTO   This dissociative state is seen among Eskimo women. The patient tears off her clothing, screams and cries and runs about wildly, endangering her life by exposure to the cold. It may result in suicidal or homicidal behaviour.

BRAIN FAG SYNDROME   This is a widespread low-grade stress syndrome described in many parts of Africa and also in New Guinea. It is commonly encountered among students, probably because of the high priority accorded to education in African society, particularly prevalent at examination times.

Five symptom types have been described as comprising brain fag syndrome:

- head symptoms: aching, burning, crawling sensations
- eye symptoms: blurring, watering, aching
- difficulty in grasping the meaning of spoken or written words
- poor retentivity
- sleepiness on studying

Guinness (1992) found the rates to be highest in rural areas serving peasant populations (34 per cent of students), compared to periurban schools (22 per cent) and schools for the professional élite (6 per cent). Sufferers of brain fag syndrome are resistant to psychological interpretation of their condition. It is suggested that brain fag syndrome is a form of depression in which depressive features are not articulated in Western psychological terms.

PSYCHIATRY AND BLACK AND ETHNIC MINORITIES IN BRITAIN

Britain is a multiracial society. In some large cities ethnic minorities represent 20 per cent or more of the total population.

Ethnic minority groups comprise two groups:

1   immigrants
2   second/third generation groups

The stresses incurred by these two groups are different. Ethnic minority groups are heterogeneous in terms of religion and cultural background.

Immigrants
People migrate for various reasons; adjustment will depend on many factors including those operating before migration, the reasons for migration and factors operating in the host society.

TYPES OF MIGRANT

- **Settlers**: likely to be prepared for a new way of life
- **Exiles**: forced migration may result in grief reaction for their old way of life. They may have suffered torture or other atrocities before migration
- **Migrant workers**: migration is likely to be time-limited, and they are less likely to put down roots in the host country. They may be supporting their family at home
- **Other**: e.g. students, business people

- Culture shock and readjustment to host society
- Often results in downward social mobility, poor housing, unemployment or job dissatisfaction, unfulfilled aspirations, and lack of opportunities
- Racial prejudice and discrimination in host society
- Loss of extended family support
- Intergenerational difficulties as children integrate, bringing cultural conflict into the home

In a three-year follow-up study of Vietnamese boat people given asylum in Norway, Hauff and Vaglum (1995) found there was no decline in psychological distress over time. One in four suffered psychiatric disorder and the prevalence of depression at three years was 18 per cent. Female gender, extreme traumatic stress in Vietnam, negative life events in Norway, and chronic family separation were the predictors of psychopathology. Thus the effects of war and persecution were long-lasting, and compounded by adversity in exile. Some studies have found that the mental health of refugees improves over time, and it is possible that adverse factors in the host environment have significant effects on the readjustment and mental health of refugees.

Mental illness among ethnic minorities

SCHIZOPHRENIA The higher than expected rates of schizophrenia among Afro-Caribbean people born in Britain have been noted since the 1960s. Studies of hospital admissions have demonstrated high rates of schizophrenia in this group compared to British whites and Asians.

The highest rates of schizophrenia in the Afro-Caribbean group occur in UK-born second-generation subjects (up to nine times that among Europeans). Differences persist even when age and socioeconomic status are taken into account.

These results have caused controversy, with criticisms of misdiagnosis due to unfamiliar culturally determined patterns of behaviour, acute psychotic reactions being mistaken for schizophrenia, or racism accounting for the observed differences. However, well-designed studies dealing with methodological problems fail to substantiate these criticisms. Harvey *et al.* (1990) studied consecutive Afro-Caribbean and white British psychotic inpatients prospectively and found no differences in the course of illness or the pattern of symptoms. This caused them to reject the hypothesis that misdiagnosis accounts for the higher rates of schizophrenia in this group.

Schizophrenia as defined by operational research criteria is more common in people of Afro-Caribbean origin living in the UK.

Sugarman and Craufurd (1994) found a lifetime morbid risk of schizophrenia in the parents of Afro-Caribbean subjects to be the same as the risks to parents of British white schizophrenic subjects (8.9 per cent and 8.4 per cent respectively). However, for the siblings of Afro-Caribbean probands the risk was 15 per cent compared to 1.8 per cent for white siblings. Among the siblings of UK-born Afro-Caribbean probands, the risk was even higher at 27.3 per cent. These observations suggest that schizophrenia in Afro-Caribbean patients is no less familial than the rest of the population (as evidenced by the similar risks to parents), but that the increased risk is caused by environmental factors capable of precipitating schizophrenia in those who are genetically predisposed to it.

The environmental factor postulated has not been identified to date. There is no evidence of increased rates of schizophrenia in the West Indies and therefore no evidence that Afro-Caribbeans carry a greater genetic loading for schizophrenia.

Admission rates for Asians are similar to Europeans, except for the 16–29-year age group, who tend to have lower psychiatric admission rates than Europeans. This gives rise to concerns that services are not reaching this particular group.

SUICIDE   Raleigh and Balarajan (1992) report suicide rates among British ethnic minority groups compared to the indigenous British white population.

Suicide rates are high among young Indian women (age-specific SMRs of 273 and 160 at ages 15–24 and 25–34 respectively), but low among Indian men (SMR 73). Suicide rates are low in Caribbeans (SMRs 81 and 62 in men and women respectively).

Suicide rates are high in East Africans (SMRs 128 and 148 in men and women respectively), and are largely confined to the younger age groups.

Immigrant groups have a higher rate of suicide by burning, with a nine-fold excess among Indian women.

High suicide rates among young Indian women are reported within India and in countries where Indian immigrants have settled. High expectations of academic and economic success, the stigma of failure, the authority of their elders and the expected unquestioning compliance of younger family members is thought to predispose to suicide in this culture. Among Indian women these pressures are accentuated by expected submission and deference to males and elders. Rates of suicide and attempted suicide in this group are not greatly different to those in the country of origin, suggesting that the increased rates are not particularly related to issues of migration. In India dowry-related self-burning is well known. The common causes of suicide by burns in young women include marital problems and interpersonal difficulties with other family members.

In contrast, suicide rates among older Indian women are low, which is thought to accord with the greater respect given to them by virtue of their age.

CHILD AND ADOLESCENT PSYCHIATRIC PRESENTATIONS   Second generation Afro-Caribbean children presenting to child and adolescent psychiatric services differ in their patterns of presentation when compared to British white children of comparable age and socioeconomic status.

Psychotic and autistic disorders are over-represented in Afro-Caribbean children compared to whites, with psychotic disorders present in 3.4 per cent and 0.8 per cent respectively, and autistic disorders present in 3.4 per cent and 0.6 per cent respectively. Studies also find that the autistic children of immigrant parents are more likely than their white counterparts to be severely or profoundly mentally handicapped. Mental handicap is also over-represented in Afro-Caribbean children (19 per cent vs 11 per cent).

Afro-Caribbean children present with a significantly higher rate of conduct disorder (35 per cent vs 25 per cent) and a significantly lower rate of emotional disorder (18 per cent vs 27 per cent) when compared to white counterparts.

Use of psychiatric services by ethnic minorities
Young, male, black, schizophrenic Afro-Caribbeans have high psychiatric admission rates compared to white British, and a higher rate of compulsory admissions. In inner-city London the ratio of black Afro-Caribbeans to whites among admissions is higher than the equivalent proportion in the population (three times higher in Hammersmith and Fulham).

Part of the explanation for this is the higher rates of schizophrenia in black Afro-Caribbeans. Bebbington et al. (1994) concluded that ethnicity was not of major importance in decisions to use the Mental Health Act in two regions in London. The use of compulsion was strongly linked with challenging behaviour and diagnosis of schizophrenia, but not with ethnicity *per se*.

Dunn and Fahy (1990) studying police admissions under Section 136 MHA 1983 to a South London psychiatric hospital found an excess of Black admissions. However, clinicians judged that more than 90 per cent of detained Black and white subjects were suffering from a psychiatric disorder, and were therefore appropriately detained. The judgement of the police in this study was not biased towards apprehending Black people as a result of unconscious racist attitudes as previously suggested by some.

Cole *et al.* (1995) found that for first-episode patients the route to psychiatric care in Haringey (North London) was different to those for chronic patients. While compulsory admission was more likely for Black patients, the excess was less striking than in other studies. Black patients were no more likely to have police involvement than other patients. The most important factors in avoiding adverse pathways to care were having a supportive family or friend, and the presence of a general practitioner. Having a GP or close person avoided the need for compulsory detention, an effect seen in Black and white subjects.

Suggestions to account for the over-representation of compulsory admissions among Afro-Caribbeans include the possibility that the stigma of mental illness is greater in this community, thus resulting in delays before cases come to the attention of the services. Afro-Caribbean patients with previous psychotic episodes are more likely than their white counterparts to deny they had a problem at all; these patients are more likely to be non-compliant with anti-psychotic medication and to require compulsory readmission.

Management

COMMUNICATION   In areas with large numbers of ethnic minorities, the service should provide for interpreters to be available for translation. It is preferable that these people have training in psychiatric and sociological terms and concepts, as well as competence in both languages. **Cultural competence** is required as well as a knowledge of the language. Relatives may need to be used, but caution must be taken to ensure that the patient's best interests are being represented.

FAMILY   Involve the family and mobilize the community for support. They may assist in the process of assessment in helping to understand the context of experience and circumstances.

PSYCHOTHERAPY   Religious leaders and healers can provide important alternative sources of support.

Psychotherapy with ethnic minority groups needs to recognize a different philosophical framework and personal development. Thus the Western concern with personal autonomy and independence may not be relevant in those cultures which emphasize the interdependence of the family and the community. Culturally consonant therapy should be offered.

BIBLIOGRAPHY

Ball, R.A. and Clare, A.W. 1990: Symptoms and social adjustment in Jewish depressives. *British Journal of Psychiatry* 156, 379–83.

Bebbington, P.E., Feeney, S.T., Flannigan, C.B. *et al.* 1994: Inner London collaborative audit of admissions in two health districts. II: Ethnicity and the use of the Mental Health Act. *British Journal of Psychiatry* 165, 743–9.

Bhatia, M.S. and Malik, S.C. 1991: Dhat syndrome – a useful diagnostic entity in Indian culture. *British Journal of Psychiatry* 159, 691–5.

Cole, E., Leavey, G., King, M. *et al.* 1995: Pathways to care for patients with a first episode of psychosis. A comparison of ethnic groups. *British Journal of Psychiatry* 167, 770–6.

Dunn, J. and Fahy, T.A. 1990: Police admissions to a psychiatric hospital. Demographic and clinical differences between ethnic groups. *British Journal of Psychiatry* 156, 373–8.

Goodman, R. and Richards, H. 1995: Child and adolescent psychiatric presentations of second-generation Afro-Caribbeans in Britain. *British Journal of Psychiatry* 167, 362–9.

Guinness, E.A. 1992: Profile and prevalence of the brain fag syndrome: psychiatric morbidity in school populations in Africa. *British Journal of Psychiatry* 160 (suppl. 16), 42–52.

Harvey, I., Williams, M., McGuffin, P. *et al.* 1990: The functional psychoses in Afro-Caribbeans. *British Journal of Psychiatry* 157, 515–22.

Hauff, E. and Vaglum, P. 1995: Organised violence and the stress of exile. Predictors of mental health in a community cohort of Vietnamese refugees three years after resettlement. *British Journal of Psychiatry* 166, 360–7.

Hotopf, M. and Mullen, R. 1992: Koro and Capgras syndrome in a non-Chinese subject. *British Journal of Psychiatry* 161, 577.

Kleinman, A. 1977: Depression, somatisation and the new 'cross-cultural psychiatry'. *Social Science and Medicine* 11, 3–10.

Kleinman, A. 1987: Anthropology and psychiatry: The role of culture in cross-cultural research on illness. *British Journal of Psychiatry* 151, 447–54.

Kon, Y. 1994: Amok. *British Journal of Psychiatry* 165, 685–9.

Leff, J., Wig, N.N., Bedi, H. *et al.* 1990: Relatives' expressed emotion and the course of schizophrenia in Chandigarh: a two-year follow-up of a first-contact sample. *British Journal of Psychiatry* 156, 351–6.

Littlewood, R. 1990: From categories to contexts: A decade of the 'new cross-cultural psychiatry'. *British Journal of Psychiatry* 156, 308–27.

Murphy, J.M. 1994: Anthropology and psychiatric epidemiology. *Acta Psychiatrica Scandinavica* (suppl.) 385, 48–57.

Orley, J. and Wing, J.K. 1979: Psychiatric disorders in two African villages. *Archives of General Psychiatry* 36, 513–21.

Patel, V. and Winston, M. 1994: 'Universality of mental illness' revisited: assumptions, artefacts and new directions. *British Journal of Psychiatry* 165, 437–40.

Raleigh, V.S. and Balarajan, R. 1992: Suicide and self-burning among Indians and West Indians in England and Wales. *British Journal of Psychiatry* 161, 365–8.

Sartorius, N., Jablensky, A., Korten, A. *et al.* 1986: Early manifestations and first contact incidence of schizophrenia in different cultures. *Psychological Medicine* 16, 909–28.

Shepherd, M. 1995: Two faces of Emil Kraepelin. *British Journal of Psychiatry* 167, 174–83.

Smyth, M.G. and Dean, C. 1992: Capgras and koro. *British Journal of Psychiatry* 161, 121–3.

Sugarman, P.P.A. and Craufurd, D. 1994: Schizophrenia in the Afro-Caribbean community. *British Journal of Psychiatry* 164, 474–80.

Thomas, C.S., Stone, K., Osborn, M. *et al.* 1993: Psychiatric morbidity and compulsory admission among UK-born Europeans, Afro-Caribbeans and Asians in central Manchester. *British Journal of Psychiatry* 163, 91–9.

World Health Organization 1973: *Report of the International pilot study of schizophrenia.* Geneva: WHO.

38
Old age psychiatry

EPIDEMIOLOGY

Fifteen per cent of the population of England and Wales is aged over 65.

Age dependency ratio = population aged over 65 as a percentage of the working population. This is projected to rise over the next decade. Thus as the aged population rises there will be fewer people of working age to support them.

The elderly population of the underdeveloped world is likely to have risen at more than twice the rate of the developed world by the year 2000.

Within the elderly population, disability rises steeply with age, from 16 per 1000 who are in their sixties to 133 per 1000 who are over 80.

The prevalence of psychiatric morbidity in those aged over 65 is:

Dementia	5	per cent
Depression	13.5	per cent
Phobic disorders	10	per cent
Generalized anxiety	4	per cent
Personality disorder	1	per cent
Paranoid states	0.5	per cent
Panic disorder		Rare

The prevalence of dementia rises exponentially with age, doubling every 5.1 years. Thus the prevalence in the over sixty-fives is 5 per cent, and in the over eighties it is 20 per cent.

AGEING

The cause of ageing is not known.

Genetic theories
PROGRAMMED AGEING   Supported by the observation of **The Hayflick limit**: human diploid cells cultured *in vitro* have a finite lifespan. Upon repeated sub-culture of normal cells, mitosis ceases independently of culture conditions. This evidence supports theories of genetically programmed ageing. Cells derived from tumour tissue do not display this limit.

It is speculated that this effect is caused by the progressive loss of DNA sequences in the telomere involved in the maintenance of DNA stability and replication.

Changes in ageing probably do not involve defects in DNA, but may involve errors in the control of DNA expression: **epigenetic defects**.

Non-genetic theories
WEAR AND TEAR THEORIES   Age-related decline in organ function is thought to be

responsible for ageing. It is no longer thought tenable as a central cause of ageing; it is probably secondary to ageing.

MITOCHONDRIAL DECLINE   Across the species mitochondria show a reduction in numbers, an increase in size and structural changes in old organisms. Free radical damage to mitochondrial membranes is thought to contribute to these changes.

FREE RADICAL THEORIES   Free radicals commonly result from oxidative reactions in normal cellular processes, particularly in the inner membranes of mitochondria and during phagocytosis. The resulting damage includes lipid peroxidation which can result in cell death. In animal experiments antioxidants (free-radical scavengers) have been shown to increase life expectancy but not to increase maximum lifespan, raising doubt about the role of free radicals in the primary ageing process.

The only method proven to increase the maximum lifespan in experimental animals is calorie restriction. This mechanism is unknown but it may involve the delayed maturation of the immune system or reduced free radical damage secondary to reduced metabolic rate.

Neurobiology of ageing

In normal ageing there is a slow reduction in weight and volume of the human brain, with a proportionate increase in the size of the ventricles and subarachnoid space after the age of 50.

The brain is overprovided with nerve cells, therefore a loss of cells does not necessarily result in a loss of function. Some parts of the brain show no loss in nerve-cell numbers with normal ageing (e.g. dentate nucleus of cerebellum). Nerve-cell loss is known to occur in parts of the cerebral cortex, the pyramidal and granule cells of the hippocampus, substantia nigra and Purkinje cells of cerebellum. In normal ageing, especially after the age of 85, a shrinkage of nerve cells is known to occur in the cerebral cortex and putamen.

Nerve-cell connections are reduced in some cells with compensatory increases seen in others in normal ageing.

Lipofuscin accumulates in the cytoplasm of nerve cells from childhood.

Tau protein, involved in linking neurofilaments and microtubules, accumulates in a small proportion of ageing nerve cells particularly in the hippocampus and entorhinal cortex, resulting in neurofibrillary tangles. Senile plaques are made up of a core of extracellular amyloid surrounded by abnormal collections of neuritic processes. In the normal ageing brain these are found in the neocortex, amygdala, hippocampus and entorhinal cortex.

Rod-shaped Hirano bodies are found near the hippocampal pyramidal cells. These comprise the microfilament actin. Accompanying their presence is a granulovacuolar degeneration in the pyramidal nerve cells.

Abnormal intracellular inclusions called Lewy bodies are found in the substantia nigra and locus ceruleus in some normal old people. They comprise a spherical body in the cytoplasm of a nerve cell. They have a laminated appearance with a dense granular core and fibrillary material radiating to the periphery.

In normal old brains amyloid can be found deposited in the walls of blood vessels. Deposits are usually small, widespread, in superficial cortical and leptomeningeal vessels overlying the cerebral lobes. Amyloid is also deposited in irregular patches in the normal ageing cerebral cortex. It is called beta amyloid (A4 amyloid) and is the same as that located at the centre of senile plaques.

All the above neuropathological changes occur in Alzheimer's disease but to a much greater extent.

PSYCHOLOGY OF AGEING

Cognition

INTELLECTUAL FUNCTIONING   Intelligence peaks at the age of 25. It levels off until the age of 60 to 70, and declines thereafter. Many studies have demonstrated an accelerated decline in cognitive functioning in those who are closest to their death. This has been referred to as the **terminal drop**, and poor health may be the cause.

Using the WAIS-R, a classic pattern of intellectual decline is seen, with performance IQ declining more rapidly than verbal IQ. Factors thought to account for this pattern include:

- speed of processing: makes some contribution to the age-related decline but is not the whole explanation
- familiarity/novelty: tasks that have been learnt over a lifetime, relying on overlearned abilities are most resistant to age-related changes (crystallized intelligence). Tasks requiring the less practised processing of new information are most sensitive to age-related decline (fluid intelligence)

Although intelligence declines with age, there are considerable individual differences.

PROBLEM-SOLVING   The ability to abstract a concept and apply it to a new situation declines with age, most prominently after the age of 70. The elderly have more problems if tasks are presented in an abstract manner.

CREATIVITY   Scientific creativity peaks in the thirties, whereas artistic creativity peaks in the fifties. Humans seem to be most creative when they are producing the greatest volume of work: **intellectual vigour.**

Psychomotor speed

Reaction times increase with age, with most slowing occurring in the central processing of information. Older people are less able to maintain a state of readiness, and less likely to choose flexible active information-processing than younger people.

Memory

SHORT-TERM MEMORY   Short-term memory as tested by the digit span does not change with age.

WORKING MEMORY   Memory tasks requiring monitoring or complex decision-making are performed more poorly in the elderly than in the young. Decline is increased with the complexity of the task or increased memory load.

LONG-TERM MEMORY   The retrieval of information in the elderly is impaired; thus uncued recall shows an age-related decrement, but cued recall reduces the extent of the decrement. Memory is more durable if it is encoded at a semantic level, rather than at a phonological or orthographic level. Older subjects are less likely to code at the semantic level. Memory performance in the elderly is best if the meaning is easily extracted.

Memory of source is impaired in the elderly, which is thought to be related to deficits in frontal lobe functioning.

Memory of distant events becomes poorer the more remote the patient is from the event.

Retention of knowledge is retained with age. Knowledge-based skills are relatively preserved into old age.

Importance of loss

People experience unique problems after the age of 65. Activities are limited by declining physical strength and some suffer debilitating illness. Loss of employment with retirement may result in feelings of reduced self-worth and low self-esteem. The ageing individual increasingly suffers the loss of partners, family and friends through death.

Erikson describes the psychosocial changes that individuals negotiate as they develop. The last of these **integrity versus despair**, is concerned with the way the individual approaches death. A well-lived life is more likely to result in a sense of integrity and wholeness at this time of reflection upon life achievements. Those with regrets and thoughts of opportunities missed are more likely to approach death with a sense of despair.

Personality changes

Most studies of personality in older age support the concept of the stability of personality with age.

Adjustment to ageing can be explained by different models which may apply in different individuals. The **activity theory** entails the successfully adjusted individual as being fully engaged with life, with interests and social contact. The **disengagement theory** suggests that the individual focuses increasingly on their inner world as they adjust to diminished family and social roles

High anxiety levels in the elderly are correlated with physical ill health.

Most chronic neurotic conditions improve in old age.

Anxiety-prone personalities arise from a more biological origin, whereas insecure personalities arise more from early environmental events. Dysthymic personalities seem to persist into old age.

SOCIAL AND ECONOMIC FACTORS IN OLD AGE

Attitude

Popular Western culture devalues old age, with women perceived more negatively than men. Children are least likely, and young/middle-aged adults are most likely to devalue the old.

Most elderly people are able to lead independent lives, are financially secure and are not lonely. However, the common perception of the elderly is as dependent, confused, lonely, rigid, depressed and passive people.

The majority of old people cope well with ageing, reporting high life satisfaction, good cognitive skills, openness to new experience and a positive view of themselves. These are considered to display an **integrated** personality. Those that cope less well display either **passive-dependent** or **disintegrated** personalities.

Factors that influence a person's view of themselves include personality, gender, health and socioeconomic status.

Deviance from social norms generally decreases with age, while the prevalence of stigmatizing conditions increases.

Status in the elderly

As people age the number of social roles they occupy decreases. This may reduce their social worth. Much of the decline in the status of the elderly is associated with their reduced socioeconomic circumstances.

The status of elderly people is high in preliterate societies and low in modern societies. The factors thought to contribute to this effect include the reduction in the usefulness of the elderly as repositories of knowledge, the break-up of the extended family and the reduced importance of land inheritance.

In modern society industrial capitalism is thought to have contributed to the declining social status of the elderly mainly through the imposition of a retirement age and stigmatizing age-related financial provision. The proportion of over 65-year-olds with a wage has steadily declined through this century through State-imposed retirement for all, irrespective of their ability to work. This has lead to poverty and the stigmatization of the old, with a loss of work role and work-related life satisfaction.

Retirement and income
State pensions were introduced in the early twentieth century following work by Booth revealing impoverishment among the elderly.

Retirement in itself is not a cause of increased morbidity. The main problem experienced in retirement is substantial income reduction. In addition to the loss of earnings there is the loss of status, companionship, and job satisfaction. The relative value of pensions today has fallen compared to 50 years ago.

Accommodation
The likelihood that elderly people will live alone, away from their families, depends on a number of factors, and is relatively common in Britain. The ageing population is living longer and is thus more likely to live alone at some stage in their later years. Increasing home ownership increases the chances that the elderly will live alone for longer.

For health reasons large proportions of the very old live in institutional care or with relatives or friends. Old people living alone make more use of statutory services than those living with others.

Disengagement theories which hold that older people gradually withdraw from society in preparation for death have now lost favour. Instead, **activity theories** encourage the maintenance of social interaction and role. Elderly people do maintain a high level of social contact with others. Unhappiness is associated with a lack of friends in a social network.

Sociocultural differences
The experience of ageing is affected by:

GENDER   Ageing women are more stigmatized than ageing men. They are more likely to live alone and are more likely to be poor.

SOCIAL CLASS   Almost half of pensioners from Social Classes I and II have money in addition to the State pension from private pension schemes and savings, compared to only 5 per cent of those in social classes IV and V.

ETHNICITY   There are competing theories about the effect of ethnicity and ageing:

- **Age as leveller hypothesis**: argues that because all old people are socially disadvantaged the relative disadvantage experienced by ethnic minorities reduces in old age
- **Double jeopardy hypothesis**: argues that disadvantages are exacerbated with age

Problems experienced by the ageing ethnic minority subject are no different to those facing all ethnic minority groups. Language difficulties are common, and lack of income is most common in Asian people who have joined their families and lack pension entitlement.

PSYCHOPHARMACOLOGY OF OLD AGE

Pharmacokinetics and pharmacodynamics

AGE-RELATED CHANGES IN DRUG HANDLING   Changes with ageing that may affect pharmacokinetics include:

- ↓ total body mass
- ↓ proportion of body mass that is composed of water
- ↓ proportion of body mass that is composed of muscle
- ↑ proportion of body mass that is composed of adipose tissue
- ↑ gastric pH
- ↓ rate of gastric emptying
- ↓ blood flow in splanchnic circulation
- ↓ gastrointestinal absorptive surface
- changes in plasma protein concentration: this may be the result of illness
- ↓ metabolically active tissue
- ↓ hepatic biotransformation
- ↓ glomerular filtration rate
- ↓ renal tubular function

CLEARANCE   This is the major determinant of steady-state plasma drug concentration. Reduced renal clearance is particularly important with respect to lithium. The reduction of renal clearance is predictable with age but the reduction with age of hepatic clearance is not as straightforward. All other psychotropic drugs are cleared by hepatic biotransformation, which is variably reduced with age.

DISTRIBUTION   This is determined by the drug's relative solubility in lipid as opposed to water, proclivity for various body tissues, and plasma protein binding. Most psychotropic drugs, being lipophilic, have a relatively small plasma concentration compared to the total amount of drug in the body.

ABSORPTION   Although structural and functional changes in the gastrointestinal tract are known to occur in ageing, there is no evidence that the rate or extent of absorption of orally administered psychotropic medications are changed in the elderly.

Drug interactions

The incidence of side-effects and adverse drug reactions increases with age. The causes that may contribute to this include:

- ↑ incidence of coexisting physical illness
- ↑ number of prescriptions with age
- ↓ compliance
- changed pharmacokinetics and pharmacodynamics exposes the body to higher drug levels
- ↑ risk for acute organic brain syndrome with age

Practical considerations

ANTIPSYCHOTICS   The elderly are more sensitive to antimuscarinic (anticholinergic) side-effects. Parkinsonian side-effects are more likely in the elderly, in women, and in those with organic brain disease. The prevalence of tardive dyskinesia increases with age and is more common in women. The length of treatment is more strongly related than the absolute dose. Acute dystonias, although common in the young, are rare in the elderly.

TRICYCLIC ANTIDEPRESSANTS   With ageing there occurs:

- ↑ plasma half-life
- ↑ steady-state levels
- ↑ volume of distribution
- ↑ postural hypotension

Heart disease is a relative contraindication. Again, the elderly are particularly prone to antimuscarinic (anticholinergic) side-effects, which may result in acute brain syndromes, urinary retention, and glaucoma.

MAOIS   Extreme caution is needed if considering prescribing these to those with hypertension and cardiovascular disease.

LITHIUM   Because of lowered renal clearance, lithium doses in the elderly are approximately 50 per cent lower than in the young. Diuretics may reduce renal clearance even further, increasing the risk of lithium toxicity.

BENZODIAZEPINES   Accumulation in the elderly is not more likely to occur than in the young. The elderly are at an increased risk of delirium and falls.

DISTRICT SERVICE PROVISION

Need for specialization
In Britain the specialization of psychogeriatric services started about 30 years ago. Mentors included Post and Roth who distinguished between types of dementia and increased the academic standing of the discipline. Specialization has allowed the development of a professional identity with academic departments, journals and a section of the Royal College of Psychiatrists concerned exclusively with the problems facing the elderly.

The elderly display a number of concomitant problems. Those with mental illness often have physical illness and social problems as well. The provision of adequate care for the elderly requires liaison with primary care, geriatric medicine and social services, as well as with informal carers and voluntary agencies. Finally, without specialization, old age psychiatry would be in direct competition for resources with adult psychiatry.

Principles of service provision
The planning of services for the elderly must take into account the age distribution of the population, including the numbers of the very elderly who are most likely to need the most costly institutional care.

The elderly require:

- accurate assessment: medical, psychological, social and functional
- specialist knowledge
- least disruptive solutions
- prompt interventions
- informal carers should be considered and supported
- liaison between all aspects of service is paramount

Needs of carers
Community care of the mentally ill, especially dementia sufferers, results in significant strain on the informal carers. Families provide the most practical and emotional help to the elderly population. This is usually provided by a very close relative, such as a spouse or a daughter, and usually falls largely on one relative. Female carers outnumber males by 2:1. Most carers are willing and

wish to keep the patient at home, but the strain on them is great. The carers of demented elderly people have more problems than others, which increase with the degree of dementia. The sources of stress include:

- practical: e.g. elderly person requiring help with personal and household tasks and care
- behavioural: e.g. nocturnal disturbance, incontinence, wandering and aggression
- interpersonal
- social: e.g. restrictions on the carer's personal life

The British government's *Health of the Nation* document recognizes the important role of carers and directs services specifically to their support.

ASSESSMENT OF A REFERRAL

Psychiatric assessment
Prior to assessment establish what the referrer wishes to know, and what the patient and their carers have been told to expect. It is useful to interview an informant and it is essential in those with organic brain syndromes.

The most informative setting for the initial assessment is within the person's home. Coordination is required to ensure that informants are available. The psychiatrist should be vigilant for unrecognized physical illness presenting with psychiatric symptoms, and if this is suspected should ensure that the patient receives the appropriate medical interventions. Examination at home allows an assessment of the patient's immediate environment including their visuospatial orientation, their ability to manage independently, the assessment of local resources such as neighbours' and relatives' availability, and any evidence of the excessive use of alcohol.

If the first assessment occurs on a medical ward as a liaison visit, the medical notes should be read and the medical and nursing staff should be interviewed before seeing the patient. Carers should be contacted to supplement the information gathered on the ward.

The interview should take place in the most private conditions available.

PSYCHIATRIC HISTORY   Following the introduction of the psychiatrist, the patient should be asked whether they have any problems they would like to discuss. An assessment of how the patient deals with questioning is made throughout. The interview should be unhurried, allowing the patient to relate their family and personal history.

The details of past medical and past psychiatric history are very important, as are any medications the patient is currently taking. It is also helpful to have some understanding of the patient's premorbid personality, which is best accessed through informants.

Establish whether the patient has a history of heavy drinking either currently or at some time in their past. A history of smoking is also needed.

Mental state examination
APPEARANCE AND BEHAVIOUR   If the patient has difficulties with verbal exchange (caused by e.g. severe dementia, delirium, aphasia, severe hearing and visual impairments), then careful observation can provide much information. Poor hygiene, incontinence or inadequate nutrition gives an indication of the patient's ability to look after themselves. Distinguish whether the problem is recent or

chronic. Any evidence of physical illness such as cerebrovascular disease may also be observed.

The patient's behaviour may be suggestive of pathology. Observe for signs of psychomotor retardation or agitation, perplexity or behavioural disturbance. An inability to focus or sustain attention appropriately may be a sign of clouded consciousness.

Patients with acute or chronic brain syndromes often display a number of behaviours which can jeopardize their placement in the community. Examples of such behaviours include day/night reversal, wandering, aggression, sliding or throwing themselves to the floor, stripping off their clothes and the smearing of faeces.

SPEECH Cognitive impairment may result in circumlocution, paraphrasia and polite evasions hiding a lack of depth and detail in speech. Severe hearing impairment may be overcome by communication through gesture and/or writing.

The elderly with mixed affective states may demonstrate a 'slow flight of ideas'.

THOUGHT Early dementia may be noticeable only after a lengthy interview with a repetition of themes, a lack of internal logic, and a limitation of discussion inconsistent with the level of intelligence.

MOOD Depression is common and is often missed in the elderly.

Mania is easily missed in the elderly and should always be considered.

HALLUCINATIONS AND DELUSIONS These do not differ substantially in old age compared to the young.

COGNITIVE EXAMINATION If a patient is unable to give a reasonable account of themselves it is often helpful to conduct the cognitive assessment earlier in the interview. If they have given a history, aspects of their cognitive functioning will already have been indirectly assessed.

- **orientation** to time, place and person
- **attention and concentration**: assessed using 'serial sevens' or naming months of year backwards if numerical abilities are not good
- **immediate memory**: assessed using digit span (normal 7 ± 2).
- **short-term verbal memory**: assessed using name and address with six parts, repeated immediately to assess registration, then again after five minutes with intervening distraction to prevent rehearsal, also using Babcock sentence
- **short-term non-verbal memory**: assessed by immediate recall (registration) of a geometric shape, then recall after five minutes with intervening distraction to prevent rehearsal
- **Long-term memory**: assessed during history-taking, ask date and place of birth
- **general knowledge**: assessed by asking historical and recent commonly known facts e.g. the current Prime Minister, monarch and family, the president of the USA, the colours of the Union Jack, the names of capital cities
- **verbal fluency**: number of words beginning with T in one minute, or the number of four-legged animals in one minute
- **calculation**: assessed by asking a simple calculation such as a subtraction
- **writing**
- **spatial** including bodily **awareness**
- **recognition** of objects and faces
- **appropriate use of everyday objects**
- **naming things**: to detect nominal dysphasia
- **receptive and expressive use** of written and spoken language
- **perseveration**: suggestive of frontal lobe dysfunction

- **tests of praxis** such as drawing a square or a clock face (constructional apraxia), asking the patient to make a fist, oppose thumb and little finger, fold a piece of paper and place it in an envelope, for example
- **tests of gnosis** such as picture recognition, tactile recognition

Physical examination

All elderly patients presenting to psychiatry need a full physical examination. Check their temperature (using a low-reading thermometer) and their state of hydration if clouding of consciousness is suspected.

Primitive reflexes are found mostly in dementing patients, although they may occur transiently in acute confusional states. Examples include the palmomental reflex, grasp reflex, pout reflex, sucking reflex and glabellar tap.

Tremors and involuntary movements are more common in old age, but be alert to the possibility of a cerebrovascular event, the onset of Huntington's or Wilson's disease or, more commonly, treatment with dopaminergic preparations such as L-dopa for Parkinson's disease.

Increasing sensory impairments in old age, particularly of hearing and vision, predispose to paranoid states. Closed angle glaucoma is a contraindication to the use of drugs with anticholinergic side-effects, such as phenothiazines and tricyclic antidepressants.

Investigations

A chest X-ray is required in all sick elderly people, even if the chest is apparently clear on physical examination. Pneumonia, tuberculosis and carcinoma can all present with acute confusional states, or depression. An ECG is also required.

The prevalence of thyroid disease increases in old age. Physical signs are often unreliable in the elderly, therefore TSH screening should be performed in all. Hyperthyroidism can be mistaken for anxiety states, hypomania or delirium. Hypothyroidism can present as depression with psychomotor retardation, dementia or delirium.

Routine investigations in the hospitalized elderly should include FBC with differential WCC, ESR, U&E, creatinine, LFTs with calcium and proteins, glucose, TSH, ECG, chest X-ray, and a mid-stream urine examination.

Structural imaging

NORMAL AGEING   Progressive cortical atrophy and increasing ventricular size is seen in normal ageing.

DEMENTIA   Structure imaging is helpful in discovering the aetiology of dementia although it does not establish the diagnosis of dementia which is determined clinically.

It identifies potentially treatable intracranial lesions.

The distribution of cerebral atrophy helps to distinguish different types of dementia:

Alzheimer's disease: normal CT scans of brain do not reliably differentiate normals from those with Alzheimer's disease, with approximately 20 per cent overlap between these groups, limiting usefulness in the individual patient. Generally cortical atrophy and ventricular enlargement are greater than in controls, with increasing cognitive dysfunction correlating with increasing cerebral atrophy, but more so with increasing ventricular size. An increase in ventricular size over one year is suggestive of Alzheimer's disease.

The clinical usefulness of neuroimaging can be improved by using a temporal lobe orientation in CT scanning which allows an accurate measurement of the medial temporal lobe. Using conventional angle CT scans it is almost impossible to measure this. In Alzheimer's disease a dramatic thinning of the width of the medial temporal lobe in the region of the brainstem is seen. SPET scans also reveal significantly reduced parietotemporal perfusion in these subjects. Combining SPET scans with temporal lobe-oriented CT scans improves the diagnostic accuracy of Alzheimer's disease by an order of magnitude over that derived using clinical criteria (likelihood ratio 30 versus 2.6).

Pick's disease: gross atrophy is seen in the frontotemporal regions (knife-blade atrophy), but the diagnosis cannot be made on this evidence alone.

Huntington's disease: gross shrinkage of the caudate nucleus ('loss of shouldering') supports a clinical diagnosis of this.

Multi-infarct dementia: focal pathology suggestive of cerebrovascular infarcts and/or white matter changes suggestive of small vessel vascular disease is suggestive of this.

Normal pressure hydrocephalus: enlarged ventricles without cortical atrophy in the presence of normal CSF pressure on lumbar puncture supports this diagnosis.

Electroencephalography
In normal ageing (after the age of 60) the following changes occur in the EEG:

- slowing of alpha rhythm
- increased theta activity particularly in the left temporal region
- increased delta activity particularly in the anterior regions
- beta activity diminishes only in the very old (over 80)

DEMENTIA   In Alzheimer's disease the EEG may be normal (6 per cent) or show minor non-specific changes. The following changes may occur:

- diffuse slowing in early stages
- reduced alpha and beta activity and increased theta and delta activity as the disease progresses
- paroxysmal bifrontal delta waves are more common than in normal ageing

In Pick's disease the EEG is more likely than in Alzheimer's disease to be normal, and shows less slowing of the alpha waves.

In vascular dementia the tracing shows asymmetry and localized slow waves, with a sparing of background activity.

In Creutzfeld–Jacob disease a slow background rhythm with paroxysmal sharp waves is characteristic.

In Huntington's disease a low-voltage pattern may be seen.

DELIRIUM   Most conditions causing delirium cause slowing of the EEG tracing:

- Metabolic

  - Hepatic encephalopathy: slowing of rhythm with posterior preservation. Triphasic waves highly indicative
  - Acute renal failure: low-voltage activity with posterior slowing
  - Bursts of theta activity
  - Hypocalcaemia: slowing with bursts of spikes
  - Hypercalcaemia: runs of 1–2-second waves
  - Hyperthyroidism: acceleration of alpha rhythm
  - Hypothyroidism: low-voltage EEG

- Drugs

    - Phenothiazines: increase voltage, slow alpha activity, reduce beta activity. In overdose, paroxysmal slow waves are characteristic
    - Antidepressants: increase EEG activity but reduce alpha rhythm. In overdose widespread alpha activity and spikes
    - Benzodiazepines: increase beta waves, especially frontal. In overdose prominent fast activity unresponsive to stimuli
    - Lithium: slow alpha rhythm with occasional, sometimes focal, spikes
    - In overdose diffuse slowing, triphasic waves and paroxysmal abnormalities

Of those with delirium, 90 per cent of patients have abnormal traces. Delta activity, asymmetry in delta waves and localized spike and sharp wave complexes occur more frequently in those with intracranial pathology. Alpha activity correlates with cognitive functioning, and delta activity correlates with the length of illness.

Psychological assessment

Changes in psychological functions such as mood, personality, behaviour and cognition are often the first signs of psychiatric illness in the elderly. Various scales have been devised to provide for the accurate and objective assessment of all aspects of psychological functioning in the elderly. The simpler tests can be used by non-psychologist disciplines in their assessment and monitoring of the elderly mentally ill. Psychologists can help other disciplines in their roles, and take on the psychometric assessments of those patients with confusing or particularly demanding clinical pictures.

PSYCHOMETRIC TESTING   This quantifies the level and range of ability. Serial measures can be used to monitor the effect of interventions, or to measure progress of the patient's condition over time.

It is essential when any particular test is used in the elderly, that it has been validated in the elderly population, and that its predictions have also been validated.

EXPERIENTIAL ASSESSMENT   This tries to clarify the nature of impairment. By understanding the nature of the impairment it is possible to develop interventions which ameliorate the impairment.

PSYCHOMETRIC MEASURE OF FUNCTION ARE USED:

1. To clarify diagnosis
    Batteries of tests have been devised to distinguish between different diagnostic groups
    The **Kendrick Battery**: developed to distinguish normal, functionally impaired and demented elderly groups
    The **Geriatric Depression Scale**: 30-item self-administered rating scale, with cut-off score determining whether depressed. Extensively validated and highly discriminant
2. To predict outcome
    Various scales e.g. **Clifton Assessment Procedures for the Elderly (CAPE)** can predict survival, placement, and decline in elderly subjects. The **Kew Cognitive Map** assesses parietal lobe function and language functions in the dementing patient. This successfully predicts six-month survival (McDonald 1969)
3. To predict need
    The CAPE assesses the level of disability and thus allows for prediction of need for support services

Identification of impairments allows for interventions which may overcome the problems posed by the impairment

Assessments can be used to provide objective evidence for allocation of resources.

4   To monitor change

The **National Adult Reading Test (NART)** is used to determine premorbid IQ, thus aiding in the initial assessment of apparent cognitive impairment. Premorbid function is compared to current functioning using the **Wechsler Adult Intelligence Scale (WAIS).**

Repeating tests over time can give an estimate of deterioration, but this can be unreliable since even the elderly with dementia can show practice effects with repeated testing.

EXPERIENTIAL ANALYSIS OF FUNCTION ARE USED:

1.   To explain dysfunction

A finding in a psychometric test may conclude that a patient is unable to carry out a task, but does not try to establish why. The **decomposition of impaired performance** is used to establish which ability is impaired. A hypothesis of what the disability comprises is tested before a conclusion is reached

2.   To develop strategies for interventions

A behavioural approach may be used with an **ABC** (**a**ntecedents, **b**ehaviour and **c**onsequences) analysis before attempting an intervention.

Social assessment

This involves a detailed assessment of:

- living conditions
- personal care
- dynamics of family/carer
- support network
- financial situation
- family structure
- level of independence
- physical functioning in their environment

This is usually conducted by a social worker, but it may also be undertaken by other disciplines in the multidisciplinary team with appropriate training and supervision.

Occupational therapy assessment

Occupational therapists assess personal independence, social, recreational and leisure activities, and interpersonal functioning with a view to maximizing functioning level and independence in all aspects of daily life.

With the elderly, assessment of **activities of daily living** (**ADL**) forms the main emphasis. This provides a baseline of functioning in areas of personal hygiene and grooming, cooking, cleaning and shopping, based on interview, observation and checking performance. An important part of the assessment is to identify strengths which can be built on to overcome deficits.

The best place to conduct ADL assessments is within the patient's own home, as early in the illness as possible in order to establish baselines. ADL assessment is invaluable in helping to establish the most appropriate placement on discharge, and to determine those packages of care which are most likely to enable ongoing independent living.

PSYCHOLOGICAL REACTIONS TO PHYSICAL DISEASE

Theories of 'successful ageing' maintain that elderly people **select** a range of activities they want or need to do, then **optimize** their performance of these activities, and **compensate** for losses of physical or mental abilities.

Because of the increased prevalence of multiple pathology, adverse social circumstances and loss in old age, the understanding of the psychological consequences of physical disease must take into account physical, mental and social factors.

Adjusting to physical illness
Several factors contribute to the experience of a physical illness:

- the meaning of the illness, both generally and specifically to that patient
- the response of those close to the patient
- physical symptoms
- the social consequences of the illness
- coincidental life events and difficulties

Responses to physical illness
There are three components to coping style:

- the exercise of autonomy and independence
- the sense of personal responsibility, or locus of control
- activity versus passivity

Factors affecting psychological response to a physical illness include:

- the characteristics of the individual
- the characteristics of the physical illness

Psychiatric disorder may arise as a consequence of the stresses imposed by the physical condition, but it may also arise as a direct physical consequence of the pathological process. For example:

- hyperthyroidism may give rise to an anxiety state
- hypercalcaemia, infection, hypoxia or organ failure may give rise to delirium
- steroids may give rise to depression, elation or emotionalism
- frontal lobe lesions are likely to result in apathy

Psychiatric consequences of specific physical disorders
CEREBROVASCULAR DISEASE   Mood disorders may follow a stroke. These are mixed and effect different patients differently. General dysphoria and worry are common. Post-stroke depression and anxiety are recognized. Mania following stroke is described but is rarely seen in practice. Apathy and social withdrawal are seen in the absence of depression.

Syndromes more characteristic of stroke include emotional lability and the denial of handicap (anosognosia).

SENSORY IMPAIRMENT   Most commonly seen are impairment of hearing and/or vision. These have a dramatic impact upon the individual's ability to communicate with others which may cause social withdrawal, reduced activity and apparent cognitive decline.

They may increase the risks of depression and paraphrenia in the elderly although this is not proven.

PSYCHIATRIC DISORDERS

DEMENTIA DISORDERS

Dementia is defined as a global deterioration in brain functions in clear consciousness, which is usually progressive and irreversible. It results in the deterioration of all higher brain functions including memory, thinking, orientation, comprehension, calculation, the capacity to learn, language and judgement, and is accompanied by deterioration in emotional control, behaviour and motivation.

The dementias become more prevalent with increasing age. The most common dementia in the elderly is Alzheimer's disease, followed by multi-infarct dementia.

Alzheimer's disease

CLINICAL FEATURES   Alzheimer's disease (AD) is a diagnosis that can only be made with accuracy at post-mortem. However, it is possible to make a reasonably accurate diagnosis on the basis of clinical findings.

AD may present at any stage of the illness. Clinical features are most easily considered in stages.

Early stages: until about two years

- impaired concentration
- memory impairment
- fatigue and anxiety
- fleeting depression of mood
- exaggeration of pre-existing personality traits
- unusual incidents cause increasing concern
- occasional difficulty with word-finding
- altered handwriting
- perseveration of words and phrases

Intermediate stages

- further deterioration in above
- neurological abnormalities start to appear
- 5–10 per cent develop epilepsy
- apraxias and agnosias develop
- disorientation in time and space
- get lost in familiar surroundings
- speech problems with nominal dysphasia, receptive dysphasia, expressive dysphasia, dysarthria, reduced vocabulary
- groping for words, mispronunciation, reiteration of parts of words (logoclonia), echolalia
- reduced ability to read and write
- concurrent progressive memory loss involving recent and past events
- misidentification (e.g. mirror sign)
- emotional lability
- catastrophic reaction (extreme anxiety and tearfulness when unable to complete a task)
- motor restlessness or inertia

Late stage

- all intellectual functions grossly impaired
- considerable neurological disability
- increased muscle tone

- wide-based unsteady gait
- personality changes, often with fatuous gross euphoria
- no communication
- failure to recognize self or family
- speech replaced by jargon dysphasia

Final stage

- no personality
- no communication
- emaciated
- incontinent
- limb contractures
- death often from pneumonia and inanition

AETIOLOGY   As mentioned in Chapter 11, the neuropathological findings in Alzheimer's disease include:

- intracytoplasmic neurofibrillary tangles
- extracellular senile (argyrophilic) plaques which comprise a central core of amyloid, silica and aluminium
- granulovacuolar degeneration
- amyloid deposited in walls of blood vessels

These are found in normal ageing but are more extensive in Alzheimer's disease. Similar neuropathology is observed in the brains of those with Down syndrome (trisomy 21) who survive into middle age.

There is significant loss of neurones in the brains of Alzheimer's disease patients compared to controls. Most neuronal loss is found in the superior, middle and inferior frontal gyri, superior and middle temporal gyri and the cingulate gyrus.

The cause of Alzheimer's disease is not known but there are several theories:

- **Ageing**: there is no clear neuropathological division between Alzheimer's disease and normal ageing, leading to speculation as to whether Alzheimer's disease is a discrete disease entity or the extreme end of a normal spectrum of age-related decline. However, the distribution of neurohistological findings suggests the former. Plaques and tangles are commonly found in the ageing hippocampus, but much more rarely in the neocortex as is seen in Alzheimer's disease.

- **Neurotransmitter abnormalities**: neurotransmitter abnormalities include a wide range of changes in catecholamines and neuropeptides. Of most interest is the low cortical cholinergic activity and reduced choline acetyltransferase especially in the temporal cortex. This is thought to be secondary to the degeneration of neurones in the nucleus basalis of Meynert which provides the cortex with its cholinergic projection.

- **Genetic**: genetic factors must account for the disease in some patients. It is familial in some families, especially those in which the onset is early (under 65, presenile dementia). It is also hypothesized that late-onset Alzheimer's disease is an autosomal dominant trait with age-dependent expression and low penetrance, resulting in apparent sporadic cases. The finding of Alzheimer's disease in many patients with Down syndrome who reach middle age has focused interest on chromosome 21 on which is located the amyloid precursor protein gene. Research has demonstrated that a defect in this gene is not the cause of Alzheimer's disease, but there is increasing agreement that in both familial and sporadic Alzheimer's disease the post-translational processing of amyloid precursor protein is abnormal. Work is now ongoing to investigate other genetic modifications on chromosome 21 which may contribute to the abnormal deposition of amyloid.

■ **Environmental**: *aluminium*: the brains of those with Alzheimer's disease contain more total aluminium than those of controls. Aluminium is found in the areas of the brain most affected in Alzheimer's disease, particularly in the neurones containing tangles, and in the core of senile plaques. Some studies have reported higher concentrations of aluminium in drinking water associated with a higher prevalence of Alzheimer's disease, but these are not consistent. Those receiving haemodialysis accumulate aluminium from the dialysate. Before this was recognized patients developed severe dementia. Steps are now taken to reduce the burden of aluminium accumulation in those receiving haemodialysis. Aluminium probably accumulates in the brains of those with Alzheimer's disease secondary to the disease process rather than being directly causative. It remains possible that aluminium is a contributory factor in some cases of Alzheimer's disease.

■ **Environmental**: *head injury*: in sporadic Alzheimer's disease there is an increased risk in those who have experienced head injury within the preceding ten years.

■ **Environmental**: *infection*: it is hypothesized that an infectious agent entering via the transolfactory route may be responsible for some cases of Alzheimer's disease. Herpes simplex type 1 is known to have a predilection for those brain areas particularly affected in Alzheimer's disease and is suspected by some as a possible cause. However, this remains speculative.

MANAGEMENT Currently there is no treatment for Alzheimer's disease other than supportive help for patient and carers. A multidisciplinary team is essential as are close links with physicians, general practitioners, social services and the voluntary sector. The Alzheimer's Disease Society can provide carers with valuable information about local facilities, and often run local counselling and sitting services.

Driving should cease as soon as there is any evidence that it may be unsafe. The patient should be asked to inform the DVLC, but if they fail to do so, the doctor has a duty to inform them.

Small doses of neuroleptic medication may be needed in those patients who are agitated, distressed, aggressive or who have sleep reversal. The elderly, and particularly those with organic brain syndromes, can be exquisitely sensitive to the adverse effects of psychotropic drugs, so caution should be taken with starting doses.

Those with Alzheimer's disease are predisposed to developing depression which may require treatment with antidepressant medication, preferably using preparations with few antiadrenergic and anticholinergic side-effects (e.g. SSRIs).

Psychological approaches include the behavioural management of problem behaviours, reality orientation, reminiscence therapy and music therapy.

Those with Alzheimer's disease are more sensitive to cerebral insults and are more prone to developing superimposed acute organic brain syndromes (delirium) than healthy people. A sudden deterioration in functioning should prompt a search for superimposed potentially treatable pathology.

Specific treatments now available have limited benefit. Tetrahydroaminoacridine (THA or tacrine) has been developed to improve cognitive functioning by its effect on central cholinergic transmission. It does not affect the natural history of the condition, however, and has limited benefits clinically with high risks of hepatic side-effects. Donepezil hydrochloride is a recently introduced selective treatment for the symptoms of mild or moderate dementia in Alzheimer's disease. It is cholinomimetic

PROGNOSIS   Disease progression varies considerably from subject to subject. The younger the age of onset the more rapid the decline. In those aged under 50 the mean survival time is about seven years whereas in those aged between 55–74 the mean survival is increased to about nine years.

Poor prognostic factors include:

■ significant language impairment
■ poor cognitive functioning
■ clinical evidence of parietal lobe involvement
■ CT scan showing reduced density of left parietal region

Vascular dementia

CLINICAL FEATURES   Vascular dementia is characterized by a stepwise deteriorating course with a patchy distribution of neurological and neuropsychological deficits. There is evidence of vascular diseases on physical examination (hypertension, hypertensive changes on fundoscopy, carotid bruits, enlarged heart, focal neurological signs suggestive of cerebrovascular accident).

Three presentations occur:

■ dementia follows a stroke
■ dementia gradually develops following multiple asymptomatic cerebral infarcts
■ neuropsychiatric symptoms gradually become evident

Distinguishing between vascular dementia and Alzheimer's disease can be difficult; indeed, in a certain proportion of cases both coexist. A more insidious onset with a continuous rather than stepwise course, less insight, fewer affective symptoms and lack of hypertension or neurological signs is more suggestive of Alzheimer's disease. Vascular dementia is more likely than Alzheimer's disease to produce coexistent depression, persecutory delusions, anxiety and emotional disturbance.

Based on clinical presentation, history and CT scan findings the vascular dementias have been subdivided into:

■ Binswanger's disease
■ leuko-araiosis
■ multiple lacunar states

Binswanger's disease   This is a progressive subcortical vascular encephalopathy with CT scan revealing markedly enlarged ventricles secondary to infarction in hemispheric white matter; infarcts are observed to affect periventricular and central white matter.

Age of onset is 50–65, with a gradual accumulation of neurological signs, dementia and disturbances in motor function including pseudobulbar palsy. There is often a history of severe hypertension, systemic vascular disease and stroke.

Leuko-araiosis   This was used by Hachinski to describe CT scan appearances of reduced density of white matter. It differs from infarcts in that it affects only white matter, is patchy and diffuse and does not result in the enlargement of cerebral sulci or ventricles.

It is found in non-demented subjects as well as those with degenerative and vascular dementia.

Multiple lacunar states   These are CT scan appearances of small well localized sub-cortical infarcts. Associated with dementia characterized by dysarthria, incontinence and explosive laughing, secondary to frontal lobe disturbance.

AETIOLOGY

- **Cardiovascular disease**: there is an excess of vascular dementia in males, which is probably caused by an increased prevalence of cardiovascular disease in men. Hypertension is the most frequent risk factor among those with vascular dementia. Risk factors known to increase the risk of stroke also increase the risk of vascular dementia e.g. cigarette smoking, heart disease, hyperlipidaemia, and moderate alcohol consumption.

MANAGEMENT As well as the general management of the dementing patient and their carers as outlined above, with vascular dementia it is worth attempting to treat the underlying cardiovascular condition in order to slow or halt the progression of the condition.

The treatment of hypertension is important.

Depression may respond to antidepressant treatment.

PROGNOSIS The rate of progression to death is similar in this group to those suffering from Alzheimer's disease.

Poor prognostic factors include:

- severity of dementia
- bedridden
- urinary incontinence

Frontal lobe dementias

Dementia of frontal lobe type and Pick's disease both mainly affect the frontal and anterior temporal areas of the brain. Alzheimer's disease and vascular dementia may also have extensive frontal involvement but they are distinguishable on clinical, radiological and histopathological grounds.

In a large-scale neuropathological study over 20 years, 10 per cent of dementia cases had dementia of the frontal lobe type, and a further 2.5 per cent had Pick's disease (the Lund study 1987).

CLINICAL FEATURES This has a younger age of onset than Alzheimer's disease, with a larger proportion presenting in the under 65 age group. There is a slow insidious onset with marked frontal lobe features including disinhibition with reduced social awareness and lack of judgement. Shallowness, lability of affect, inappropriate jocularity (*Witzelsucht*) and apathy are typical. Persistent pain, hyperalgesia, and Kluver–Bucy syndrome may also occur. Obsessionality in daily routine and language difficulties characterized by reduced spontaneity, reduced output, stereotyped phrases, perseveration echolalia and finally mutism is seen. Memory loss is variable, and not as marked as in Alzheimer's disease, and agnosias and dyspraxias are less common.

CT scan reveals frontotemporal atrophy.

AETIOLOGY

- **Genetic**: clearly implicated, with half of cases showing a family history.

Little else is known about the aetiology of these conditions.

MANAGEMENT Similar to that of Alzheimer's disease.

PROGNOSIS Slow deterioration of functions. Mean duration of dementia of frontal lobe type is eight years, and of Pick's disease 11 years.

Parkinson's disease dementia

It is difficult to distinguish dementia specifically associated with Parkinson's disease from other causes of dementia which are likely to occur coincidentally in elderly people suffering from Parkinson's disease. It is estimated that dementia occurs in 15–20 per cent of those with Parkinson's disease, compared to 5–10 per cent of the normal population corrected for age.

CLINICAL FEATURES   Cognitive deficits seem to occur in most subjects with Parkinson's disease; it is possible that those considered to be suffering from dementia are simply those at the extreme end of cognitive decline in this condition.

Cognitive deficits in Parkinson's disease include:

- slowness in comprehension and response (bradyphrenia)
- impaired abstract reasoning
- memory impairment including poor retrieval and poor short-term memory especially frontal lobe working memory
- remote memory is only impaired in the late stages

Those patients with typical extrapyramidal signs of Parkinson's disease who later develop cognitive impairment, especially of a sub-cortical type, are given a diagnosis of dementia of Parkinson's disease.

AETIOLOGY   This is not known. It is known that in Parkinson's disease there is damage to the ascending monoaminergic system affecting central dopamine, serotonin and noradrenaline systems. There is also damage to substantia inno-minata, causing cortical cholinergic disruption.

All patients with Parkinson's disease have Lewy bodies in their cerebral cortex, with a subset having more Lewy bodies than most. Not all of these have dementia, although it appears that all have some evidence of cognitive decline.

MANAGEMENT   Exclude treatable pathology, such as depression or acute brain syndrome.

Treatment with anti-Parkinsonian drugs does not improve the cognitive mani-festations of the disease. Avoid anticholinergic drugs if possible.

Transplants of fetal nerve cells is experimental and may improve the outlook for those with Parkinson's disease. It is not known how helpful this will be in the treatment of dementia of Parkinson's disease.

Cortical Lewy body disease

It is not clear whether this type of dementia should be separated from the dementia of Parkinson's disease. Some patients who suffer from a condition almost indistinguishable clinically from Alzheimer's disease have diffuse Lewy bodies in the cerebral cortex on post-mortem examination. In some patients the neurohistology is mixed with features of this and Alzheimer's disease.

CLINICAL FEATURES   Memory impairment progresses into dementia and a motor disorder often suggestive of Parkinson's disease. The dementia is often like that of Alzheimer's disease but is more likely to have features suggestive of an acute brain syndrome such as a fluctuating mental state, altered conscious level and hallucinations.

Cortical Lewy body disease is diagnosed in those presenting with dementia suggestive of Alzheimer's disease, but in whom Parkinsonian features develop.

PROGNOSIS   Terminal decline.

Normal pressure hydrocephalus

CLINICAL FEATURES   Insidious onset of dementia with psychomotor retardation, unsteady gait and urinary incontinence. Onset is usually in sixties and seventies. Behavioural disturbance, hallucinations and paranoia are uncommon.

Diagnosis is made on the basis of clinical presentation, with a CT scan of brain revealing dilated ventricles (especially the third ventricle) without cortical atrophy, with normal CSF pressures.

AETIOLOGY Obstruction to outflow of CSF from subarachnoid space, but ventricular system remains in communication with subarachnoid space thus allowing CSF to flow out of ventricular system.

Associated with:

- subarachnoid haemorrhage
- cerebrovascular disease
- meningoencephalitis
- post-intracranial surgery

MANAGEMENT Shunt insertion to allow the drainage of CSF from the ventricles to the heart.

PROGNOSIS The best results are seen in those with a full clinical syndrome, a short history and an obvious cause for their condition. Mental and physical improvement is likely after surgery.

One-third of those undergoing surgery will develop complications such as:

- shunt infection and malfunction
- epilepsy
- subdural haematoma

Creutzfeldt–Jakob disease

This is a very rare cause of a rapidly progressive dementia.

CLINICAL FEATURES There may be a brief prodromal period of anxiety, depression or hallucinations. Sudden onset and rapid progression of dementia, pyramidal and extrapyramidal deficits present usually in the 50–60-year-old age group.

Physical features include limb spasticity, muscular wasting and fasciculation, tremor, rigidity, choreiathetoid movements, myoclonus, dysarthria and dysphagia. Convulsions may occur.

In addition to the above classic form, three variant forms are described:

- **heidenhain form**: prominent visual defects which may result in cortical blindness, extrapyramidal symptoms and myoclonus occur
- **ataxic form**: rapidly progressive cerebellar ataxia, with involuntary movements, myoclonic jerks. Finally muteness and generalized rigidity
- **cortical form**: parietal lobe symptoms

The EEG is always abnormal in CJD showing an increase in slow-wave activity, a reduction in alpha rhythm, and, as the disease progresses, bilateral slow spike wave discharges may accompany myoclonic jerks.

AETIOLOGY Microscopy of brain material reveals vacuolar changes in grey matter particularly in cerebral and cerebellar cortex, creating characteristic spongiform appearances. There is a loss of nerve cells and reactive astrocytosis.

- **Genetic**: about 10 per cent of cases appear to be familial
- **Infectious agent**: experimentally transmissible to laboratory animals by intracerebral inoculation, with symptoms developing years later. Similar to spongiform encephalopathies observed in animals (scrapie in sheep, bovine spongiform encephalopathy (BSE) in cows). Prion protein is responsible for transmission. This is an unusual infective agent since it does not appear to contain nucleic acid, being made up entirely of protein. It differs from normal cell-membrane-derived proteins in that it is highly resistant to degradation by cellular proteases, heat or conventional chemical disinfectants. CJD has been

transmitted in man through dural grafts, human pituitary-derived growth hormone used to treat children with growth hormone deficiency, through cross-contamination from instruments used in brain biopsy. Pathologists and those handling human brain tissue are also at increased risk of developing this condition.

A new form of CJD known as the BSE variant has been identified in humans. It has a slightly different clinical presentation with an onset in younger people, is rapidly progressive and is thought to be associated with eating or being otherwise exposed to cattle infected with BSE.

Other human diseases related to CJD in humans include kuru and Gerstmann–Sträussler syndrome. Kuru results from eating human brain and causes a cerebellar degeneration. Gerstmann–Sträussler syndrome is inherited with cerebellar ataxia forming a prominent clinical feature. Both are extremely rare.

HIV dementia
This is one of the most prominent features of HIV encephalopathy.
CLINICAL FEATURES   Initial lethargy, apathy, cognitive disturbance, reduced libido and general withdrawal. As the condition progresses evidence of dementia becomes apparent with cognitive disturbance, incontinence, ataxia, hyperreflexia and increased muscle tone.
AETIOLOGY   Although HIV infection results in complications such as opportunistic cerebral involvement of cytomegalovirus, and cerebral lymphoma, the encephalopathy of HIV is thought to be directly caused by HIV which is a neurotropic virus.

Pathology is found in the white matter of cerebral and cerebellar hemispheres and in deep grey matter. Multinucleated giant cells deriving from macrophages are found in the affected brain tissue.
MANAGEMENT   Therapeutic trials of anti-viral treatment suggest that improvement in HIV dementia may occur.
PROGNOSIS   Poor.

Huntington's disease (chorea)
A genetic disorder resulting in a condition characterized by continuous involuntary movements and a slowly progressive dementia.

There are five cases per 100 000 in the UK.
CLINICAL FEATURES   The onset is usually age 35–45, but childhood onset in 10–20 per cent. Onset insidious, with fidgety movements or non-specific psychiatric symptoms in the early stages.

Movement disorder consists of choreiform movements in the head, face and arms, ill-sustained and jerky voluntary and involuntary movements affecting all muscles, and a distinctive wide-based gait with sudden lurching.

Psychiatric disturbance is variable but common. Initial insight may result in depression. Prodromal personality changes, antisocial behaviour with substance misuse, affective and schizophreniform disorders are sometimes seen. Insight gives way to mild euphoria with explosive outbursts, irritability and rage. There is a slowly progressive intellectual impairment, with some patients profoundly demented in the final stages, whereas others remain reasonably aware.
AETIOLOGY

- **genetic**: transmission by fully penetrant single autosomal dominant gene, affecting 50 per cent of offspring (see Chapter 19 for more details)
- occasionally sporadic cases occur

Pathological appearances include a marked atrophy of head of caudate nucleus and putamen, severe generalized neuronal loss resulting in cortical atrophy which is most marked over the frontal lobes, with ventricular dilatation.

MANAGEMENT   Tetrabenazine helps to reduce movement disorder.

Antidepressants, ECT and minor tranquillisers may be helpful in the early stages, with phenothiazines in low dose in later stages to control behavioural disturbance.

Genetic counselling for family members should be offered. Gene located on chromosome 4.

PROGNOSIS   Average duration to death 12 to 16 years.

General paralysis of the insane (GPI)

Rare, but can be missed.

CLINICAL FEATURES   Develops five to 25 years after primary infection with treponema pallidum.

Onset is usually gradual with depression a dominant symptom. Slowly progressive memory and intellectual impairment. Frontal lobes are particularly involved, resulting in characteristic personality change with disinhibition, uncontrolled excitement, and overactivity which may be mistaken for hypomania. Grandiose delusions are present in only 10 per cent.

Physically there is slurred speech, a tremor of lips and tongue and Argyll Robertson pupil in 50 per cent. As the condition progresses there is increasing leg weakness leading to spastic paralysis.

Wasserman Reaction on CSF examination is always positive, with lymphocytosis, raised protein and raised globulin.

AETIOLOGY   A terminal consequence of syphilis.

There is marked cerebral atrophy with meningeal thickening, resulting from neuronal loss and astrocyte proliferation. The presence of iron pigment in microglia and perivascular space is specific for the disease. Spirochaetes are found in the cortex in 50 per cent of cases.

MANAGEMENT   Treatment is with high-dose penicillin under steroid cover to prevent Herzheimer reaction.

PROGNOSIS   Following treatment, mental symptoms may diminish.

DELIRIUM

This is a state of fluctuating global disturbance of the cerebral function, abrupt in onset and of short duration, arising as a consequence of physical illness or toxic effects.

Epidemiology

It is most common at the extremes of life both in the very young and the elderly. This may be caused by reduced cerebral reserve, a concurrence of multiple physical problems and a higher prevalence of polypharmacy in the elderly.

It affects 10–25 per cent of over-65-year olds admitted to medical wards. Those with dementia are particularly vulnerable to developing superimposed delirium.

CLINICAL FEATURES

- rapid onset with fluctuating course
- tends to be more marked at night particularly in conditions of poor illumination
- lucid intervals occur

- awareness is always impaired, alertness tends to fluctuate and can be both increased or decreased
- orientation is always impaired, particularly for time
- recent and immediate memory is impaired with poor new learning and lack of recall for events occurring during the delirious period; however, knowledge base remains intact
- thinking is slowed or accelerated
- misperceptions, particularly visual, are common
- hallucinations and delusions may occur
- heightened anxiety and fear are often prominent
- the sleep–wake cycle is always disturbed with daytime drowsiness and nocturnal insomnia
- physical illness or drug intoxication is usually present

Aetiology

Although delirium presents with global disturbance of cognitive function, certain neurological pathways seem to be specifically involved. Autonomic disturbance implicates the brainstem. Cholinergic and adrenergic pathways are also thought to mediate delirium.

Any physical insult can result in delirium particularly in a predisposed individual. In the elderly the following causes are the most common:

- hypoxia
- infection
- metabolic disturbance
- iatrogenic
- CNS disease
- epilepsy

Management

Delirious patients should be fully investigated physically. The treatment of delirium is the treatment of the underlying condition.

Hydration and nutrition should be monitored. Vitamin supplements, particularly thiamine, should be administered if there is any possibility of previous alcohol abuse or malnutrition.

Confusion is minimized if the delirious patient is nursed as consistently as possible by the same staff, in a well-illuminated environment. The patient should be aided in their orientation by providing environmental cues such as signposting and repeating information slowly and regularly.

Drugs known to exacerbate delirium should be avoided if possible. Sleep reversal may respond to small doses of temazepam or thioridazine. Disturbed behaviour not amenable to other interventions, such as gentle reassurance, may respond to treatment with a neuroleptic. Haloperidol is the most frequently used in this situation because it is effective and safe.

PROGNOSIS 30–40 per cent of delirious patients on medical wards die of the underlying condition. However, those that recover have a good prognosis, and only 5 per cent go on to develop dementia.

AFFECTIVE DISORDERS OF OLD AGE

DEPRESSION

Epidemiology

Depressive symptoms affect between 11 and 16 per cent of the population over 65 years of age; about 3 per cent suffer major depression.

Female first admissions for affective illness peak at age 80, then fall off, whereas male first admissions continue to climb until the end of life, overtaking women at the age of 85.

The prevalence of depression declines with advancing age despite the above findings. This may be because of a survivor effect with fewer young depressed surviving to old age, or it may imply that depression in older age is more likely to require inpatient admission.

Clinical features

Elderly depressives present with much the same features of depression as younger people, but the following may be more common in the elderly:

- hypochondriacal preoccupations
- psychomotor retardation or agitation
- paranoid and delusional ideation
- neurovegetative symptoms
- depressive pseudodementia
- behavioural disturbance (e.g. food refusal, aggressive behaviour, shoplifting, alcohol abuse)
- minimization/denial of low mood
- complaints of loneliness
- complaints disproportionate to organic pathology and pain of unknown origin
- onset of neurotic symptoms

Because the elderly commonly suffer from coexistent physical disorders affecting neurovegetative functioning, the diagnosis of depression can prove more difficult than in the young. A careful history usually suffices to address this difficulty. **The Geriatric Depression Scale** is helpful since it focuses almost entirely on cognitive rather than physical symptoms of depressive disorder and is easy to administer.

Aetiology

GENETIC   The genetic contribution to depressive illness reduces with age. The risk of depression in first-degree relatives is lowered with the increasing age of onset of depression in the proband. The risks to relatives are also lower if there has been only a single episode, whereas they are increased with recurrent depression in the proband.

NEUROBIOLOGICAL   Felix Post (1968) suggested that subtle cerebral changes may make ageing persons increasingly liable to affective disorders.

A subgroup of elderly depressives have ventricular enlargement on a CT scan of the brain. They are characterized as being older, with a later age of onset, more neurovegetative symptoms, and a higher death rate at two years than elderly depressives without ventricular enlargement. CT scan appearances in late onset depressives are more comparable to those with Alzheimer's disease than those with early onset depression or normal controls. Thus early and late onset depression may be different disorders, and late onset depression may have a stronger association with neurological dementing disorders than early onset depression.

Depressed patients with ischaemic brain lesions have more vascular risk factors and less family history of mood disorders than those without.

In a proportion of elderly depressives, subtle brain disease is a risk factor.

PHYSICAL ILLNESS   Depression can present secondary to a variety of physical conditions, and may sometimes be the first indication of ill-health. The following are the main causes of secondary depression which is more common in the elderly:

- occult carcinoma, particularly of lung and pancreas
- chronic obstructive airways disease (COAD)
- cerebrovascular accident (CVA)
- myocardial infarction (MI)
- hypercalcaemia
- Cushing's disease
- hypo- and hyperthyroidism
- alcoholism
- pernicious anaemia
- iatrogenic: steroids, beta-blockers, methyl-dopa, reserpine, clonidine, nifedipine, digitalis, L-dopa, tetrabenazine
- infections: brucellosis, neurosyphilis, influenza

PERSONALITY   It is suggested that personality dysfunction is associated with some late-life depression.

ENVIRONMENT   Murphy (1982) found an association between the onset of depression and severe life events occurring significantly more commonly in the previous year compared to healthy controls. These included physical illness, separation, bereavement, financial loss and enforced change of residence.

Management

The depressed elderly should be treated in much the same way as depressed younger people, with antidepressants in an adequate dose for an adequate duration. The choice of antidepressant will depend on concurrent physical morbidity, and the dose is generally lower, particularly when commencing a new drug.

Although tricyclic antidepressants are not absolutely contraindicated in the elderly, they have cardiotoxic properties and cause sedation and confusion in some. Thus lofepramine is often preferred. Alternatively trazodone and SSRIs are sometimes better tolerated.

Deluded depressed patients require the addition of a neuroleptic.

ECT remains the most effective treatment for depression and is the treatment of choice in those with life-threatening depression. It is generally well tolerated, although memory problems may follow, so unilateral electrode placement is sometimes considered preferable. It is contraindicated in those with raised intracranial pressure, and is inadvisable within three to six months of a cerebrovascular accident, pulmonary embolus or myocardial infarction. However, the anaesthetist's views should be sought in any patient over whom there is particular concern. The liable consequences of inadequately treated or resistant depression should be weighed against the potential adverse effects of a general anaesthetic and ECT. Monoamine oxidase inhibitors should be discontinued at least 10 days prior to giving ECT.

About two-thirds of cases resistant to first-line therapy show an improvement with lithium augmentation. Generally this is well tolerated, although the levels need careful monitoring in those with impaired renal function or those on diuretics.

Psychotherapy can be considered, although this should usually be in addition to drug therapy.

Socially isolated elderly depressed patients are at a high risk of committing suicide, and so it is important that they are treated energetically.

Prognosis

Depression of old age is a heterogeneous condition and therefore has a heterogeneous outcome.

Seventy per cent of elderly depressives recover within a year but 20 per cent subsequently relapse. The death rate is higher for late-life depressives than for non-depressed patients.

Chronicity in late-life depression is more common in those with:

- active medical illness
- high severity of depression
- melancholic features
- delusions
- cognitive impairment
- morphologic brain abnormalities

The development of a transient dementia syndrome during a depressive episode, the onset of first depressive episode in very old age and abnormalities in brain morphology may be predictors of dementia in the elderly with major depression.

MANIA

Epidemiology

In most elderly suffering from mania, the age of onset is usually in young adult life. However, in the elderly population, the onset of the first manic episode is bimodally distributed with peaks at age 37 and 73. Mania in the elderly is relatively uncommon, comprising about 5 per cent of elderly psychiatric admissions.

Aetiology

GENETIC   Late onset cases appear to have less genetic loading than younger onset cases, with fewer elderly onset manic patients giving a family history of affective disorder compared to their younger counterparts.

ORGANIC   Secondary mania is that arising in a patient with no previous history of affective disorder, soon after a physical illness such as cerebral tumour or infection. However, evidence suggests that this is more likely to arise in those genetically predisposed to a bipolar affective disorder by virtue of a family history of such.

Patients with late onset mania have a greater number of large subcortical hyperintensities on brain magnetic resonance imaging compared to controls. It is thought that some cases of late onset mania are a subtype of secondary mania attributable to changes in the brain's deep white matter.

CLINICAL FEATURES   These are similar to younger adults but it is thought that the following features are more common in elderly manic patients:

- garrulousness
- slow flight of ideas
- cognitive impairment

- irritable surliness
- mixed affective states
- depression following soon after mania recovers

Management

Most patients require treatment in hospital. Treatment is with neuroleptics and/or lithium, with the addition of carbamazepine if this is not fully effective.

If unresponsive or intolerant to this combination, ECT can be effective for manic or mixed affective states.

Lithium prophylaxis is advisable in the longer term.

Prognosis

This is the same as the prognosis of bipolar disorder. Recurrence is usual and therefore mood stabilizers are advisable in the longer term.

LATE-LIFE PSYCHOSES

Paraphrenia

This is a term introduced originally by Kraepelin in 1909 to describe a psychotic condition characterized by the relatively late age of first onset, chronic delusions and hallucinations, the preservation of volition and the lack of personality deterioration.

The term quickly lost favour until Roth in 1955 reintroduced it to describe late paraphrenia, a condition with age of first onset after 60, well-organized delusions with or without hallucinations, with a well-preserved personality and affective response.

ICD-9 allowed the diagnosis of paraphrenia, but this has been dropped from ICD-10. In ICD-10 late onset disorders are not differentiated from early onset disorders, therefore most paraphrenia is coded under schizophrenia or delusional disorders.

Epidemiology

Good epidemiological studies in this area have not been completed. It is estimated that in Camberwell there is an annual incidence of late paraphrenia of 17–26 per 100 000.

There is a well-established preponderance of females over males in late paraphrenia.

Late paraphrenics are more likely to be unmarried, and have a lower fecundity than controls.

Clinical features

Despite recent developments in the ICD-10 classification of late-life psychosis, evidence suggests that some late onset delusional disorders are distinct from schizophrenia, and the use of the term late paraphrenia therefore persists.

Osvaldo et al. (1995) studied the psychopathology of late paraphrenics and found the following:

- all had at least one type of delusion. These most frequently involved persecution and self-reference; delusions of thought broadcast, sin, guilt, and grandiosity were also present
- 46 per cent had at least one Schneiderian first-rank symptom

- 83 per cent had some hallucinatory experience, most commonly auditory, but also visual, somatic, and olfactory
- thought disorder and catatonic symptoms were almost never seen
- inappropriate affect was not seen
- negative symptoms were seen frequently but were mild
- other psychiatric symptoms such as worry, irritability, poor concentration, self-neglect and obsessive features were all seen more commonly in late paraphrenics than in controls

Aetiology

GENETIC   There is an increased risk of schizophrenia in the first-degree relatives of paraphrenics but it is less than the risk to the relatives of younger onset schizophrenics.

Paraphrenia is partly genetically determined, but the part played by inheritance requires further study.

PERSONALITY   In a subset of paraphrenic patients there is a history of those who have long-standing paranoid personalities which are thought to predispose to the development of paraphrenia in old age.

SENSORY IMPAIRMENT   Hearing impairment is associated with the development of paranoid symptoms. The characteristics most strongly associated with late paraphrenia are the early age of onset of hearing impairment, long duration and profound hearing loss. Auditory hallucinations are most consistently associated with hearing loss. It is thought that deafness may exert its action through increased social isolation, withdrawal and suspiciousness. Late paraphrenia has also been associated with visual impairment.

BRAIN DISEASE   Compared to normal controls, late paraphrenics have significantly larger cerebral ventricles and are more cognitively impaired.

Miller et al. (1991) in an MRI study of non-demented late paraphrenics found that organic brain pathology was common. In a group selected to exclude obvious organic pathology the following abnormalities were found:

- 42 per cent had structural brain abnormalities, with white matter lesions particularly evident in temporal, occipital and frontal areas
- 58 per cent had neuromedical illness, such as tumours and metabolic disorders
- 25 per cent had evidence of silent cerebral vascular disease, most commonly associated with hypertension
- neuropsychological testing revealed deficits in intellectual, frontal lobe and verbal memory functions

Management

Assessment and management are usually best undertaken in the patient's home where the psychopathology is most likely to be evident. Time must be spent developing a rapport and trying to engage with the patient.

If sensory impairment is present there is evidence that the condition can improve upon treatment of the deficit e.g. a hearing aid for the deaf.

The treatment of metabolic disorders or other physical conditions may bring about an improvement in the mental state. The treatment of hypertension may prevent a deterioration if this is caused by silent cerebrovascular disease.

Day-centre attendance may be helpful in increasing socialization.

MEDICATION   Neuroleptic medication may bring about an improvement. A substantial minority show no significant response, and about one-quarter show a full response to treatment. Treatment response is associated with improved compliance, the use of depot medication, an involvement of a CPN and lower medication doses.

Prognosis
Variable. Some patients make little or no response to treatment, others make a full response. Long-term contact with psychiatric services is required.

ANXIETY DISORDERS

Epidemiology
PHOBIAS Quite evenly distributed across the age groups, with lower rates in the over-75-year group compared to the 65–75 year group. Most common psychiatric disorder in elderly women in a community sample. Specific phobias are more common than agoraphobia or social phobia. One-month prevalence for phobic disorders is approximately 10 per cent.

GENERALIZED ANXIETY DISORDER Prevalence increases with age and is more common in women. One-month prevalence for GAD is approximately 4 per cent.

PANIC DISORDER Rarely encountered in the elderly. One-month prevalence for panic disorder in <1 per cent.

Anxiety disorders are often chronic, but about one-third of cases in the elderly have an age of onset after the age of 65.

Clinical features
These are generally similar to those seen in younger adults but the following are more common in the elderly:

- anxious preoccupation with physical illness, finance, crime and family
- subjectively impaired sleep which may be a normal part of ageing
- somatic symptoms of anxiety may be misattributed to physical causes
- abuse and over-prescription of sedative drugs

Aetiology
ENVIRONMENT Early parental loss is associated with phobic disorders in younger and older adults.

PHYSICAL ILLNESS Anxiety disorders and neuroses are associated with increased mortality and increased cardiovascular, respiratory and gastrointestinal morbidity.

The onset of agoraphobia after the age of 65 is often associated with a physical insult such as a myocardial infarction, surgery or a fracture.

Anxiety symptoms can be caused by a number of physical disorders, and a full physical examination should form a part of the assessment of the elderly anxious patient. Causes include:

- cardiovascular: e.g. myocardial infarction, cardiac arrhythmia, postural hypotension
- respiratory: e.g. pulmonary embolism, asthma, hypoxia, COAD
- endocrine: e.g. hyper/hypothyroidism, hypoglycaemia, phaeochromocytoma
- neurological: e.g. epilepsy, cerebral tumour, vestibular disease
- drug-induced: e.g. caffeine, sympathomimetics, sedative withdrawal

CO-MORBIDITY There are high levels of co-morbidity with other psychiatric conditions, particularly depression. Late onset cases of anxiety are almost always associated with depression, either a primary or a secondary association.

Management

Although there is less formal evaluation of therapies for anxiety disorders in the elderly, there is evidence that they do respond to psychological interventions including behavioural, cognitive and anxiety-management training.

Benzodiazepines and other sedatives are not generally indicated in the treatment of persistent anxiety disorders, particularly not in the elderly because of the problems of tolerance, dependence, confusion and falls.

Some anxiety disorders will respond to treatment with an antidepressant, particularly the SSRIs which are specifically helpful in depression associated with anxiety, and panic disorder.

Neuroleptics are sometimes helpful for their anxiolytic properties, but caution is required when prescribing any sedative in the elderly.

SUICIDE AND ATTEMPTED SUICIDE IN OLD AGE

Suicide is over-represented in the elderly. The elderly comprise 15 per cent of the UK population, yet they account for 25 per cent of all completed suicides, and only 5 per cent of attempted suicides. Ninety per cent of those completing suicide in old age are depressed, and two-thirds of those attempting suicide in old age have a psychiatric disorder. Suicide rates increase with age until very old age when they seem to tail off, more so for women.

The suicide rate is greater in men than in women; men are more likely to use a violent method and to use alcohol.

The depressed elderly who complete suicide tend to suffer from a moderate, often first episode depression with the clinical picture often comprising agitation, hopelessness, guilt, insomnia and hypochondriasis. The times of highest risk include bereavement and their anniversaries, the first few weeks after antidepressant treatment when the patient develops the ability to enact their thoughts prior to full recovery, and in the first few weeks after discharge from hospital. Eighty per cent of those completing suicide see their general practitioner before their death.

The incidence of physical illnesses in completed elderly suicides is higher than expected. Chronic pain is often a contributory factor, particularly post-herpetic neuralgia. Living alone, a widowed or separated status, and alcohol abuse are also risk factors.

Cultural factors probably play a role since suicide rates among some elderly populations, such as elderly Indian people, are extremely low.

Thus suicidal elderly patients should always be taken seriously. Depression should be adequately treated, isolation ameliorated if possible and pain should be properly managed.

PERSONALITY IN OLD AGE

Introversion increases with ageing. At an extreme level this can result in the 'senile squalor' or **Diogenes syndrome** in which the elderly recluse lives a limited life in advanced squalor with extreme hoarding of rubbish. Alcohol or frontal lobe dysfunction may play a part in this condition, although characteristically the syndrome is unaccompanied by any psychiatric disorder sufficient to account for the state in which the patient lives. Thus it is usually inappropriate to invoke the Mental Health Act; Section 47 of the Public Health Act is usually used to deal with these situations if required.

The prognosis is poor with almost inevitable relapse. Daycare may help, and institutional care is often required.

PSYCHOTHERAPY WITH OLDER ADULTS

Individual psychodynamic therapy

Traditionally psychoanalysts have been sceptical about the treatment of people over the age of 50. Freud himself argued that older adults were too far removed in time from the formative childhood experiences, that there was too little time left to work with problems, and that older adults were too rigid to allow therapeutic change. A minority of psychotherapists work with older adults, demonstrating that these views are still pervasive. However, a view also exists that these notions do not derive from evidence, rather from conflicts within therapists regarding ageing and dealing with older subjects.

Older adults can be treated with psychodynamic therapy. Conditions suitable for treatment include neurotic and personality disorders rooted in unconscious, unresolved childhood conflict.

Adaptations in therapy

Patients treated include those suffering from depression, phobias, anxiety neurosis and hysteria. Psychosomatic disorders in patients over the age of 60 are not considered treatable with psychotherapy.

It is suggested that the treatment of choice for neurotic disorders in the 55–75-year-age group is one to two 50-minute sessions per week for between several months to two years. In those with reactive crises short term, low frequency dynamic therapy of five to 20 sessions is indicated until the age of about 80.

Older adults have completed their psychosexual and psychosocial development, but still have to cope with psychosocial tasks such as retirement, loss of partner, ill health and impending death. They also have to struggle with unresolved unconscious psychological conflict and intergenerational difficulties.

With age the ego adapts by deploying increasingly mature defence mechanisms. The superego similarly adapts. However, the unconscious id is largely unchanged with time. Inner psychological conflict can persist from childhood.

Transference and counter-transference

Early in therapy with elderly patients the transference and counter-transference is likely to be reversed compared to therapy with younger patients. With the younger patient the therapist unconsciously assumes the position of a powerful parent. With the elderly patient the transference is likely to be reversed whereby the therapist experiences the unconscious transference of their own parental relationships. It is essential that supervision is provided such that the therapist is aware of these issues as they arise in therapy. Similarly early in therapy the patient is likely to transfer past experiences with those younger than themselves, such as their children, but as the therapy progresses they will develop the more classical transference relationships.

Common themes

In older age an increasing number of threatening and loss events occur. The therapist must work with the patient to mourn the losses, thus freeing the patient to continue to take up new opportunities and relationships. Decreasing independence and increasing dependence are often central themes in therapy. Coming to terms with the past and changed relationships and power structures are also relevant.

For the isolated elderly person, group work may be more appropriate than individual therapy.

BEREAVEMENT

Mood disorders associated with bereavement are prevalent in later life and are associated with morbidity and chronicity similar to other late-life depression. In a study of late-life widows, 24 per cent are depressed at two months after the loss, 23 per cent at seven months, and 16 per cent at 13 months. Risk factors for depression at 13 months include a past history of mood disorder, intense grief or depression early after the loss, and few social supports.

SLEEP DISORDERS

Forty per cent of older adults complain of chronic sleep problems, and use a disproportionate amount of night-time sedation, often on a long-term basis.

The cause of sleep disturbance in the elderly is multifactorial. Assessment therefore requires a careful history, with selective investigation.

Primary sleep disorders

These include sleep apnoea and nocturnal myoclonus, both of which are age-related.

SLEEP APNOEA   Sleep apnoea is an extremely common disorder affecting a quarter of independently living old people, and higher proportions of those in institutional care. However, the presence of sleep-related breathing disturbance in the absence of daytime sleepiness or impaired daytime functioning is probably not clinically significant.

Sleep apnoea is associated with increased morbidity and mortality. It is associated with daytime fatigue, memory problems, hypertension and cardiac arrhythmias. It is further associated with the increased risk of a stroke, even after controlling for other risk factors such as hypertension, cardiac arrhythmia and obesity.

CIRCADIAN RHYTHMS   Some sleep disturbance in old age is associated with changes in the systems that regulate circadian rhythm.

In older age the body's circadian rhythms lose their strength with a breakdown in timing and amplitude. Proposed interventions include:

- fitness training
- evening bright light exposure
- melatonin supplementation in those deficient

All these methods have brought about an improvement but are of only limited usefulness. Fitness training and bright-light exposure require a lot of time and effort and are continued after research trials in a minority of subjects. Melatonin is not commercially available in reliable formulations, and in some can cause depression.

Secondary sleep disorders

The significant numbers of complaints of disturbed sleep are secondary to other conditions such as medical or psychiatric illness, drug and alcohol use, behavioural and environmental factors.

It is essential that the primary problem is identified and treated, rather than treating the secondary sleep disturbance. The use of hypnotics should be avoided whenever possible.

Sleep disturbance is typically associated with poor physical health and depression.

In some elderly the apparent sleep disturbance is simply the unrealistic expectation that they should sleep for as long and as soundly as when they were younger. This often responds well to reassurance. In other patients attention to issues of **sleep hygiene** is required. This involves addressing behaviour such as the excessive use of caffeine-containing drugs, and environmental conditions improving the conduciveness to sleep, such as ensuring the bedroom is peaceful and dark, without stimulation, and keeping regular sleep hours without daytime napping.

ALCOHOL AND DRUG PROBLEMS

Alcohol abuse reduces with ageing, especially in men. About 3 per cent of over-75-year-olds in a general practice survey drank above the safe limits.

Reasons for this apparent decline in alcohol abuse with age include the selective death of early onset alcoholics, reduced tolerance to the effects of alcohol secondary to reduced liver enzymes and increased sensitivity of the ageing brain to sedatives, increased poverty in old age, and reduced opportunities to drink in elderly social circles.

New cases of alcoholism in old age tend to be more neurotic with less evidence of personality disorder than in younger onset cases. Physical ill health and psychiatric illness may be a trigger to excessive alcohol use in old age.

Drug abuse

Illicit drug abuse is not a great problem in the elderly, but addiction to prescribed benzodiazepines, opiates and other analgesics, barbiturates and laxatives is problematic. In the USA where the very elderly comprise 12 per cent of the population, they are responsible for the consumption of 50 per cent of prescribed hypnotics.

Doctors need to take care in their prescribing, to prevent the initiation of prescribed drug addiction. It is often worth attempting to wean even elderly persons from their drug of addiction, since abstinence can greatly improve the quality of life. However, there is a group, particularly the very elderly, who are better left on the drug if they strongly object to withdrawal.

PSYCHOSEXUAL DISORDERS

Normal sexual behaviour in old age

Sixty per cent of married couples aged 60 to 75 and 25 per cent of those over 75 are sexually active. One-fifth of men aged over 80 have sexual intercourse at least once a month. Thus sexual activity and sexual interest continue into old age.

The determinants of sexual activity in old age include:

- age
- sex: men are more sexually active than age-matched women
- married status
- own physical health
- physical health of partner
- enjoyment of sex

Loss of, or illness in, a partner is a common reason for the cessation of sexual activity in the elderly.

PHYSIOLOGICAL CHANGES WITH AGEING   The female genitalia atrophy with age particularly after the menopause. Blood flow is also reduced during arousal resulting in reduced vaginal lubrication. However, regular sexual intercourse or masturbation protects the female genitalia from these changes. Clitoral sensitivity and orgasm do not change with ageing.

In the male erections are slower to develop and require more tactile stimulation than in youth. The erection is less firm and persistent than in youth. The plateau phase can be prolonged longer and although ejaculation is less forceful, orgasm remains unaltered. The refractory period is much longer than in youth.

Sexual problems in old age
Physical illness may impair sexual activity because of:

- fear of the risk involved in sexual intercourse: e.g. myocardial infarction
- difficult or painful intercourse: e.g. arthritis
- impaired responsiveness of genitalia: e.g. neuropathy
- reduced feelings of sexual attractiveness: e.g. post-mastectomy or colostomy
- reduced sexual desire: e.g. dementia
- drug effects: e.g. antidepressants, antipsychotics, antihypertensives, thiazide diuretics, benzodiazepines

Elderly people in residential homes or hospitals should be provided with the privacy required to continue sexual expression with a consenting partner or by masturbation if they wish. The attitudes of staff and family may need to change through a process of education and discussion.

MEDICOLEGAL ISSUES IN OLD AGE PSYCHIATRY

Elder abuse
The abuse of elderly persons by their carers has received increasing attention since the 1970s. Its prevalence is difficult to estimate and depends on the definition of abuse which can range from irritability and verbal abuse, to sexual and physical abuse.

Among patients referred for respite care to geriatric wards in London, there was a high morbidity for dementia. Almost half of the carers admitted to some form of abuse, verbal more commonly than physical. Verbal abuse was associated with poor pre-morbid relations between patient and carer, and depression and anxiety in the carer. Physical abuse was associated with poor communication by the patient and high alcohol consumption in the carer. Few patients admitted to any abuse by their carers.

Management of financial affairs
Mental disorder from whatever cause can restrict a person's ability to deal with money, pay bills or buy or sell property. This can affect people in any age group

but is more common in the elderly, particularly among those suffering from dementing conditions. Various options exist to help deal with the financial affairs of people unable to do so themselves because of mental disorder. See Chapter 20 in which advocacy, appointeeship, the powers of attorney, the Court of Protection and testamentary capacity are considered. The effect of psychiatric disorders on driving capability is also considered in that chapter.

BIBLIOGRAPHY

Brun, A. 1987: Frontal lobe degeneration of the non-Alzheimer type. I: neuropathology. *Archives of Gerontology and Geriatrics* 6, 193–208.

Department of Health 1991: *Epidemiological overview of the health of elderly people.* London: Central Health Monitoring Unit.

Jacoby, R. and Oppenheimer, C. (eds) 1991: *Psychiatry in the elderly.* London: Oxford University Press.

Kay, D.W.K., Beamish, P. and Roth, M. 1964: Old age mental disorders in Newcastle upon Tyne. Part I: A study of prevalence. *British Journal of Psychiatry* 110, 146–58.

McDonald, C. 1969: Clinical heterogeneity in senile dementia. *British Journal of Psychiatry* 115, 267–71.

Miller, B.L., Lesser, I.M., Boone, K.B. *et al.* 1991: Brain lesions and cognitive function in late-life psychosis. *British Journal of Psychiatry* 158, 76–82.

Murphy, E. 1982: Social origins of depression in old age. *British Journal of Psychiatry* 141, 135–42.

Lindesay, J., Briggs, K. and Murphy, E. 1989: The Guy's/Age Concern survey: Prevalence rates of cognitive impairment, depression and anxiety in an urban elderly community. *British Journal of Psychiatry* 155, 317–29.

Osvaldo, P., Almeida, R., Howard, R.J. *et al.* 1995: Psychotic states arising in late life (late paraphrenia): psychopathology and nosology. *British Journal of Psychiatry* 166, 205–14.

Osvaldo, P., Almeida, R., Howard, R.J. *et al.* 1995: Psychotic states arising in late life (late paraphrenia): the role of risk factors. *British Journal of Psychiatry* 166, 215–28.

Post, F. 1968: The factor of ageing in affective illness. In Coppen, A. and Walk, A. (eds), *Recent developments in affective disorders.* Ashford: Headley Brothers, 105–16.

Schneider, L.S. 1993: Treatment of depression, psychosis, and other conditions in geriatric patients. *Current Opinion in Psychiatry* 6, 562–7.

Zisook, S. and Peterkin, J.J. 1993: Mood disorders and bereavement in late life. *Current Opinion in Psychiatry* 6, 568–73.

39
Forensic psychiatry

EPIDEMIOLOGY OF OFFENDING

Relationship with age
In the UK the peak age of offending is 14 years in girls and 17–18 years in boys. Half of all indictable crimes are committed by people aged under 21 years. By the age of 30 years, 30 per cent of males in the UK have been convicted of an indictable offence.

Sex ratio
The sex ratio of convicted males to females in the UK is approximately 5:1.

JUVENILE DELINQUENCY

Definition
Juvenile delinquency is law-breaking behaviour by 10- to 21-year-olds.

Aetiology
The aetiology is multifactorial and is not associated with an established psychiatric disorder. Factors associated with the development of delinquency include:

- unsatisfactory child-rearing
- ↓ IQ
- conduct disorder in childhood
- parental criminality
- large family size

Management and prognosis
Factors that may improve the prognosis with respect to adult criminality include:

- counselling
- establishing a good relationship with a parent or counsellor
- improvement in the home environment
- a good experience in school
- a good peer group
- successful employment
- a good relationship or marriage

Approximately 50 per cent have stopped their delinquent behaviour by the age of 19 years.

CRIMINAL RESPONSIBILITY

Age of commencement
In England and Wales criminal responsibility starts at the age of 10 years. In Scotland it starts at the age of 8 years.

DOLCI INCAPAX   Criminal responsibility is partial (**Dolci Incapax**) between the ages of 10 and 14 years. After the age of 14 years an individual is legally responsible for their actions unless caused by:

- a mistake
- an accident
- duress
- necessity
- responsibility being affected by mental disorder

ACTUS REA   This is an unlawful act.

MENS REA   This is guilty intent, and is required in addition to an unlawful act for certain offences, such as murder and rape.

MENTALLY ABNORMAL OFFENDERS

Epidemiology
The prevalence of mental abnormality in all offenders is estimated to be 1 per cent. The prevalence of mental abnormality in those in prison in the UK is estimated to be up to 33 per cent.

Forensic psychiatric assessment and court reports
These should include:

- a full history and mental state examination
- obtaining an objective account of the offence
- obtaining an objective account of previous offences
- additional information from relative, friends, social workers, probation officers, etc.
- a review of previous psychiatirc and other relevant records

Table 39.1 details a model psychiatric court report.

Outcome of sentencing
The outcome of sentencing of mentally abnormal offenders in England and Wales is shown in Table 39.2.

Mental disorder
Mental disorders that may be associated with offending include:

- schizophrenia: mostly associated with minor offending secondary to deterioration in personality and social functioning
- depressive disorder: under-represented in offenders; associated with homicide and shoplifting
- epilepsy: over-represented in prisoners but offending in epileptics is rarely ictal
- morbid delusional jealousy (Othello syndrome): associated with repetitive and serious injury to the spouse/partner

Alcohol and drugs that have been taken voluntarily do not, in general, lessen the

Table 39.1 Model psychiatric court report

Para 1	**Introduction** Inform the court of when and where the patient was seen, at whose request, what information was available, e.g. statements related to the case, who were the informants, and sometimes what information was not available. State the current offences(s) with date for which charged.
Para 2	Inform the court of his past medical history and of the result of medical examination, e.g. 'Physical examination revealed no abnormality'.
Para 3	Report the important, relevant points of the family history, including family psychiatric disorder and criminality.
Para 4	**Personal history** Report the important points of his personal history, i.e. his physical development, e.g. birth, milestones, bedwetting (enuresis), schooling (e.g. bully/bullied, truancy), occupational history (which will include difficulties sustaining employment or with colleagues at work).
Para 5	Report his sexual and marital history: be reasonably discreet as the report may be read in open court.
Para 6	Report details of his personality in terms of his social interaction, his emotions, his habits, e.g. drinking, gambling, drugs.
Para 7	Report past forensic history, e.g. past convictions. This is, however, inadmissible.
Para 8	Report past psychiatric history (dates, diagnoses, relevant details and relationship of mental disorder and treatment to offending).
Para 9	Report circumstances leading to current offence(s) and the defendant's state of mind at the time of the offence. Restrict discussion to the phenomena observed, e.g. 'For the time of the offence he gives a history of tearfulness, loss of hope, poor sleeping', etc., 'These are symptoms of the mental illness of depressive disorder', etc.
Para 10	Report the result of the interview: 'He showed/did not show evidence of mental illness or mental impairment'. Then give a brief outline of the evidence, e.g. 'He muttered to himself, looked around the room as though hallucinating' etc., or list symptoms detected and say 'these are symptoms of the severe mental illness of schizophrenia' etc. Information in paragraphs 1–10 should be factual, verifiable and ideally agreed by all, even if others' opinions of these facts differ from your own.
Para 11	The final paragraph should express your opinion. The court will be interested particularly in your opinion regarding: ■ Is the defendant fit to plead and stand his trial? ■ Is he suffering from a mental disorder, i.e. mental illness, a form of mental impairment or psychopathic disorder? ■ Where appropriate, comment on issues of responsibility, e.g. not guilty by reason of insanity; diminished responsibility in cases of homicide. ■ If suffering from mental disorder, can arrangements be made for his treatment in the National Health Service (arrange this if you think they can). Make suggestions to the court about which Mental Health Act order would be appropriate, e.g. Sections 37/41 in England and Wales, or suggest treatment as a condition of a Probation Order, e.g. 'In my opinion this man suffers from the severe mental illness schizophrenia, characterized by delusions (false beliefs) and hallucinations (voices, or visions). I consider he would benefit from treatment in a psychiatric hospital. I have made arrangements for a bed to be reserved for him at X hospital under Section 37 of the Mental Health Act 1983 if the court considers that this would be appropriate. I additionally recommend, if

the court so agrees, that he be made subject to restrictions under Section 41 of the Mental Health Act 1983 to protect the public from serious harm and to facilitate his long-term psychiatric management, including specifying the conditions of his discharge from hospital, e.g. of residence and compliance with out-patient psychiatric treatment.' As an alternative: 'In my opinion this man does not suffer from mental illness, mental impairment nor psychopathic disorder and is not detainable in hospital under the Mental Health Act 1983. He has an anxious and dependent personality disorder, requires considerable support and would benefit from group psychotherapy as an out-patient. The court may consider that it would be an appropriate disposal to help this man if he were to attend an out-patient group under my direction at X Health Centre as a condition of probation.

Comment should be made on any mitigating circumstances, e.g. marital/work stress, and on the prognosis. Express any doubts you may have as to the likelihood of benefit from treatment.

If you have no psychiatric recommendation, say so, e.g. 'I have no psychiatric recommendation to make in this case'.

Finally, if essential information is lacking or, if time is not sufficient to make the necessary arrangements for a hospital bed, then do not hesitate to state your findings up to date, state what you would like to do, and ask for a further period of remand.

Reproduced with permission from Puri, B.K., Laking, P.J. and Treasaden, I.H. 1996: *Textbook of psychiatry* Edinburgh: Churchill Livingstone.

Table 39.2 Outcome of sentencing of mentally abnormal offenders

- The law takes its course, e.g. a fine, prison
- Conditional or absolute discharge, possibly with voluntary psychiatric treatment
- Probation order, with or without condition of psychiatric treatment (e.g. under Section 3 of the Powers of the Criminal Courts Act 1973 in England and Wales)
- Detention under the Mental Health Act, e.g. under Section 37 with or without a Section 41 Restriction order under the Mental Health Act 1983 of England and Wales

Reproduced with permission from Puri, B.K., Laking, P.J. and Treasaden, I.H. 1996: *Textbook of psychiatry.* Edinburgh: Churchill Livingstone.

individual's full legal responsibility. While amnesia is not a legal offence, its underlying cause may well be.

Fitness to plead

A mentally disordered offender is unfit to plead if, at the time of the trial (but not necessarily at the time of the offence) they are unable to carry out one or more of the following:

- instruct counsel
- appreciate the significance of pleading
- challenge a juror
- examine a witness
- understand and follow the evidence of court procedure

McNaughten Rules

To be found not guilty by reason of insanity, it has to be proved to a court that at the time of the offence the offender laboured under such defect of reason that they met these Rules, namely:

- that by reason of such defect from disease of the mind, they did not know the nature or quality of their act
- they did not know that what they were doing was wrong

Diminished responsibility

In the case of a charge of murder, a defence of diminished responsibility (Homicide Act 1957) may be brought in, whereupon it has to be shown that at the time of the offence the offender suffered from:

- such abnormality of mind, whether caused from a condition of arrested or retarded development of mind or any inherent causes or induced by disease or injury, as substantially impaired their mental responsibility for their acts

Infanticide

In England and Wales infanticide is a type of unlawful homicide in which:

- a woman by any wilful act caused the death of her child under the age of 12 months, but at the time of the act or omission the balance of her mind was disturbed by reason of her not being fully recovered from the effect of giving birth to the child, or the effect of lactation consequent upon the birth of the child

Automatism

In this rare plea, usually in cases of homicide, the defendant pleads that at the time of the offence their behaviour was automatic.

DANGEROUSNESS

Dangerous individuals are people who have caused or who might cause serious harm to others. Its features include:

- repetition
- incorrigibility
- unpredictability
- untreatability
- infectiousness

The best predictor of future dangerous behaviour is the individual's past behaviour. Shorter term prediction is better than longer term prediction. Dangerousness is associated with the availability of weapons, morbid jealousy, and the sadistic murder syndrome.

CIVIL ASPECTS

Testamentary capacity

This is considered in Chapter 21.

Tort

A mentally disordered person is considered incapable of committing a tort (a civil wrong to an individual or to the reputation or estate of an individual) unless the disorder did not preclude an understanding of the nature or probable consequences of the act.

Contracts

A contract requires free full consent and is void if an individual was of unsound mind at the time of making the contract.

Marriage

Being a contract, it is void if an individual had a mental disorder at the time of marriage such that the nature of the contract was not appreciated at that time. A marriage may be annulled for any of the following reasons:

- the partner has a mental disorder at the time of marriage so as not to appreciate the nature of the contract
- one partner did not disclose that they suffered from epilepsy or a communicable venereal disease
- either party was under 16 years at the time of marriage
- pregnancy by another male at the time of marriage was not disclosed
- there was non-consummation
- one of the partners was forced to agree to the marriage by duress

BIBLIOGRAPHY

Faulk, M. 1988: *Basic forensic psychiatry.* Oxford: Blackwell.
Treasaden, I.H. 1996: Forensic psychiatry. In Puri, B.K., Laking, P.J. and Treasaden, I.H. *Textbook of psychiatry.* Edinburgh: Churchill Livingstone.

Index

beta adrenoreceptor blocking drugs 418
  anxiolytic action 169
bias in measurement 67
Binswanger's disease 410
black and ethnic minorities, cross-cultural
  psychiatry 388–91
Black report (1980) on socioeconomic
  inequalities in health 70–1
blood–brain barrier 163
body build, and personality 339
body image disorders 92–3
bonding 25–7
Bowlby's attachment theory 25–7
boxplots 54–5
brain fag syndrome 388
brain syndromes, acute 5
brain vesicles
  diencephalon 107
  mesencephalon 107
  metencephalon 107
  myelencephalon 107
  prosencephalon 106
  rhombencephalon 107
  telencephalon 106
brain–steroid and brain–thyroid axes, affective
  disorders 274
brainstem cholinergic pathway 122
breastfeeding, drugs 308–9
British National Formulary (BNF), official
  guidance 180–1
Broca's area, speech and language 19
Broca's nonfluent, aphasias 92
brucellosis 418
bulimia nervosa 377–82
  differentiatial diagnosis 381
buspirone
  effects 169
  side-effects 179

caffeine 242
CAGE questionnaire, problem drinking 234
California Psychological Inventory (CPI) 24
cannabinoids 235, 246
cannabis (grass, hash, ganja, pot) 246
Cannon–Bard theory, emotion 10
canonical correlation analysis 62
CAPE, level of disability/prediction of
  needs 404–5
Capgras syndrome 263
carbamazepine
  action 169
  monitoring 176
  in personality disorders 350
carbohydrate metabolism disorders 190
cardiovascular disease, aetiology 411
case identification 192
case registers 193
catatonic disorders, organic, defined 219

catechol-O-methyltransferase (COMT) 150,
  151
CATEGO, classification of schizophrenia 250
Cattell's trait theory, classification of personality
  disorders 338
censorship, Freudian theory 95–9
central nervous system (CNS)
  biology 106–213
  disease, delirium 92, 416
central tendency
  mean, mode and median 51
  outliers 54
cerebral palsy, incidence 366, 367
cerebral tumours 126–7
cerebrospinal fluid (CSF) 106
cerebrovascular accident (CVA) 418
cerebrovascular disease, psychiatric
  consequences 406
chaining 3
challenging behaviours 368
chi-square test 58–9
childhood onset disorders
  black and ethnic minorities 390
  classification 210, 353–5
  conduct disorders 358–9
  depression 355
  elective mutism 359–60
  encopresis, non-organic 363–4
  enuresis, non-organic 362
  hyperkinesis 357–8
  neurotic and stress-related disorders 284
  school refusal 355–7
  tic disorders 360–1
children
  fear development 34–5
  finalism 32
  intellectual development 31–2
  precausal reasoning 32
  preoperational stage 32
  sexual abuse 29
  sexual behaviour 36
  syncretism 32
  temperament 30
    differences 30
  Weschler intelligence scale: revised (WISC-
    R) 23–4
  see also adolescence; infants
chlorpromazine
  in anorexia nervosa 377
  photosensitization 174
cholecystokinin 152
cholinergic receptors 148
chromosomal abnormalities, associated
  conditions 188–9
chromosomes 182
chronic obstructive airways disease
  (COAD) 418
circadian rhythms 425
  sleep disorders 425